ALLERGY AND IMMUNOLOGY OF THE EYE

...nell h. friedlaender M.D.

...Clinical Professor of Ophthalmology,
...ent of Ophthalmology;
...nt Research Ophthalmologist,
...is I. Proctor Foundation for Research in Ophthalmology,
...iversity of California, San Francisco, California

ALLERGY AND IMMUNOLOGY OF THE EYE

HARPER & ROW, PUBLISHERS
Hagerstown

Cambridge
New York
Philadelphia
San Francisco

London
Mexico City
Sao Paolo
Sydney

1817

The author and publisher have exerted every effort to ensure that drug selection and dosage set forth in this text are in accord with current recommendations and practice at the time of publication. However, in view of ongoing research, changes in government regulations, and the constant flow of information relating to drug therapy and drug reactions, the reader is urged to check the package insert for each drug for any change in indications and dosage and for added warnings and precautions. This is particularly important when the recommended agent is a new and/or infrequently employed drug.

79 80 81 82 83 84 10 9 8 7 6 5 4 3 2 1

ALLERGY AND IMMUNOLOGY OF THE EYE. Copyright © 1979 by Harper & Row, Publishers, Inc. All rights reserved. No part of this book may be used or reproduced in any manner whatsoever without written permission except in the case of brief quotations embodied in critical articles and reviews. Printed in the United States of America. For information address Medical Department, Harper & Row, Publishers, Inc., 2350 Virginia Avenue, Hagerstown, Maryland 21740.

Library of Congress Cataloging in Publication Data
Friedlaender, Mitchell H
    Allergy and immunology of the eye.
    Includes bibliographies and index.
    1. Eye—Diseases and defects—Immunological aspects. 2. Allergy. I. Title. [DNLM: 1. Eye diseases—Immunology. 2. Hypersensitivity.
WW140 F911a]
RE48.F74   617.7′1   79-9333
ISBN 0-06-140843-3

TO MY FAMILY

contents

preface

In 1958, a time when modern-day immunology was still in its embryonic stages, Theodore and Schlossman's book OCULAR ALLERGY was published. During the past 21 years the field of immunology has veritably burgeoned, and today immunology touches every specialty within clinical medicine. New concepts have arisen which have begun to shed light on once-obscure diseases, many of which affect the visual system.

Immunologic mechanisms in ophthalmic disease have gained wide attention, and a book which updates immunologic concepts within ophthalmology has been greatly needed for many years. (Interest among ophthalmologists is long overdue, since for many decades the eye has been a site favored by immunologists for the study of immunologic phenomena.) In the future, immunologic study of ophthalmic disease will continue to expand, and a basic understanding of immunologic principles will become essential for those in training as well as for practicing clinicians. Basic scientists can also learn much about the clinical manifestations of immunologic processes by studying immunologic phenomena which occur in the eye.

ALLERGY AND IMMUNOLOGY OF THE EYE is intended to bring together an understanding of immunologic principles at work in conditions affecting the eye, and the varied clinical manifestations of these conditions. The first three chapters review the basic principles of general and ophthalmic immunology. Subsequent chapters cover the clinical entities in which these immunologic mechanisms are thought to play a significant role. It is intended that the reader will gain an understanding of the basic principles of immunology as well as a more specific understanding of the special and enlightening immunologic features of ocular tissues. If this goal is accomplished, this book will have served a useful purpose.

I wish to express my gratitude to several individuals who assisted me in researching, writing, and editing ALLERGY AND IMMUNOLOGY OF THE EYE. My outstanding teachers, Drs. Phillips Thygeson, H. Bruce Ostler, and G. Richard O'Connor provided great inspiration and many helpful suggestions for improving the clarity and the quality of this book. Drs. Joseph Michelson, Khalid Tabbara, Edward Howes, and Stewart Sell were kind enough to review chapters and to offer useful comments.

I would also like to thank Mrs. Lucy Lee and Mr. Richard Cyr for their valuable help with library work, Peggy Costa and Barbara Goldsmith for their proficient transcribing and typing, and the staff of the Medical Division of Harper and Row for their patience, hard work, and dedication.

M.H.F.

ALLERGY AND IMMUNOLOGY OF THE EYE

ONE
ONE
ONE principles of general immunology

HISTORY OF THE CONCEPT OF IMMUNITY

Immunology is generally thought of as a modern-day discipline which has evolved only recently. The concept of immunity, however, dates back many centuries and its route is marked by several important milestones leading to our present-day understanding of immunology (Fig. 1-1). As far back as the eleventh century, Chinese physicians noted that inhalation of smallpox crusts prevented the occurrence of this dreaded disease. Variolation, the intradermal inoculation of powdered scabs, became widely used in the Middle East. During the eighteenth century the technique reached England, where Lady Mary Wortley Montagu popularized this primitive practice. In 1798, Edward Jenner, while still a medical student, greatly advanced the embryonic science of immunology when he discovered that milkmaids who contracted cowpox became resistant to smallpox infection.

Modern-day methods of preventive immunization against smallpox and other infectious diseases resulted largely from the efforts of Louis Pasteur. Pasteur developed the germ theory of disease, which led to the *in vitro* culture of microorganisms. Thus, material became available for the production of vaccines. Pasteur found that old cultures of cholera organisms, when given to fowl, produced no disease, yet the animals became resistant to subsequent infection with cholera. Inoculation with living attenuated organisms could thus produce resistance to infectious disease.

Robert Koch discovered the tubercle bacillus while investigating the bacterial etiology of infectious disease. In 1880, while attempting to develop a vaccine for tuberculosis, he observed the phenomenon of delayed hypersensitivity. Roux and Yersin, in 1885, showed that the diphtheria bacillus produces a potent exotoxin. Von Behring and Kitasato used this toxin to inoculate animals and to produce a toxin-neutralizing substance known as antitoxin. This antitoxin, when given to uninoculated animals, conferred protection against the harmful effects of the diphtheria bacillus. Thus, the important therapeutic technique of passive immunization was introduced.

At the turn of the century, two divergent immunologic theories were developing. The **humoral** theory, proposed by Paul Ehrlich, stressed the importance of the biochemical products, or **antibodies,** elaborated by certain cells. At about the same time, Metchnikoff developed the theory of **cellular immunity,** which emphasized the host's cellular response to foreign substances. Ehrlich proposed, in his side-chain theory, that receptors exist on cell surfaces and that when these receptors interact with toxins, excess receptors are shed into the circulation as antibody. Metchnikoff felt that wandering phagocytes are the body's primary defense system. We now recognize that phagocytic cells can respond nonspecifically to foreign substances but may also participate with lymphocytes in specific cellular immune reactions. The theories of both Metchnikoff and Ehrlich were essentially correct and both theories were laborated and interconnected over the next several decades. Although

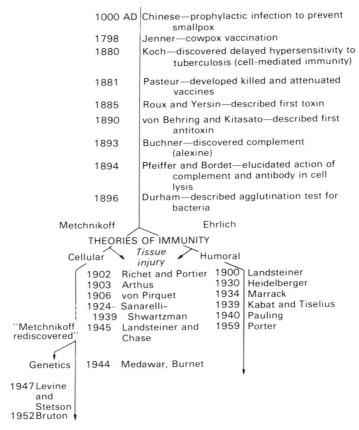

FIG. 1-1. Important milestones in the history of immunology. (Bellanti JA: Immunology, Philadelphia, WB Saunders, 1971, p 4)

today's concepts differ somewhat from those of Ehrlich and Metchnikoff, cellular and humoral immunity are now known to be the two major immunologic mechanisms by which the body maintains an adequate and proper defense system.

TYPES OF IMMUNITY

Immunology is the study of **immunity,** a term derived from the Latin *immunis,* meaning "free from burden." In one sense, immunity refers to the protection of the host from infection or reinfection by a microbial agent. The scope of immunity has been broadened, however, to include also the harmful or unpleasant effects resulting from interaction of a foreign substance with the host's defenses. To this type of response we apply the terms **allergy** and **hypersensitivity. Allergy** is the term coined by

von Pirquet, who hypothesized that both the beneficial and harmful responses of the host to a foreign substance were manifestations of a common biologic mechanism. We now use the broader term **immunity** to denote a generalized reactivity of a host to a foreign substance as well as its protective status against these substances.

Immunity may be innate or acquired. **Innate immunity** refers to those immune properties which are genetically determined. **Acquired immunity** refers to immunity developed through some type of immunization process.

Protective immunization may be acquired by use of a **vaccine,** a substance which immunizes a host. It usually is a preparation of killed or attenuated microorganisms. Immunization may be spoken of as active or passive. In **active immunization,** exposure to an organism or administration of a vaccine causes the host to develop immunity, a process which may take several weeks. This active form of protection, however, lasts for several months or even years. In **passive immunization,** serum from an immunized donor is passively transferred to a recipient and offers immediate but short-lived protection.

Immunity may also be considered as nonspecific or specific. **Nonspecific immunity** allows the host to differentiate between the host's own constituents and outside invaders, but this mechanism does not require the specific immunologic recognition of foreign substances. Nonspecific immunity includes the barrier functions of the skin, certain antimicrobial substances in the serum and external secretions, and nonspecific phagocytosis. **Specific immunity** depends on the immunologic recognition of foreign substances, known as antigens, and the reactions to these substances by humoral or cellular immune mechanisms, as will be discussed. **Specificity,** or specific recognition of a foreign substance is a key feature of the immune system.

LYMPHOID CELLS

In carrying out the function of the immune system, an extensive cell system, known as the **lymphoreticular system,** has evolved. Its cells are found throughout the body, with large collections located in the thymus, lymph nodes, and spleen (see Lymphoid Organs). An important component of this cell system is the lymphoid series of cells. This group includes both lymphocytes and plasma cells. The main function of the plasma cell is the production of **antibody,** a protein which reacts with a foreign substance, or **antigen.** The lymphocyte also has the ability to react specifically with an immunizing substance (antigen) and to elaborate certain cell products in consequence. Thus, two different types of **immune responses** may occur: one involving antigen and antibody, and another involving antigen and specifically sensitized lymphocytes.

Two different populations of small lymphocytes are known to exist (Fig. 1-2). Both are derived from bone marrow stem cells. **T lymphocytes** are lymphocytes that have been processed by the thymus or are in some way dependent upon the thymus. The thymus is responsible for specific **cellular (or cell-mediated) immune responses** which are mediated by **T lymphocytes,** and if a thymectomy is performed on an animal during the neonatal period, these cell-mediated responses fail to develop. **B lymphocytes** are dependent on the

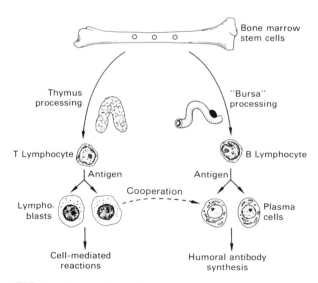

FIG. 1-2. Processing of bone marrow stem cells by the thymus to form T lymphocytes and by the bursa or "bursal equivalent" to form B cells. (Roitt IM: Essential Immunology, Oxford, Blackwell, 1974, p 48)

bursa of Fabricius, a gut-associated lymphoid organ in birds, and on the so-called "bursal equivalent" in man. The location of the bursal equivalent in man is not known; however, it is in the fetal liver that immunoglobulin-producing cells are recognized earliest. The bursa, or its equivalent, appears to be responsible for **humoral immunity** (*i.e.,* immune responses mediated by antibodies). Both populations of lymphocytes, when appropriately stimulated, undergo morphologic changes and divide. The T lymphocytes undergo transformation to a blast form after which they are **sensitized,** that is, capable of recognizing a specific antigen; B lymphocytes differentiate into plasma cells which form antibody.

T CELLS

T cells (Fig. 1-2), the lymphocytes which are processed by the thymus, occupy the thymus-dependent areas of lymphoid tissue. The use of antithymus serum, cytotoxicity tests, and other techniques allows T cells to be identified.

T cells are capable of mediating many diverse types of immunologic reactions. These include immunity to many viruses, bacteria, and fungi; contact allergy; graft and tumor rejection; and certain types of autoimmune disorders. Subpopulations of T cells have been identified in recent years: **suppressor** or **regulator** T cells actively suppress an immune response; **helper** T cells cooperate with B lymphocytes in antibody formation.

T cells may be identified by the presence of markers on their surfaces known as **alloantigens.** Alloantigens are genetically determined. They can be identified with the use of specific antiserums, and have been widely studied in inbred strains of mice. Several different systems of alloantigens have been studied in this manner. The thy antigen on mouse T cells is an example. One of the most useful of these markers has been the Ly alloantigen system. These markers are glycoproteins found only on the surface of lymphocytes and they can be used to identify certain functional subpopulations of T lymphocytes. Five different Ly alloantigens have been identified, each with two different antigenic specificities, or alleles. Ly-1

is determined by a gene on chromosome 19 of the mouse, and Ly-2 and Ly-3 by genes on chromosome 6. In the peripheral blood of mice, 50% of T lymphocytes possess Ly-1, 2, and 3; 30% have Ly-1 only, and 7% have Ly-2 and 3. It appears that cells possessing only Ly-1 express helper functions with respect to antibody formation and delayed hypersensitivity while cells with Ly-2 and 3 suppress immune responses and may also be cytotoxic. Cells possessing Ly-1, 2, and 3 seem to be precursors of the other cell types and are not functionally committed cells. T cells of different Ly types appear to interact and cooperate with one another in a variety of immunologic activities, including antibody formation, cytotoxicity, immunosuppression, delayed hypersensitivity, and killing of microorganisms by macrophages.

Certain thymus-derived factors seem to be associated with T cell maturation and these factors may restore T cell responses in neonatally thymectomized animals. One of these factors, known as thymopoietin, causes bone marrow cells to develop into T lymphocytes.

After stimulation by a sensitizing antigen, the T lymphocyte undergoes transformation into a blast cell. These cells are pyroninophilic and actively synthesize new DNA, as evidenced by uptake of tritiated thymidine. The sensitized T lymphocyte elaborates a number of soluble substances, known as **lymphokines,** which may serve as the mediators of some T cell functions (see Lymphokines, Ch. 2).

B CELLS

B cells are derived from the bursa of Fabricius in birds and from the gastrointestinal tract or fetal liver in other animals. B cells possess surface immunoglobulin on their cell membranes, by which they can be identified. Most B cells have immunoglobulins IgM and IgD on their surfaces. Upon appropriate stimulation, B cells proliferate and differentiate into antibody-secreting plasma cells.

Antibodies are proteins synthesized by plasma cells after stimulation by an antigen. Antibodies have the capability of reacting specifically and uniquely with the configuration that was responsible for their formation. In the human, antibody is associated with five major classes of proteins known as **immunoglobulins,** designated IgG, IgA, IgM, IgD, and IgE. Each has a distinct chemical nature and a specific biologic role. IgG is the most abundant of the immunoglobulins and provides the bulk of immunity against infectious agents which have a blood-borne dissemination, including bacteria, viruses, parasites, and fungi. Antibodies and immunoglobulins are discussed in detail later in this chapter.

HUMAN T AND B CELLS

For differentiating human T and B cells, the rosetting test with sheep erythrocytes is a useful technique. Some 80%–100% of human T cells will form rosettes with normal sheep erythrocytes. Each of these rosettes appears as a central lymphocyte with four or more red blood cells attached to its surface (Fig. 1-3). B cells will not form rosettes with normal sheep erythrocytes. If, however, the red cells are first coated with antibody and if complement is then added, rosetting of B cells, but not T cells, will take place.

T cells comprise 60%–75% of all lymphocytes in the peripheral blood, spleen, and lymph nodes; B cells account for 20%–30%. In lymphoblastic leukemia most of the leukemic cells are T cells, while in chronic lymphatic leukemia most are B cells. Lymphomas may contain either B or T cells. T cells are decreased in patients with cancer, lepromatous leprosy, and certain other diseases.

A third population of lymphocytes exists, which do not have B or T cell markers. These lymphocytes are known as **null cells.** Null cells may simply be immature T cells that have not yet been exposed to thymus tissue. Null cells may play a role in various rheumatoid diseases. A cell which may be identical to the null cell is the **killer** cell or **K** cell which appears to be responsible for certain forms of cell-mediated cytotoxicity.

LYMPHOID ORGANS

Lymphocytes are found in the lymph nodes, spleen, thymus, and gastrointestinal tract. All lymphoid organs have a similar structure. The organs are encapsulated and divided into lobules by connective tissue strands. Blood is supplied by a single artery and drained by veins and lymphatics. The parenchyma consists of a cortex, or peripheral zone, and a medulla, or central zone.

Lymph nodes (Fig. 1-4) serve as filters for the lymphatic drainage. The cortical region of

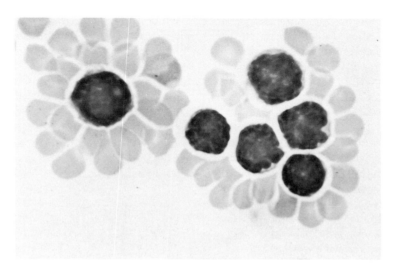

FIG. 1-3. Rosettes formed by sheep erythrocytes surrounding T lymphocytes. (Courtesy of Dr. S. Barrett).

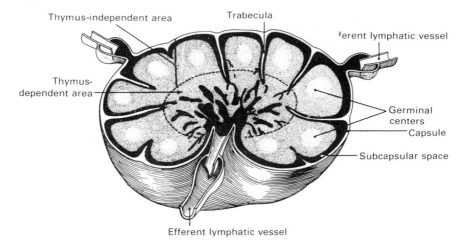

FIG. 1-4. Structure of lymph node showing thymus-dependent and bursa-dependent areas. (Bellanti JA: Immunology, Philadelphia, WB Saunders, 1971, p 33)

the lymph node contains tightly packed nodules of lymphocytes, known as primary follicles, and more loosely packed nodules surrounded by a rim of tightly packed lymphoid cells, known as secondary follicles. Each primary follicle has a central zone of immature cells known as the **germinal center.** The paracortical areas are strips of lymphoid tissue lying between the follicles. These paracortical areas are considered to be thymus-dependent areas; thymectomy in neonatal animals leads to depletion of lymphoid cells in these areas. The follicular areas, on the other hand, are bursa-dependent: they become depleted of lymphocytes in birds if the bursa of Fabricius is removed. The medulla of the lymph node contains a network of draining sinusoidal channels, and rows of lymphocytes known as **medullary cords.**

The spleen (Fig. 1-5) also contains lymphoid follicles. These are not confined to the cortical areas but are distributed throughout the parenchyma. Lymphoid follicles occupy the area known as the white pulp, while the vascular region, containing many red blood cells, is known as red pulp. The spleen does not contain lymphatic vessels, but, rather, has an extensive arterial and venous drainage.

The thymus (Fig. 1-6) contains a cortical area and a medulla; however, it has no lymphoid follicles. Rather, the cortex consists of packed lymphocytes. The thymus processes T lymphocytes, which, as was said, are the mediators of cellular immunity.

The gastrointestinal system contains lymphoid tissue in the Peyer's patches, appendix, and tonsillar areas. Lymphocytes in these areas are arranged as follicles, and some thymus-dependent follicles are present in these tissues. The tonsils form a ring of lymphoid tissue around the oral cavity (Waldeyer's ring). The gastrointestinal lymphoid tissues are important in the development of the secretory immunoglobulin system, and in the synthesis of immunoglobulin A.

The bone marrow contains stem cells and other blood precursors. Both B and T lymphocytes are derived from bone marrow stem cells. Bone marrow lymphocytes circulate to other organs where they undergo differentiation into B and T lymphocytes: those migrating to the thymus differentiate into T cells, while those going to the gut-associated lymphoid tissue differentiate into B cells.

EFFECT OF LYMPHOID TISSUE STIMULATION

An immune response is the specific recognition of a foreign substance by the body's immune system and the formation of antibody or

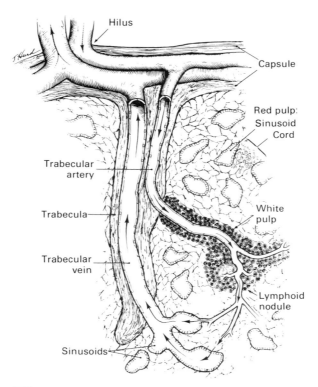

FIG. 1-5. Schematic drawing of spleen. (Bellanti JA: Immunology, Philadelphia, WB Saunders, 1971, p 35)

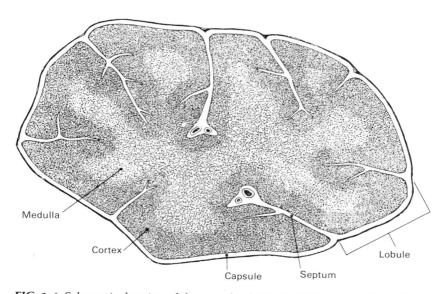

FIG. 1-6. Schematic drawing of thymus gland. (Bellanti JA: Immunology, Philadelphia, WB Saunders, 1971, p 36)

sensitized lymphocytes in response to this recognition.

When an immune response occurs, certain morphologic changes take place within the lymphoid tissue. In antibody production, antigen is taken up by macrophages located in the medullary areas of the lymph nodes and spleen. These cells become elongated and are closely associated with lymphocytes in the lymph node cortex or the splenic white pulp. Lymphoid follicles develop around the macrophages containing antigen, and within a few days the progenitors of the antibody-forming plasma cells are detectable in the circulation. Plasma cells can be found in the germinal centers and medullary cords about 7 days after active immunization. There they persist for several weeks and produce antibodies.

If delayed hypersensitivity (a cell-mediated immune response) is stimulated instead of antibody production, the changes in the lymph node occur in the paracortical areas rather than in the cortex. The paracortical areas undergo expansion, and a few days after active immunization, large pyroninophilic blast cells appear in the paracortical regions. These cells undergo division and small lymphocytes (T cells) are released into the draining lymph (see also Lymphocyte Transformation, Ch. 2).

Blast transformation of T cells can also be induced by certain agents known as **mitogens.** These include substances such as phytohemagglutinin (PHA) and concanavalin A. Mitogens may also stimulate the B cell system. The mechanism of mitogenic activity is unknown; however, it is known that this type of activation bypasses the usual antigen-specific stimulation.

How antigen is processed in delayed hypersensitivity is unknown. It may occur in the lymph nodes, or in peripheral areas such as the skin. T lymphocytes do not readily bind antigen to their surfaces. Although receptors can be demonstrated on the surface of T lymphocytes, they are scarce and only partially accessible. Presumably, macrophages assist in processing the antigen or presenting it to the T lymphocyte. B cells, on the other hand, possess immunoglobulin receptors on their cell surfaces which are detectable by immunofluorescence and other techniques. These receptors behave as antibody and are capable of binding antigen. In the B cell, this binding leads to transformation into a plasma cell and the production of antibody.

Several theories have evolved to explain the processing of antigen and the interaction between the cells involved in the immune response. Macrophages concentrate antigen and in some way present the antigen to the lymphocyte, perhaps by transferring information regarding the antigen to the lymphocyte. Moreover, T and B cells apparently interact and cooperate in the formation of antibody. The interactions of T and B lymphocytes and macrophages *in vivo* has not been well defined, and the mechanism of these interactions is presently unknown.

IMMUNOLOGIC MEMORY

As just described, when the immune system is stimulated, lymphatic tissue undergoes differentiation and proliferation. This may result in **humoral immunity,** with proliferation of plasma cells and production of antibody, or **cellular immunity,** with proliferation of specifically sensitized T lymphocytes (*i.e.,* lymphocytes capable of specific recognition). Both types of immunity may also be produced simultaneously in response to a particular antigen. The resultant antibodies or specifically sensitized T cells have the capability of reacting with the antigen responsible for their production. Furthermore, reintroduction of the same antigen into the system at a later time results in a more rapid and greater proliferation of plasma cells or of lymphocytes known as **memory cells** (Fig. 1-7). These memory cells may be either T or B lymphocytes. This secondary response, known as the **anamnestic response,** is due to the presence of memory cells produced by previous antigenic stimulation.

A feedback mechanism exists for the control of antibody production. During either the primary or the anamnestic response, high levels of antibody are produced, followed by a tapering off of antibody levels. Such regulatory

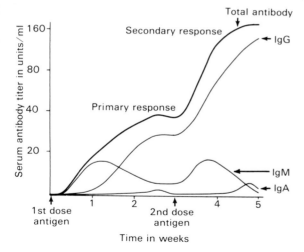

FIG. 1-7. Primary and secondary (anamnestic) antibody response. Note shorter latency period and higher concentration of antibody during secondary response. (Köngshavn PAL, Hawkins D, Shuster J: The biology of the immune response. In Freedman SO, Gold P (eds): Clinical Immunology, Hagerstown, Harper & Row, 1976, p 35)

mechanisms are important in controlling the immune system when continued antigenic stimulation takes place. The mechanism by which feedback takes place is unknown, but it may be related to suppressor cells or to inhibition by specific antibody.

EFFECTOR MECHANISMS

Two types of effector mechanisms exist which mediate the several kinds of immune responses. One, known as **humoral immunity,** is mediated by antibody. The second, known as **cell-mediated** or **cellular immunity,** is mediated by specifically sensitized T lymphocytes. A third response, a state of nonreactivity known as **immune tolerance,** may also develop after immune stimulation of B or T lymphocytes (Fig. 1-8).

HUMORAL IMMUNITY

Antibodies may interact with antigens under a variety of circumstances. These interactions occur within the blood stream, on mucosal surfaces, or within various tissues of the body. The effects of such interactions may be beneficial or harmful to the host; in the latter situation we say that a state of **allergy** or **immediate hypersensitivity** exists. Humoral immunity accounts for the body's responses to a variety of microorganisms as well as for the production of many allergic conditions and disease entities. The humoral immune system is closely linked embryologically with lymphoid tissue commonly known as gut-associated lymphoid tissue (GALT). In birds, the bursa of Fabricius is responsible for processing the cells involved in humoral immunity. In man the analogous lymphoid tissue may be located in the bone marrow, fetal liver or GI tract.

CELL-MEDIATED (CELLULAR) IMMUNITY

The second major effector mechanism which participates in the immune response involves specifically sensitized lymphocytes directed against foreign antigens. Cellular immunity is monitored by the thymus, and responses are mediated by the thymus-dependent T lymphocytes. The term **delayed hypersensitivity** had also been used as a synonym for

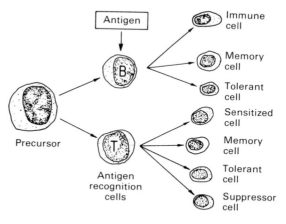

FIG. 1-8. Response of B and T cells to antigen. B and T lymphocytes may respond immunologically in several ways. B lymphocytes may develop into antibody-producing plasma cells, B memory cells or tolerant B cells. T lymphocytes may become sensitized, memory, tolerant, or suppressor T cells. (Sell S: Immunology, Immunopathology, and Immunity, Hagerstown, Harper & Row, 1975, p 117)

cellular immunity, and this mechanism is discussed under that heading in Chapter 2. However, some authors feel that this term should be restricted to the undesirable or tissue-damaging responses induced by T cells. Cell-mediated immunity encompasses other important biologic responses, including recovery from many infectious diseases, surveillance against neoplasia, and rejection of foreign grafts and malignant cells.

IMMUNE TOLERANCE

A state of unresponsiveness to a specific antigen may be induced under certain circumstances. This phenomenon, known as immune tolerance, prevents the host from responding to a foreign substance with antibody or sensitized T cells. Again, this response is specific. It may be produced by presenting the host with an antigen that is not easily catabolized, such as pneumococcal polysaccharide. It may also be induced with unusually high or low doses of antigen, and may at times be induced by administration of antigen by the oral or intravenous route. A host also maintains nonreactivity to his own bodily tissues because of immune tolerance: presumably, antigens that the host encounters *in utero* or at birth, before the immune surveillance system is fully developed, will henceforth be recognized as "self." Sometimes an abnormality in the immune surveillance system, or possibly an alteration in the host's own antigens, results in the recognition of certain host tissues as foreign. This situation leads to an immune reaction against the body's own tissues and is the basis of so-called autoimmune disease. (See also Immune Tolerance, Ch. 2.)

ANTIGENS

PHYSICAL AND CHEMICAL PROPERTIES

An **antigen** is a substance capable of eliciting an immune response. Some authors prefer the term **immunogen** and reserve the term **antigen** for a substance which combines only with antibody. In common parlance, however, the terms antigen and immunogen are used virtually interchangeably.

In order for a molecule to immunize, that is, to be antigenic, it must first be genetically foreign to the host. However, not all foreign substances are capable of stimulating a specific immune response. Inert substances such as carbon, for example, will only induce a nonspecific phagocytic response. Antigens tend to be large molecules, with molecular weights of 10,000 or more. Still, some smaller molecules with molecular weights in the range of 1000 have been shown to be antigenic. While there is a lower limit of molecular weight below which substances are unlikely to be antigenic, there seems to be no upper limit in size. Usually antigens are proteins but they may also be polysaccharides or combinations of proteins and polysaccharides (Table 1-1). Normally, lipids and nucleic acids are not antigenic; however, they may become antigenic if combined with proteins or polysaccharides.

Haptens are small molecules which induce an immune response only after combining with a protein. The hapten–protein complex may then function as a complete antigen, and a specific immune response will be directed against the hapten or the hapten and carrier protein.

Insoluble particles such as red blood cells

TABLE 1-1. CHEMICAL TYPES OF ANTIGENS

Type	Source
Protein	Serum proteins, microbial products (toxins), enzymes
Lipoprotein	Serum lipoproteins; cell membranes
Polysaccharides	Capsules of bacteria (pneumococcus)
Lipopolysaccharides	Cell walls of gram-negative bacteria (endotoxins)
Glycoproteins	Blood group substances A and B
Polypeptides	Hormones (insulin, growth hormone), synthetic compounds
Nucleic acids	Nucleoproteins, single-stranded DNA

(Bellanti JA: Immunology. Philadelphia, Saunders, 1971, p 98) may possess many different antigenic groups, which are known as **antigenic determinants.** (These antigenic determinants may be found in soluble as well as in particulate antigens.) Those determinants which are most readily accessible to antibody or lymphocytes tend to be closer to the outer surface of the molecule. In very complex macromolecules, certain amino acids or groups of amino acids are antigenically more potent than others. Further, a higher degree of variability in amino acid composition tends to confer a greater antigenicity upon a molecule.

A variety of factors influence the immunogenicity of an antigen. These include solubility, molecular configuration, charge, and accessibility of the determinant groups. A substance which can be degraded and phagocytized by the host is more likely to elicit an immune response. (If the antigen is eliminated, the immune response has been beneficial. If the antigen persists, the mechanisms of immunity may lead to immunologic tissue injury.) Chemical properties are also important. Most organic substances, with the exception of lipids, can be immunogenic. The vast majority of immunogens are protein in nature; often these proteins are combined with carbohydrates, lipids, or nucleic acids. Polysaccharides, such as the capsular components of the pneumococcal bacteria, or lipopolysaccharides, such as endotoxins, are biologically important antigens. Glycoproteins can be antigenic; these include the blood group antigens A and B, associated with transfusion reactions. For many years nucleic acids were considered nonimmunogenic; however, in certain diseases such as systemic lupus erythematosus, an immune response to the patient's own nucleic acids may develop and lead to tissue damage.

BIOLOGIC PROPERTIES

It is well known that live, attenuated, vaccines confer greater protection than killed or inactivated preparations; this may be due to the removal of important determinant groups during the preparation of a killed vaccine. Also, an immune response to a particular antigen may vary from one species to the next. Thus, the mouse develops a good immune response to the isolated pneumococcal polysaccharide capsule while the rabbit does not. Even within a species there may be variations in the immunologic response to a given antigen. The dose and route of introduction of an antigen are also important factors. A very low dose or a very high dose of an antigen may actually produce tolerance. Similarly, antigens given by the oral or intravenous route may lead to immunologic unresponsiveness. On the other hand, parenteral administration of the same antigen may produce a potent immune response. Ordinarily, however, the immunogenicity of an antigen can be assessed by the antigen's ability to stimulate an immune response. The type of immune response which develops depends on the nature of the antigen. Specific antibody may be produced in response to one type of antigen while specifically sensitized T lymphocytes develop in response to a different antigen. Some antigens can elicit both a humoral and a cellular immune response.

EXOGENOUS ANTIGENS

The antigens which confront the host in the environment are varied in nature. They include, for example, microorganisms, drugs, airborne pollens, and pollutants. These **exogenous antigens** under certain conditions may cause an infectious or allergic disease (Table 1-2). Bacterial cell walls, for instance, are known to contain a number of antigenic substances. The exterior structure of virus particles can also serve as a rich source of exogenous antigens.

ENDOGENOUS ANTIGENS

Antigens found within the host are known as **endogenous antigens.** They may be subdivided into heterologous, homologous, and autologous antigens (Table 1-2).

Heterologous Antigens

Those antigens which are shared by phylogenetically unrelated species are known as **heterologous** antigens. These antigens, also known as **heterogeneic** or **heterophilic,** reflect

TABLE 1-2. CLASSIFICATION OF ANTIGENS

Type	Example	Clinical Significance
Exogenous	Viruses, bacteria, pollen	Susceptibility to infection, immunologically mediated disease (asthma)
Endogenous		
Heterologous	Heterogenetic antigens	Pathogenesis of certain diseases, *e.g.,* glomerulonephritis, rheumatic fever
Autologous	Organ-specific antigens	Autoimmune diseases
Homologous	Blood group antigens, histocompatibility antigens (HLA)	Hemolytic disease of the newborn, transfusion reactions, transplantation immunity

(Bellanti JA: Immunology. Philadelphia, Saunders, 1971, p 75)

a very similar chemical structure which is present in the cells and tissues of entirely unrelated species. The Forssman antigen is a heterologous antigen found in the tissues of humans, guinea pigs, horses, cats, birds, and fish. Following infectious mononucleosis in humans, an antibody response directed against the Forssman antigen may develop. This is the so-called heterophil antibody response that is a helpful diagnostic test for this disease. Some other cross-reacting antigens are also useful in diagnosing certain disease states. Cardiolipin, for example, which is present in beef heart and plants, is also found in spirochetes; it is the basis of several serologic tests for syphilis. A common antigen is shared by the group A β-hemolytic streptococcus and human heart muscle. It is believed that cardiac damage in rheumatic fever is due to the cross reactivity of antibody and this heterologous antigen.

Homologous Antigens (Isoantigens, Alloantigens)

The most important group of endogenous antigens are the **homologous antigens.** These are genetically controlled determinants which are specific to a given species, and serve to differentiate one individual from another within that species. In man, these **isoantigens,** or **alloantigens,** include antigens found on red blood cells, white blood cells, and platelets, and the histocompatibility antigens. When an individual is immunized with an isoantigen from another person, an immune response may take place and occasionally leads to a disease state. A well-known example is the reac-

tion to an incompatible blood transfusion. Red blood cells contain a variety of isoantigens; however, only the ABO and Rh systems seem to be of major importance. This may be due either to the immunogenicity of these antigens or to their frequency in the population.

Landsteiner, in 1900, demonstrated the major isoantigens on human red blood cells. By placing red blood cells from one individual into another individual's serum *in vitro*, he showed that red blood cell agglutination would sometimes take place. He was able to determine that individuals of blood type A possess anti-B antibodies (isoagglutinins) and those of blood type B possess anti-A antibodies. Those of blood type O have both anti-A and anti-B antibodies, while individuals of group AB have neither anti-A nor anti-B isoagglutinins. The type of blood group that an individual possesses is under genetic control. Three allelic genes control the expression of these antigens. The A and B genes are dominant over the O gene. Individuals who possess the O gene, while not possessing either A or B isoantigens, do possess an O antigen, known as H substance, which is a heterogeneic antigen found in a variety of species.

Another important isoantigen of the red blood cell is the Rh antigen. Even in the presence of ABO compatibility, a variation in the Rh system may lead to significant incompatibility, and a severe hemolytic reaction. This is the basis for the disease of newborn infants known as erythroblastosis fetalis. In this disease, the paternal isoantigens on red blood cells of the fetus enter the maternal circulation. The antibodies formed as a result may be transferred back to the fetus in a subsequent pregnancy and produce severe hemolysis. There are approximately 30 Rh antigenic types, but the most critically significant one is that controlled by the D gene locus. When a mother who is D negative (Rh−) is carrying a D-positive (Rh+) fetus, it is possible for maternal sensitization to occur, and subsequent Rh+ fetuses may be in danger of developing hemolytic disease of the newborn.

Histocompatibility Antigens. Histocompatibility antigens are isoantigens found on the surfaces of most cells, including white blood cells and platelets. They are important clinically because they form the basis for graft rejection in organ transplantation. These antigens are lipoproteins which are found on plasma membranes of tissue cells. When donor histocompatibility antigens are transplanted to a host (recipient) not possessing these antigens, an immune response may be induced and the donor tissue cells rejected. If tissue compatibility exists between the isoantigens of the donor and the host, the transplanted tissue will not be rejected as foreign but will be accepted as a graft. Complete histocompatibility is not essential for successful transplantation. The acceptance of a graft depends on the degree of antigenic similarity between the recipient and the donor, the nature of the transplanted tissue itself, and the immune responses of the host.

In humans, the major histocompatibility system is known as the HLA (human leukocyte antigen) system (Table 1-3). HLA antigens are found on the surface of all nucleated cells. The HLA antigens are determined by a series of four genes located on chromosome 6. These gene loci are known as HLA-A, HLA-B, HLA-C, and HLA-D, and each controls several different antigenic specificities. Over 95% of the possible specificities can be recognized by serologic methods. Table 1-3 lists the current recognized HLA antigens. Those listings in

TABLE 1-3. COMPLETE LISTING OF RECOGNIZED HLA SPECIFICITIES*

HLA–A	HLA–B		HLA–C	HLA–D	HLA–DR
HLA–A1	HLA–B5	HLA–Bw42	HLA–Cw1	HLA–Dw1	HLA–DRw1
HLA–A2	HLA–B7	HLA–Bw44	HLA–Cw2	HLA–Dw2	HLA–DRw2
HLA–A3	HLA–B8	HLA–Bw45	HLA–Cw3	HLA–Dw3	HLA–DRw3
HLA–A9	HLA–B12	HLA–Bw46	HLA–Cw4	HLA–Dw4	HLA–DRw4
HLA–A10	HLA–B13	HLA–Bw47	HLA–Cw5	HLA–Dw5	HLA–DRw5
HLA–A11	HLA–B14	HLA–Bw48	HLA–Cw6	HLA–Dw6	HLA–DRw6
HLA–Aw19	HLA–B15	HLA–Bw49		HLA–Dw7	HLA–DRw7
HLA–Aw23	HLA–Bw16	HLA–Bw50		HLA–Dw8	
HLA–Aw24	HLA–B17	HLA–Bw51		HLA–Dw9	
HLA–A25	HLA–B18	HLA–Bw52		HLA–Dw10	
HLA–A26	HLA–Bw21	HLA–Bw53		HLA–Dw11	
HLA–A28	HLA–Bw22	HLA–Bw54			
HLA–A29	HLA–B27				
HLA–Aw30	HLA–Bw35				
HLA–Aw31	HLA–B37				
HLA–Aw32	HLA–Bw38				
HLA–Aw33	HLA–Bw39				
HLA–Aw34	HLA–B40				
HLA–Aw36	HLA–Bw41				
HLA–Aw43					
	HLA–Bw4				
	HLA–Bw6				

* The following is a list of those specificities which have arisen as clear cut splits of other specificities:
HLA–A9 into HLA–Aw23, HLA–Aw24
HLA–A10 into HLA–A25, HLA–A26
HLA–B5 into HLA–Bw51, HLA–Bw52
HLA–B12 into HLA–Bw44, HLA–Bw45
HLA–Bw16 into HLA–Bw38, HLA–Bw39
HLA–Bw21 into HLA–Bw49, HLA–Bw50
Historically, HLA–Aw19 has included HLA–A29, HLA–Aw30, HLA–Aw31, HLA–Aw32 and HLA–Aw33.
(Nomenclature for factors of the HLA system. Tissue Antigens, 11:84, 1978)

which a small w appears have been provisionally identified but are still being studied in workshops around the world. The antigens designated DR are closely associated with the D locus but it is not certain at this time whether or not they are actually products of this locus.

Every individual may be characterized by HLA typing, which identifies his HLA phenotype. Owing to the multiplicity of allelic genes, the possible HLA phenotypes are numerous. In pretransplantation tissue typing (see Transplantation Immunology, Ch. 11), the closer the HLA match between the donor and the recipient, the better are the chances for a successful transplant. A possibility exists that HLA antigens are genetic markers rather than real transplantation antigens: possibly, strong transplantation antigens are closely linked with the HLA markers on the genetic material. This concept has led to an intensive search for the association of certain HLA antigens with specific disease entities in which an abnormal immune response is thought to occur.

Tumor Antigens. Tumor cells contain antigens which are either products of oncogenic viruses or fetal antigens normally found on cells during early development (Fig. 1-9). When a cell undergoes malignant transforma-

tion, a variety of surface membrane changes take place, and membrane antigens may be altered from their normal state. These altered antigens are referred to as **tumor-specific transplantation antigens (TSTAs).** Examples of TSTAs include the following: Epstein–Barr (EB) virus–related antigens are found on lymphoblastoid cells. Antibodies to these antigens are present in patients with Burkitt's lymphoma, nasopharyngeal carcinoma, and other diseases. S (sarcoma) antigens are found in human sarcomas, and antibodies to S antigens are present in sarcoma patients, their relatives, and close contacts. Two types of melanoma antigens are found in patients with malignant melanomas. One is an intracellular antigen found in all melanomas. Antibodies to this antigen are present in the serum of melanoma patients. A second type of antigen is found on the surface of melanoma cells and is likely to be a TSTA. Fetal antigens, such as α-fetoprotein, may be reactivated during the malignant process. This antigen is found in the serum of patients with embryonal cell carcinoma or hepatoma. The carcinoembryonic antigen (CEA) has been found in patients with carcinoma of the digestive tract. γ-Fetoprotein has been detected in all histologic types of tumors as well as in benign neoplasms. (See also Tumor Antigens, Ch. 12.)

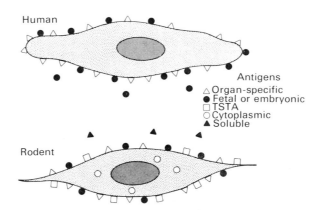

FIG. 1-9. Schematic representation of tumor cell antigens. These antigens have been identified in humans and other animals. (Reproduced with permission from Beyers VS and Levin AS: Tumor Immunology. In Fudenberg HH, Stites DP, Caldwell JL, Wells JV, (eds). Basic and Clinical Immunology, Los Altos, Lange, 1976, p 243)

Autologous Antigens

Under normal circumstances the antigens of the host's own bodily constituents are recognized as self and are nonimmunogenic. In autoimmune disease, however, these autologous antigens may in some way be changed so that the host mounts an immunologic attack on his own tissues.

ADJUVANTS

Antigens are frequently injected along with certain substances which enhance the immune response. These substances, known as **adjuvants,** in some way stimulate the immune system. The mechanism by which adjuvants work is not clear; however, they may increase the surface area of the antigen, provide a slow, sustained release of the antigen from a depot, or activate macrophages and other cells. The most commonly used adjuvant is a water and oil emulsion known as **Freund's adjuvant.** Complete Freund's adjuvant contains killed mycobacteria in addition to mineral oil, water, and an emulsifier; incomplete Freund's adjuvant contains no mycobacteria. Complete Freund's adjuvant induces a stronger and more persistent response to an antigen. Other adjuvants which are useful in immunology include *Corynebacterium parvum, Bordetella pertussis,* alum (potassium aluminum sulfate), aluminum hydroxide, and killed microorganisms such as staphylococci and streptococci.

ANTIBODIES

Antibodies are protein molecules produced by plasma cells. In the human, antibody activity is associated with five major classes of proteins known as the **immunoglobulins.** Nearly all antibodies are immunoglobulins. Antibody has the ability to react specifically with the antigen, or immunogen, responsible for its formation. The result of this interaction is varied. The antibody may neutralize the effects of a toxin, produce cell lysis, or lead to an allergic or hypersensitivity reaction.

GENERAL PROPERTIES

During the late 1930s, Tiselius and Kabat demonstrated by electrophoresis that antibody activity was associated with the γ-globulin fraction of human serum. During the 1950s, Porter found that by treating antibody with the enzyme papain, he could split the molecule into three pieces (Fig. 1-10). Two of these fragments retained antibody activity, while the third possessed the antigenic features of γ-globulin. Porter later proposed a model of the immunoglobulin molecule consisting of four polypeptide chains. Because of the heterogeneity of the immunoglobulins, it was long thought that unravelling their structure was impossible. However, the finding that very homogeneous immunoglobulin substances are associated with multiple myeloma made it possible to learn a great deal about these mole-

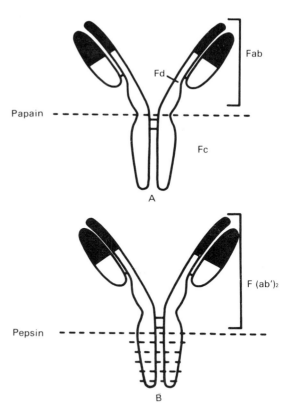

FIG. 1-10. Enzymatic cleavage of antibody molecule by (A) papain and (B) pepsin. (Van Oss CJ: The Immunoglobulins. In Rose NR, Milgrom F, Van Oss CJ (eds): *Principles of Immunology,* New York, Macmillan Publ. Co. Inc., p 130)

cules. Edelman, during the early 1960s, demonstrated that immunoglobulins were multichain structures. He and other investigators were able to unravel the amino acid sequence of immunoglobulin molecules obtained from the urine of patients with multiple myeloma. Further studies of immunoglobulins have helped to clarify the chemical nature and biologic functions of these molecules.

In man, there are five known classes of immunoglobulins (Table 1-4), designated as IgG, IgA, IgM, IgD, and IgE. The prefix **Ig** is an abbreviation for immunoglobulin; the symbol γ has sometimes been used in its place, indicating the electrophoretic mobility of these proteins. Each class of immunoglobulins has a specific chemical structure and biologic role.

Structural Features

Basically, all immunoglobulin molecules contain four polypeptide chains: two heavy chains, each having a molecular weight of 55,000–75,000, and two light chains with molecular weights of about 23,000. There are five structurally distinct types of heavy chains, one for each class of immunoglobulins. The heavy chains are designated as γ chains for the IgG molecule, μ for IgM, α for IgA, δ for IgD, and ϵ for IgE. Two different types of light chains also exist. These, designated κ and λ chains, are found in immunoglobulin molecules of each class. Any immunoglobulin molecule has light chains of either the κ or λ type. In addition, some of the major types of immunoglobulins have heavy-chain subgroups.

Heavy chains are attached to one another and to the light chains by disulfide bonds. Since there are five different kinds of heavy chains and two different kinds of light chains, ten possible combinations of heavy and light chains may be found in any individual. The basic four-chain structure may be written as a formula describing the makeup of heavy and light chains. Thus, $\gamma_2\kappa_2$ would represent an IgG molecule containing two γ heavy chains and two κ light chains, while $\gamma_2\lambda_2$ would be an IgG molecule containing two γ chains and two λ chains.

Antibody molecules are highly specific, owing to variations in their primary amino acid sequence at the amino terminal end of the molecule. The variability involves the distal half of the light-chain sequence and the distal quarter of the heavy-chain sequence. This "variable region" of the immunoglobulin molecule is the site where antigen binding occurs. The opposite end of the molecule, the carboxy terminal, is a much more constant part of the immunoglobulin.

The three-dimensional structure of immunoglobulins has been studied by electron microscopy and x-ray crystallography. The IgG molecule is Y-shaped and the antibody combining sites are located at the ends of the arms of the Y. The area where the arms and body of the Y intersect is called the hinge region. The distance between the arms of the Y may vary, depending on whether or not the IgG molecule has combined with antigen. IgM has a star shape, or pentameric form, composed of five Y-shaped IgG-like units.

In addition to the amino acid sequence which forms its primary structure, the immunoglobulin molecule has higher orders of structure. These include the secondary structure or coiling of the individual peptide chains, the tertiary structure or folding of the polypeptide coils, and the quaternary structure or the association between the folded chains.

The polypeptide chains have a considerable amount of helical coiling. Thus, the peptide chains are pinched into a series of loops, each containing approximately 60 amino acids. Two loops are formed in each light chain and four in each heavy chain. Disulfide bonds are located at these pinched-off areas.

Biologic Features

IgG is the most abundant immunoglobulin, and accounts for most of the antibody directed against infectious agents. IgA is the second most abundant immunoglobulin and has an important function in the secretory immune system. IgM is the largest of the immunoglobulins and is an efficient agglutinator of particulate antigens. It is the first immunoglobulin to appear in the development of the primary immune response. The function of IgD is still uncertain, but recent investigation has shown

TABLE 1-4. PROPERTIES OF IMMUNOGLOBULIN CLASSES

	IgG	IgA	IgM	IgD	IgE
Normal adult serum concentration (g per 100 ml)	1.0–1.4	0.2–0.3	0.04–0.15	0.003	1–7×10^{-5}
Major body distribution	Intravascular and extracellular fluid	Intravascular and internal secretion	Mainly intravascular	Mainly intravascular	Skin; respiratory and GI tracts
Electrophoretic mobility	γ	Slow β	Between β and γ	Between β and γ	Slow β
Sedimentation coefficient (in Svedberg units)	7S	7S (11.5S for secretory IgA)	19S	7S	8S
Molecular weight	160,000	170,000 (400,000 for secretory IgA)	900,000	185,000	200,000
Molecular weight of the heavy chains (M of Light chains + 23,000)	55,000	62,000	65,000	70,000	75,000
Nomenclature of heavy chains	γ	α	μ	δ	ϵ
Molecular formula	$\gamma_2\kappa_2, \gamma_2\lambda_2$	$\alpha_2\kappa_2, \alpha_2\lambda_2$	$\mu_{10}\kappa_{10}, \mu_{10}\lambda_{10}$	$\delta_2\kappa_2, \delta_2\lambda_2$	$\epsilon_2\kappa_2, \epsilon_2\lambda_2$
Normal heavy/light chain ratio	2/1	5/4	3/1	1/6	?
Subclasses	IgG1, IgG2, IgG3, IgG4	IgA1, IgA2	IgM1, IgM2	—	—
Allotypes	Gm	Am	—	—	—
Carbohydrate (%)	2.3	5–10	5–10	13	10
Synthetic rate (g/day/70 kg)	2.3	2.7	0.4	0.03	?
Half-life (days)	23	6	5	3	3
Tendency to polymerize or aggregate	+	+	+	?	?
Complement binding	+	—	+	—	—
Rheumatoid factor binding	+	—	—	—	—
Placental transport	+	—	—	—	—
Skin sensitization Heterologous	+	—	—	—	—
Skin sensitization Homologous	—	—	—	—	+

(Rose NR, *et al* (eds): Principles of Immunology. New York, Macmillan, 1973, p 126) that IgD is present on the surface of lymphocytes in the newborn infant. IgE occurs in very minute quantities; it is felt to play a prominent role in the development of atopic allergy.

Within each of the classes of immunoglobulins, different subclasses may exist. These subclasses are differentiated by minor differences in antigenic reactivity and immunochemical analysis. Four subclasses exist for the IgG molecule and two for IgA. Two subclasses may also exist for IgM.

IMMUNOGLOBULIN G

Structure

IgG is the most abundant immunoglobulin in serum, with a concentration of 1.0–1.4 g/100 ml. It has a half-life of approximately 23 days, longer than that of any other immunoglobulin. Its electrophoretic distribution is over the entire range of the γ-globulins (Fig. 1-11). The molecular weight of IgG is approximately 160,-000 and its sedimentation coefficient is 7S (Svedberg units). IgG is a symmetric structure having two heavy chains and two light chains joined together by disulfide bonds (Fig. 1-12).

Biologic and Immunologic Properties

IgG is the only immunoglobulin that crosses the human placental barrier. Thus, it provides the maternal antibodies that lend protection to the newborn infant during the first few months of life. IgG plays an important role in almost all immune defense reactions, including defense against microbial infections. IgG and IgM are the only two immunoglobulins which will normally fix complement, doing so after interaction with an appropriate antigen. IgG is the major antibody formed during the secondary or anamnestic response. It also forms **blocking antibodies,** which can combine with allergens and prevent their interaction with mast-cell–bound IgE. Antibodies which passively bind to the skin of animals of other species (heterocytotropic antibodies) are also of the IgG class. IgG antibodies are the most efficient antibodies in the precipitation reaction, but are somewhat less efficient agglutinators (see Serologic Tests in Diagnosis).

The IgG molecule can be split into fragments by the use of certain enzyme preparations (see Fig. 1-10). Papain splits the heavy chains of IgG, leaving three fragments. One, which contains most of the antigenic determinants of IgG, is known as the Fc fragment. The two other fragments, which retain the ability to combine with antigen, are known as Fab fragments. A second enzyme, pepsin, degrades the heavy chain of IgG below the main disulfide bonds which hold the two heavy chains together. This leaves two fragments: a bivalent piece with antibody activity known as the F(ab')$_2$ fragment, and the carboxy terminal half of the IgG heavy chain. The latter fragment undergoes virtually complete digestion, which destroys the antigenic determinants and complement-binding ability of the molecule. The heavy and light chains can be separated by reduction with mercaptoethanol, which breaks the disulfide bonds. Besides the Fab and Fc fragments, another portion of the IgG molecule has been named. The Fd fragment consists of the heavy-chain portions of the Fab fragments (Fig. 1-13). This portion of the IgG molecule has great biologic significance, since it contributes to the antigen-binding site of the IgG molecule.

Immunoglobulin molecules other than IgG can also be cleaved by enzymes. However, the area of cleavage is not always the same as with IgG. Still, the different parts of the various immunoglobulin molecules are designated according to the system used for IgG (*e.g.,* Fab, Fc, and Fd).

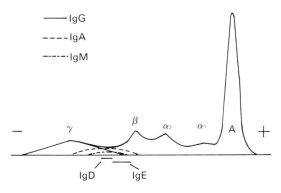

FIG. 1-11. Electrophoretic distribution of the immunoglobulins. **A.** Albumin (Van Oss CJ: The Immunoglobulins. In Rose NR, Milgrom F, Van Oss CJ (eds): Principles of Immunology, New York, Macmillan Publ. Co. Inc., p 125)

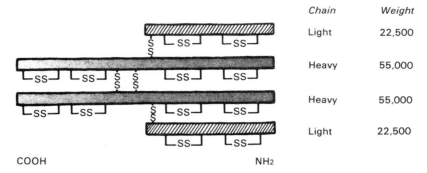

Chain	Weight
Light	22,500
Heavy	55,000
Heavy	55,000
Light	22,500

COOH   NH2

FIG. 1-12. Schematic representation of IgG molecule showing light and heavy chains connected by disulfide bonds. A similar structure is applicable to other immunoglobulins. (Bellanti JA: Immunology, Philadelphia, WB Saunders, 1971, p 104)

IgG Subclasses

Four subclasses exist for the IgG molecule—IgG1, IgG2, IgG3, and IgG4. These four subclasses vary slightly in their physical and chemical properties, making possible their separation by gel electrophoresis. They represent respectively 75%, 15%, 7%, and 3% of the total serum IgG. Certain functional differences exist in the different subclasses. For instance, IgG4 does not fix complement; IgG2 does not cross the placenta as easily as the other subclasses, and does not occur as heterocytotropic antibody. IgG3 has a shorter half-life than the other subclasses, and when present in large amounts gives rise to a hyperviscosity syndrome. The structural differences which account for the separate subclasses of IgG reside in the heavy chains and in the location of the major disulfide bonds.

Aggregation of IgG

After treatment with heat or alcohol, some IgG molecules will form aggregates. Mild treatment with alcohol results in the formation of 10S IgG dimers. Heating IgG to 63° C for 10 min or more leads to formation of larger aggregates of 20S–40S. These aggregates have some of the same properties as untreated IgG when it combines with specific antigen. Aggregated IgG fixes complement and combines with rheumatoid factor (see under Immunoglobulin M) in the absence of antigen. Apparently, heating and aggregation lead to configurational changes and exposure of se-cluded regions in the Fc region which contain reactive sites. Only about 20% of human IgG is capable of aggregation. The IgG3 subclass is particularly prone to aggregation.

IgG Allotypes

Genetic markers have been identified on the chains of immunoglobulin molecules. Allotypes of immunoglobulins are antigenic specificities which differ among individuals of the same species. These antigenic differences are detected by the agglutination of antigen-

Fd

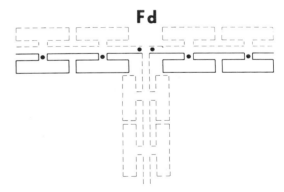

FIG. 1-13. Location of the Fd fragment of an IgG molecule. Molecular location of the **Fd** fragment of IgG is indicated by the solid line. It is that portion of the heavy chain located in the Fab fragment. This region of the heavy chain has great biologic significance since it shares in the antigen-binding site. The light chains and the Fc portion of the heavy chain are represented by dashed lines. (Bellanti JA: Immunology, Philadelphia, WB Saunders, 1971, p 110)

coated red blood cells in the presence of specific antibody found in typing sera. Using this technique, up to 25 different specificities of IgG have been found, associated with the γ chain. These are known as Gm specificities, or Gm factors, and are only found on the γ chain. Various Gm factors are associated with the different subclasses of IgG. At least three allotypic specificities have been identified on the κ light chain of each immunoglobulin class. These, known as Inv factors, are determined by single amino acid substitutions. Allotypic differences are of interest because of their varying distribution within the population. For instance, Gm(3), Gm(21), and Gm(22) are rarely found in the black population.

IMMUNOGLOBULIN A

General Properties

IgA is the second most abundant class of immunoglobulins in the serum. Its normal concentration is 0.2–0.3 g/100 ml. IgA has a molecular weight of approximately 170,000 and its sedimentation coefficient is 7S. Like IgG, it is composed of two heavy chains (in this case, α chains) and two light λ or κ chains.

Electrophoretically, IgA is a slow β-globulin. Most of the IgA in serum exists in a monomeric form, but a small proportion exists as dimers, trimers, and tetramers. In the polymeric form, the 7S subunits are held together by a third polypeptide chain known as the J chain (Fig. 1-14). Two subclasses exist for the IgA molecule, IgA1 and IgA2.

Biologic and Immunologic Properties

IgA appears to be important in the body's defense against viral infections. IgA antibodies probably coat viruses and prevent them from penetrating target cells. IgA does not fix complement or rheumatoid factor. It does, however, function in agglutination and immune precipitation. It does not appear to play a role in allergic reactions, and does not cross the placenta.

Secretory IgA

IgA is the principal immunoglobulin found in tears, saliva, nasal secretions, colostrum, and bronchial and gastrointestinal secretions. The form of IgA in these external secretions is di-

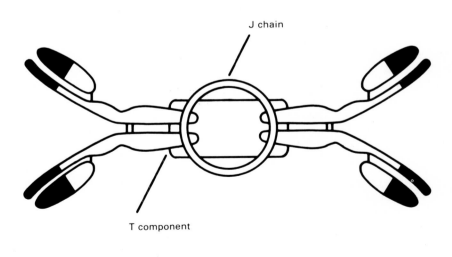

J chain

T component

100 Å

FIG. 1-14. Structure of IgA molecule. Dimeric structure is held together by a J chain. Secretory piece (T component) is also indicated. (Van Oss CJ: The Immunoglobulins. In Rose NR, Milgrom F, Van Oss CJ (eds): Principles of Immunology, New York, Macmillan Publ. Co. Inc., 1973, p 135)

meric, the two constituents being bound together by a J chain and also by a component known as **secretory piece** or **T component**. Secretory IgA is produced locally at mucosal surfaces. Secretory piece is synthesized by epithelial cells, and in humans it is bound to the α chains by disulfide bonds. Secretory piece may facilitate the transport of IgA through mucosal surfaces. It also makes the IgA molecule more resistant to enzymatic degradation, which may aid in preserving its structure in external secretions, since these are rich in proteolytic enzymes. Secretory piece does not bear any close structural relationship to the immunoglobulins. In fact, it is even present in agammaglobulinemic humans in whom IgA cannot be found. The molecular weight of secretory IgA is about 400,000 and it has a sedimentation coefficient of 11.5S.

IMMUNOGLOBULIN M

General Properties

IgM has a concentration in serum of 0.04–0.15 g/100 ml. It has a molecular weight of 900,000 and a sedimentation coefficient of 19S. It migrates electrophoretically between the γ- and β-globulins. Because of the molecule's large size, it is restricted almost entirely to the intravascular space.

Structure

IgM molecules contain five monomeric units joined together by disulfide bonds (Fig. 1-15). Electron microscopic studies have shown that IgM is a star-shaped polymer consisting of five Y-shaped units, each having the shape of an IgG molecule. These subunits contain two μ

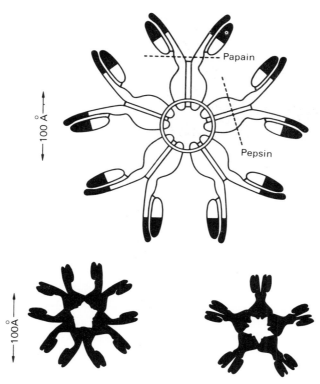

FIG. 1-15. Structure of an IgM molecule. Molecule is a pentameric structure with a J chain joining the subunits. Like IgG, it can be cleaved by pepsin and papain. (Van Oss CJ: The Immunoglobulins. In Rose NR, Milgrom F, Van Oss CJ (eds): Principles of Immunology, New York, Macmillan Publ. Co. Inc., 1973, p 137)

chains and either κ or λ light chains; the κ light chains predominate 3:1. Two subclasses of IgM may exist. One molecule of IgM has 10 antigen-binding sites, and may bind five to ten antigen molecules depending on the size of these molecules. J chains have been found in association with IgM as well as secretory IgA. Their probable function is to solidify the carboxy terminal ends of two chains and tighten them in a pentagonal structure.

Biologic and Immunologic Properties

IgM is an efficient agglutinator of particulate antigens such as red blood cells and bacteria. It is also capable of fixing complement with a high degree of efficiency. IgM seems to be of great importance in the primary immune response. When an antigen is introduced into an organism, IgM and IgG can be detected at about the same time; however, the level of IgM antibody peaks within a few days and then declines more rapidly than the level of IgG. IgM is the first immunoglobulin detectable on the surface of B lymphocytes after birth. IgM and IgD are found on the surface of most human and mouse B lymphocytes and may serve as antigen receptors which signal B cells to differentiate. IgM-like antibodies are the predominant and often the only antibodies found among primitive animal forms. IgM antibodies are important in the body's defense against bacterial infections, and they are the antibodies formed against polysaccharide antigens. They form the natural antibodies to blood group antigens, as well as the cold agglutinins. IgM antibodies do not cross the placenta, and their levels in the newborn develop rather slowly. Elevated serum levels of IgM in infants therefore suggest congenital or perinatal infection.

Rheumatoid Factor

Rheumatoid factor (RF) is an immunoglobulin, usually of the IgM class, although IgG and IgA rheumatoid factors have also been found in small amounts. Rheumatoid factor reacts with human IgG that is either aggregated or altered in some other way. The resulting 22S complexes can often be demonstrated in rheuma-

toid arthritis patients. Rheumatoid factor can be detected by agglutination of particles, such as erythrocytes or latex particles, that have been coated with IgG (see Passive Hemagglutination). Rheumatoid factor is thought to react with antigenic determinants of IgG that are normally buried within the molecule. If the IgG molecule is denatured, unfolding may reveal these antigenic sites.

IgM Fragments

Papain and pepsin treatment of IgM results in fragmentation similar to that occurring with IgG. Papain cleaves the molecule above the amino terminal disulfide bonds, yielding ten monovalent Fab μ fragments and a large Fc μ fragment. Pepsin treatment yields bivalent F(ab)$_2$ μ pieces but no Fc piece.

IMMUNOGLOBULIN D

Relatively little is known about IgD. It is present in very low concentrations in serum (approximately 0.003 g/100 ml), and is distributed mainly within the intravascular space. Its molecular weight is 185,000 and it has a sedimentation coefficient of 7S. The structure of IgD is similar to that of IgG, although the δ chain is somewhat heavier than the γ chain.

IgD antibody activity has rarely been identified; however, some cases of penicillin allergy seem to involve IgD. Like IgM, IgD has also been found on the surfaces of human lymphocytes, and may serve as some type of receptor for antigen. IgD is particularly prominent on the lymphocytes of newborn infants, and appears after IgM. It has been found on the surface of leukemic cells in patients with chronic lymphatic leukemia. The significance of these observations is unclear at the present time.

IMMUNOGLOBULIN E

IgE is present in trace amounts in serum, with concentrations in the range of 70μg/100 ml. It has a molecular weight of 200,000 and migrates electrophoretically as a slow β-globulin. Structurally, IgE is similar to IgG except that it contains 2 ϵ heavy chains. IgE levels in allergic individuals may be increased as much as tenfold, and this immunoglobulin is of great importance in patients with atopic allergy. IgE has the ability to fix and **sensitize** certain cells and tissues, including mast cells. When a specific allergen interacts with mast-cell–bound IgE, the mast cell degranulates and releases its vasoactive contents (Fig. 1-16). This chain of events initiates certain aspects of the allergic reaction. Since IgE sensitizes human mast cells and leukocytes in skin and other tissues, it is known as **skin-sensitizing** or **homocytotropic antibody.** The term **reagin** has also been applied to IgE antibodies. IgE loses its skin-sensitizing ability after being heated to 56° C, but retains its antibody activity.

IgE does not cross the placenta nor does it fix complement or rheumatoid factor. In fact, complement does not seem to be required for immediate hypersensitivity reactions involving homocytotropic antibody. Some IgE antibody is probably formed locally in the respiratory and gastrointestinal mucosal surfaces. In this respect it is part of the external secretory system of antibody. IgE deficiency has been reported in association with IgA deficiency in some individuals with impaired immunity. Aside from a role in allergic disease, IgE may function in the organism's defense

against infections, particularly those caused by parasites.

ANTIBODY SPECIFICITY

Antibody is produced in response to an antigen, and can react specifically with that antigen. This property of specific reactivity with an antigen is known as **specificity.** It is determined by the primary amino acid sequence of the antibody molecule. The part of the antibody molecule concerned with reactivity is the **antigen-binding site,** or **antibody combining site.** The antibody specificity in this region, the Fab region (Fig. 1-10), is determined by the amino acid sequence of both the heavy and light chains. It is the first 110 amino acids of the amino terminal end of the molecule which form the variable region dealing with antibody activity.

MYELOMA PROTEINS

Much information regarding the structure and function of immunoglobulins has come from the relatively homogeneous immunoglobulins produced by plasma cell neoplasms such as multiple myeloma and macroglobulinemia (see Ch. 12). Myeloma proteins representing

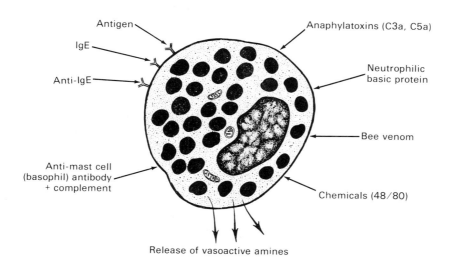

FIG. 1-16. Effect when IgE attaches to tissues such as mast cells or basophils. Stimulation of these receptors (as well as stimulation by other agents) leads to release of vasoactive substances. (Bellanti JA: Immunology, Philadelphia, WB Saunders, 1971, p 226)

each of the major classes of immunoglobulins and the four subclasses of IgG have been identified. In addition, some myelomas produce only light chains, some only heavy chains, and some only Fc fragments of γ chains. Light chains may be detected in the urine of myeloma patients as Bence Jones proteins. These proteins have been the basis of a diagnostic test for myeloma for many years, but were only recently recognized as light chains.

ONTOGENY OF IMMUNOGLOBULINS

The human fetus begins to produce immunoglobulin at about the 20th week of gestation. Despite this, the levels are relatively low at birth except in the presence of perinatal infection. The newborn, however, is protected by maternal IgG, which crosses the placenta and supplies the newborn with adult levels of IgG. This maternal IgG is rapidly dissipated, and in 2 or 3 months the infant is left with very low levels of immunoglobulin. By this time, however, the infant has been exposed to a variety of antigens and begins to synthesize IgM and IgG. At the age of 4 months, IgM levels may even surpass adult levels. IgG gradually reaches adult levels by the age of 5 years. IgA increases at a slower rate, reaching normal serum concentrations by adulthood.

THEORIES OF ANTIBODY FORMATION

There are two basic types of theories about antibody formation, the selective and the instructive. The **selective theory** was first proposed by Ehrlich in 1900. He suggested that antibody-producing cells contain receptors which combine with the antigens that fit best. After combining with antigen, the cells then secrete large quantities of antibodylike receptors.

One selective theory is the **clonal selection theory** of Burnet. This postulates that many antibody-forming cells exist, each capable of synthesizing its own antibody. When antigen reacts with one of these cells, a clone of cells is formed which all synthesize the same antibody. According to this theory, many cells with different antibody specificities are produced through random somatic mutations

during a period of hypermutability early in the individual's development. During this early period, "forbidden clones" of antibody-forming cells, that is, cells capable of making antibody against the individual's own antigens, are wiped out. Thus, the individual becomes tolerant to his own antigens. The **germ line theory** proposes that each antibody-forming cell has the potential of synthesizing all conceivable antibodies, but that once an antigen–antibody interaction occurs, the production of all unrelated antibodies is suppressed.

One **instructional theory** proposes that uncommitted and amorphous globulins become folded about a specific antigen which serves as a template for cells which then produce similar antibodies. Another instructional theory suggests that antibodies are synthesized one amino acid at a time, using preformed proteins as a template. While the selective theories are considered more tenable at the present time, these theories have many aspects which are closely related to the instructive theories.

THE COMPLEMENT SYSTEM

The complement system consists of at least 11 serum proteins which are found in normal serum. Components of the complement system react sequentially with antigen–antibody complexes, resulting in the activation of components which create inflammation and cellular injury. The complement sequence is frequently activated in cytotoxic or cytolytic immune reactions, and in reactions associated with antigen–antibody complexes. The components of the complement system are designated numerically, in the order of their discovery rather than their sequence of interaction. The eleven known serum proteins of the complement system are termed C1q, C1r, C1s, C2, C3, C4, C5, C6, C7, C8, and C9. Most of these components are present in serum in very small quantities (less than 10μg/ml). Several of the components can be quantitated by immunochemical assays. C3 is the most abundant component of complement in human serum, being present in concentrations of approximately 1.0 mg/ml. This level is 10 times greater than that of any other component except for C4, which is present in one-third the amount of C3. C3 is therefore the most commonly measured component of the complement system.

HEMOLYSIS AND COMPLEMENT FIXATION

A classic indicator of complement activity is a system using sheep erythrocytes (an antigen) coated with rabbit antibody, forming an antigen–antibody complex. When fresh guinea pig serum, a source of complement, is added to the mixture, lysis of the red blood cells occurs. Soluble or particulate antigen–antibody complexes may also be formed by the combination of proteins or other antigens with specific antibody. These complexes are capable of fixing complement and reducing the complement concentration of normal serum. Complement activation may lead to the generation of certain chemotactic substances. If the antigen–antibody complex is membrane-bound, complement activity will produce ultrastructural holes in the cell membrane of approximately 100 A in diamter.

MOLECULAR EVENTS

The sequence and result of complement interaction with an antigen–antibody complex are illustrated in Fig. 1-17. In this illustration, the antigen is an erythrocyte (E). In the presence of antibody (A) an antigen–antibody complex is formed (EA). This complex fixes the first component of complement, C1. C1 actually consists of three subunits (C1q, r, and s). These form a trimolecular aggregate which in the presence of calcium is a proesterase. Thus, a complex, EAC1a, containing activated C1 (C1a) and possessing esterase activity, is formed. This complex can bind C4, forming EAC1a4. This complex reacts with C2 and forms EAC1a42a. When C4 and C2 enter the sequence, they become bound to the cell membrane. Since C2a can easily convert to an inactive form (C2i), the process may be halted at this stage and regeneration of EAC1a4 can occur.

The next step in the sequence involves the addition of C3, also known as $\beta_1 C$. (It has been estimated that several hundred molecules of C3 are bound to the cell membrane for every molecule of IgG in an EA complex.) C3 binds to the complex, forming EAC1a42a3. Several biologic and chemical events occur as a result of this complex formation. Two biologically active materials derived from C3 are released during this stage, low-molecular-weight chemotactic factor, and anaphylatoxin. Low-molecular-weight chemotactic factor (molecular

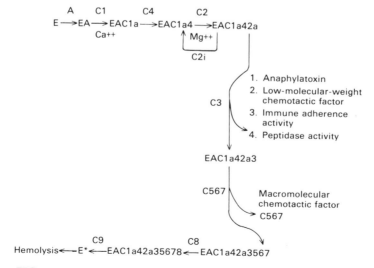

FIG. 1-17. Schematic representation of the complement sequence. See text for explanation. (Reichlin M: Complement Fixation. In Rose NR, Milgrom F, Van Oss CJ: Principles of Immunology, New York, Macmillan Publ. Co. Inc., 1973, p 85)

weight, 6000) attracts leukocytes to the site of the reaction. An anaphylatoxin has three distinct actions: 1) it causes contraction of smooth muscle, 2) it increases vascular permeability, and 3) it causes release of histamine from mast cells. The biologic result of chemotactic factor and anaphylatoxin release is acute inflammation with accumulation of neutrophils and compromised vascular integrity. In addition, the phenomenon of **immune adherence** may take place. This process involves the attachment of C3-coated antigen to erythrocytes or platelets, resulting in large aggregates that can be removed by the reticuloendothelial system. It should be pointed out that this event occurs *in vitro* and may have no relation to *in vivo* events. The addition of C3 to the complement sequence also gives stability to the complex, allowing time for the next steps in the complement sequence to occur.

C5, C6, and C7 are added in rapid succession to the complement sequence. In fact, these three components form a trimolecular complex which, when activated, becomes chemotactic for neutrophils. Some information is known about the interaction of C7 with neutrophils. Three of the leukocyte enzymes must be available for chemotaxis to occur. One of these enzymes, a proesterase, must be activated to an esterase by the C567 complex in order for the leukocytes to respond. Besides the chemotactic activity generated by C567, a cleavage product of C5, known as C5a, has anaphylatoxic as well as chemotactic properties.

C8 and C9 are added to the sequence, forming EAC1a42a356789, and cell lysis occurs. Cells do not become permanently damaged until C9 is added. The completion of the complement sequence leads to the generation of 100-A holes in the involved cell membrane.

ALTERNATE PATHWAY OF COMPLEMENT ACTIVATION

An alternate pathway exists for activating the complement sequence at the C3 stage, bypassing the early events of the classic pathway just described. The alternate pathway allows for activation of the complement system without the participation of an antigen–antibody reac-

tion. This activation of the C3 shunt may be triggered by a protein or by a broad system of substances known as **properdin**. The properdin system includes enzymes which attach to cell walls and activate the complement sequence beginning at C3. The properdin system represents a nonimmune way of activating the complement sequence. The C3 shunt may play a role in certain disease states such as bullous pemphigoid and glomerulonephritis. The alternate pathway and properdin system may also function in the defense against certain pathogens prior to the formation of circulating antibody.

ANTIBODY STRUCTURE AND COMPLEMENT FIXATION

Immunoglobulins in their monomeric form will not fix complement. Usually more than one IgG molecule must be associated with an antigen in order for complement fixation to occur. A structural change takes place between two adjacent IgG molecules, allowing them to act jointly upon one molecule of C1. By contrast, a single molecule of IgM is capable of binding complement. This is probably due to the fact that IgM is pentavalent, and adjacent subunits can act like two IgG molecules. This property of IgM may explain its great efficiency in fixing complement. Of the subclasses of IgG, only IgG4 does not fix complement. IgA and IgE do not fix complement either, and little is known about the complement-fixing activity of IgD. The complement-binding site of the immunoglobulin molecule involves both the Fc and Fab regions. The Fc fragment may provide binding sites for C1 and other early components of the sequence. The Fab region may provide binding sites for C3, C4, and the later components.

COMPLEMENT FIXATION *IN VITRO*

Complement fixation has been widely used for many years as an indicator of antigen–antibody reactions. Serums can be tested for antibody reactivity by mixing dilutions of antigen with dilutions of serum and adding a fixed amount of complement. If complement activity disappears, as judged by the effect of adding sensitized sheep erythrocytes to the mixture, then antigen–antibody interaction has occurred. This technique is useful in the diagnosis of bacterial, viral, and fungal disease. It also forms the basis for certain serologic tests for syphilis.

COMPLEMENT FIXATION *IN VIVO*

The measurement of serum complement is useful in the diagnosis of certain disease states in which antigen–antibody complexes are formed. These complexes fix complement and cause a reduction in the level of free serum complement. This situation is seen in serum sickness, acute poststreptococcal glomerulonephritis, systemic lupus erythematosus, and subacute bacterial endocarditis. Complement activity can also be assayed in synovial fluid taken from patients with rheumatoid arthritis. In active rheumatoid disease, there is marked depression of synovial fluid complement levels. Low levels of serum complement may also be found during renal allograft rejection.

C1-esterase inhibitor, a normal serum protein which prevents activation of the first component of complement, is deficient in patients with hereditary angioedema. A C2 deficiency has been demonstrated in patients who have defective *in vitro* immune adherence and bacterial lysis. C3 and C5 deficiencies have been associated with repeated bacterial infections and decreased phagocytosis.

The complement system may be regarded as a complex series of substrates from which mediators of the inflammatory response can be generated. Its function is basically protective. It can coat foreign particles and lead to their destruction or phagocytosis. The complement system may also be involved in phagocytosis or destruction of cancer cells. Complement may produce an adverse effect if antibodies are formed against an individual's own tissue components. In systemic lupus erythematosus, anti-DNA antibodies are formed against an individual's own nucleic acid, and complement fixation leads to vascular and connective tissue lesions. Thus, the complement system can be activated in a variety of ways and can participate in responses which are beneficial or harmful to the individual.

ANTIGEN–ANTIBODY INTERACTION

Antigen reacts with antibody in a manner which is specific yet reversible. The reversibility of the antigen–antibody bond depends on how tightly the two molecules are bound. If the degree of binding is strong, the antibody is considered a high-affinity antibody. This implies a precise lock-and-key type of physical and chemical interaction. If the fit is poor and the antigen–antibody complex can be readily dissociated, the antibody is considered to be one of low affinity. Generally, an antibody molecule has two binding sites, one on each Fab fragment. The IgM molecule is an exception, however, having ten antigen-binding sites. Antigens may have many more binding sites, with valences of 10–50 per molecule, and sometimes more than 200.

The binding between antigen and antibody may be considered as primary, secondary, or tertiary. The initial combination of antigen and antibody, which is rarely detectable, is considered the primary antigen–antibody interaction. Secondary antigen–antibody interaction leads to precipitation, agglutination, complement-dependent reactions, neutralization, and cytotropic effects. These *in vitro* reactions form the basis of laboratory tests for the detection of specific antibody. Tertiary antigen–antibody interactions include *in vivo* events leading to immune-mediated tissue damage.

The forces which bind antigen to antibody are not stable trivalent bonds but weaker forces which allow dissociation of the complex to occur. Van der Waals forces and hydrogen bonds are probably the most important factors in binding. Electrostatic forces may also be involved if the molecules are ionically charged. Hydrophobic interactions may also contribute to the energy of the bond. These forces are usually maximal at a physiologic pH and ionic concentration. At pH values less than 4 or greater than 10.5, the collective forces may weaken and complexes can dissociate.

SPECIFICITY OF ANTIGEN–ANTIBODY BINDING

Antigen–antibody interaction is highly specific, and very minor changes in molecular structure will greatly reduce or even abolish this interaction. Antibody affinity for a given antigen may also vary throughout the immunization process. Thus, when an animal is first immunized against a hapten bound to a protein, the affinity of the first antibodies produced is lower than that of antibody formed at later intervals. If a complex antigen is used for immunization, not only is the initial antibody of lower affinity, but it also has greater specificity for that antigen. In other words, there is little cross reactivity with other closely related antigens at this stage. Antibody produced at a later time, however, may cross react with other closely related antigens. It is thought that the initially produced antibodies are directed against only a few of the most dominant antigenic determinant groups of the complex antigenic structure. These antibodies may also be directed against the tertiary structure of the antigen. Antibody formed at a later time may be directed against more antigenic determinants, some of which become exposed as the antigen is degraded. Thus, in the later phases of immunization, a wide variety of antibodies may be produced, some of which cross react with other antigens.

IN VITRO REACTIONS

The primary interaction of antigen and antibody in the test tube may be undetectable or may lead to visible secondary consequences such as precipitation or agglutination. In vitro tests which take advantage of these physical properties are used for assaying antibodies. Antibodies tend to be classified according to the nature of their interaction with a specific antigen. However, Zinsser proposed the **unitarian theory** of antibody reactivity, which maintains that antibody should not be divided into agglutinating, complement-fixing, or precipitating types, because under different circumstances the same antibody could perform all these functions.

TITRATION

Titration is a method of quantitating the amount of antibody in a given sample. Usually, a given amount of test antigen is added to a group of progressively more dilute samples of the patient's serum. In a precipitin reaction, the test antigen is usually a soluble protein or polysaccharide. In agglutination reactions, the test antigen is a suspension of red blood cells, bacterial cells, or other particulate matter. A given amount of test antigen is usually incubated at 37° C with the various dilutions of serum and the tubes are observed for evidence of precipitation or agglutination. Usually, the greatest dilution of serum with a visible reaction is considered the titer. This may, for example, be a 1/16, 1/32, or 1/64 dilution. In a complement-fixation reaction, a constant number of sheep red blood cells and an adequate amount of complement are mixed with increasing dilutions of serum. The endpoint or titer is the last tube that shows complete hemolysis or the last tube showing 50% hemolysis by spectrophotometry.

SEROLOGIC TESTS IN DIAGNOSIS

A positive serologic test for the presence of an antibody to an infectious agent indicates only that the individual has had contact with that organism at some time in the past. To help establish that the organism was involved in the disease process under study, an acute-phase serum sample should be obtained and compared with convalescent serum taken late in the illness. The absence of detectable antibody during the early phase of an illness, its appearance during the course of the illness, and its eventual decline would be highly suggestive of an infectious illness. Isolation of a microorganism by culture would be confirmation of an ongoing infection, and is highly desirable information to obtain.

It should be pointed out that different techniques of antibody detection will produce different patterns of appearance and disappearance of antibody. For example, in brucellosis agglutinating antibodies are found in the early stages of the infection and low levels persist for many years. Precipitating antibodies appear later in the disease and disappear much sooner. In viral and rickettsial diseases, complement-fixing antibodies appear later in the disease and subside sooner than those antibodies measured by neutralization. These discrepancies may be explained by the fact that microbial antigens are complex structures consisting of many different antigenic determinants that are detectable at different levels of sensitivity by various serologic methods. Antibodies formed against these determinant groups differ in structure and function, and therefore they also vary in their detectability.

Precipitation Reactions

Precipitation reactions involve the interaction of a soluble antigen and antibody molecules to form insoluble precipitates. The antibody itself is referred to as a **precipitin.** It is usually bivalent, whereas the antigen is frequently multivalent. When the concentrations of antigen and antibody reach optimal levels, and conditions of temperature, pH, and ionic strength are proper, formation of a lattice structure takes place (Fig. 1-18). During this process, unbound combining sites on the antibody molecules attach to receptors on the antigen molecules, and a lattice network is formed. A specific cross linking between antigen and antibody molecules grows increasingly in size until it finally forms a precipitate because of its size and weight. The optimal antigen–antibody ratio is considered that ratio at which soluble antigen and antibody will precipitate fastest. In order for lattice formation to occur, it is necessary that antibody be present in excess amounts. If, on the other hand, antigen is present in excess amounts and antibody molecules are present in limited numbers, little or no precipitate will form. This is because antibody molecules, when present in small amounts, react with antigen to form soluble complexes.

Precipitation reactions may be carried out in capillary tubes, in which the antigen solution is layered on top of antibody-containing serum. A precipitate forms at the interface of the two solutions, where optimum concentrations of antigen and antibody exist. The Ouchterlony double-diffusion procedure is an important technical application of the precipitation reaction (Fig. 1-19). In this technique, antigen and antibody preparations are placed in separate wells in an agar gel. The soluble reactants diffuse toward each other through the gel and lines of precipitation form in the areas where optimal concentrations of the two components meet.

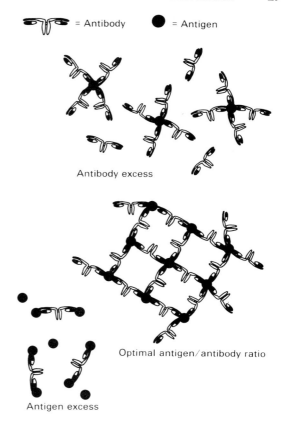

= Antibody   ● = Antigen

Antibody excess

Optimal antigen/antibody ratio

Antigen excess

FIG. 1-18. Formation of antigen–antibody lattice network. Lattice formation depends on antigen and antibody concentrations. In antibody excess, free antibody and complexes are present. In antigen excess, free antigen and complexes form. If concentrations of antigen and antibody are optimal, lattice formation and precipitation occur. (Van Oss CJ: Precipitation and Agglutination. In Rose NR, Milgrom F, Van Oss CJ (eds): Principles of Immunology. New York, Macmillan Publ. Co. Inc., 1973, p 32)

The precipitin reaction is helpful in establishing the identification of unknown antibodies or antigens. If two different antigens, A and B, are being tested, they will diffuse at different rates through the agar. Therefore the concentrations at any given point will be different. If antigen A is placed in one well and antigen B in a second well, and an antibody mixture containing anti-A and anti-B is placed in a third well, a precipitin reaction can be observed. The region where the optimal proportions of an A–anti-A reaction is reached will differ from the region where the optimal proportions of a B–anti-B reaction occur. This will

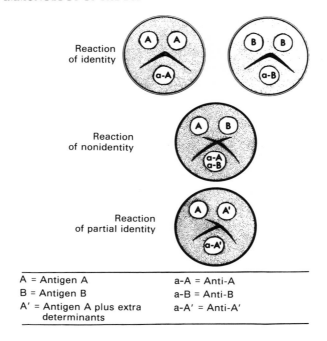

Reaction of identity

Reaction of nonidentity

Reaction of partial identity

A = Antigen A	a-A = Anti-A
B = Antigen B	a-B = Anti-B
A' = Antigen A plus extra determinants	a-A' = Anti-A'

lead to a crossing of the two precipitin bands and a **reaction of nonidentity.** If, on the other hand, both antigens being tested are the identical antigen A, then antigen from the two wells will diffuse at exactly the same rate, and the optimal proportions for precipitation will be reached at the same location. This produces a **reaction of identity.** If the two antigens are different, but share common antigenic determinants, a **reaction of partial identity** with a characteristic spur formation will be seen. Figure 1-19 shows these three types of reactions.

Variations of the standard precipitin test are commonly used in immunologic testing. One of the techniques, known as radial immunodiffusions (Fig. 1-20), incorporates specific antibody into an agar gel. Antigen in various concentrations is placed in wells cut in the agar, and the area of precipitate formed around each antigen well is measured. Higher concentrations of antigen diffuse further from the well before the ringlike precipitates of optimal antigen–antibody concentration are reached. The measured areas may then be compared with standardized preparations, and

levels of the antigen being tested may be determined. This method is also used to determine levels of serum complement and immunoglobulin.

Immunoelectrophoresis

Immunoelectrophoresis is a technique in which serum is separated into its differently charged components by an electrical field in an agar gel. Once this separation has taken place, antiserum is put in long troughs parallel to the electrophoresis pathway and is allowed to diffuse toward the electrophoretic fractions. Precipitation lines are formed where antibody has interacted with the various proteins of serum (Fig. 1-21). Electrophoretic separation makes the identification of individual antigen–antibody reactions possible.

Agglutination Reactions

Another method for detecting antibody in serum is agglutination. In this process, anti-

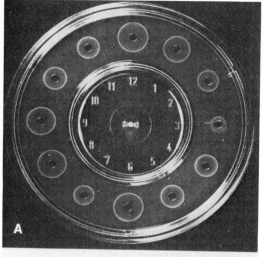

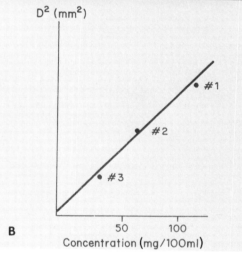

FIG. 1-20. Radial immunodiffusion method for evaluation of serum complement levels. A. Wells 1, 2, and 3 contain known concentrations of complement. B. The squares of the diameters can be plotted on a graph and from this the concentration of complement in the other wells can be determined. (Bigley NJ: Immunologic Fundamentals. Copyright © 1975 by Year Book Med. Pub., Inc., Chicago. p 91 Used by permission.)

gens are attached to red blood cells or insoluble particles. When specific antibody is added to the mixture, these insoluble particles form larger aggregates or clumps. Agglutination is a more sensitive test for antibody than precipitation since much less antigen is needed to obtain a visible reaction in agglutination. In precipitation reactions, the antigen molecules are smaller and are spread homogeneously throughout the entire mixture. A relatively high concentration of antibody is required to obtain a lattice network and visible precipitation. A precipitation reaction may require 500 times more antibody than an agglutination reaction.

Agglutination reactions occur when immunoglobulin molecules form bridges, or cross linkages, between two or more insoluble particles. These immunoglobulins attach to antigenic determinants on the surfaces of cells or particles. It should be kept in mind that the particulate antigens are several hundred times larger in size than the immunoglobulin molecules. The ability to form cross linkages successfully depends on the valence of the immunoglobulin. IgM, with ten combining sites, is a much better agglutinator than IgG, which has only two combining sites. Not all IgG antibodies are capable of cross linking and agglutinating cells or particles, although they may be capable of combining with antigen. Those antibodies which are unable to form cross linkages and cause agglutination have been referred to as incomplete, but more properly are termed nonagglutinating antibodies. Other factors, including the avidity of the antigen sites, their number, and their spacing, must also be taken into account. If very high concentrations of antibody are being tested, the binding sites on the cells may become totally occupied with antibody so that no free combining sites can be found. Thus, all the antigenic sites become tied up and because no cross linkages can take place, no agglutination occurs. Under these circumstances the IgG antibodies are called **blocking antibodies.** Usually when the antiserum is appropriately diluted, this phenomenon disappears and agglutination takes place.

Direct Hemagglutination. This technique is used in blood banking for typing erythrocyte antigens. Erythrocytes containing a known blood group antigen are added to a sample of serum. If red cells containing blood group A antigen are added to serum containing anti-A antibodies, agglutination will take place. If the serum contains anti-B, but no anti-A antibodies, no agglutination will take place.

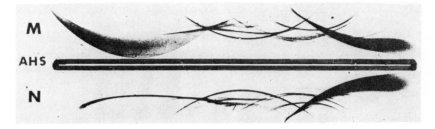

FIG. 1-21. Immunoelectrophoresis of serum from patient with IgG myeloma. Immunoelectrophoresis of human sera: IgG myeloma protein compared with normal serum IgG. Top, Immunoelectrophoretic pattern of huma IgG myeloma serum (**M**); note the extensive amount of precipitate in the arc on the left in the presence of anti-human serum (**AHS**). Bottom, immunoelectrophoretic pattern of normal human serum (**N**) in the presence of anti-human serum. (Bigley NJ: Immunologic Fundamentals. Copyright © 1975 by Year Book Med. Publ., Inc. Chicago. p 92. Used by permission.)

Passive Hemagglutination. Red cells can be used passively as indicators of a reaction. The cells are coated with antigens such as carbohydrates or proteins by coupling with bis-diazotized benzidine, chromium chloride, or glutaraldehyde. When a specific antigen–antibody reaction takes place, the red blood cells agglutinate. This principle is made use of in the assay for rheumatoid factor. Rheumatoid factor is an IgM antibody directed against human IgG (see under Immunoglobulin M). Particles such as latex may be coated with denatured heavy chains of human IgG. When serum containing rheumatoid factor is added, the IgM in the serum agglutinates the coated latex particles, forming a visible precipitate (see Fig. 8-9). The VDRL (Venereal Disease Research Laboratory) test for syphilis is a flocculation test of this kind in which the patient's serum is tested for a reaction with a particulate cardiolipin material; aggregation indicates a positive test.

Coombs Test. Red blood cells from patients with autoimmune hemolytic anemia often have immunoglobulin attached to their cell membranes, even after careful washing. Adding an anti–human globulin serum (Coombs serum) to the cells and incubating the mixture at 37° C for 30 min will cause red cell agglutination to take place (Fig. 1-22). A positive **direct Coombs test** will be seen in acquired hemolytic anemia and in erythroblastosis fetalis.

In the **indirect Coombs test,** serum antibodies to erythrocyte antigens are measured. Frequently, maternal antibody to an infant's red blood cells are looked for. The serum being tested is used to coat red blood cells with antibody. If antibody to an erythrocyte antigen is present in the serum, an antigen–antibody interaction takes place, but no agglutination occurs. If Coombs serum (anti–human globulin) is added, agglutination may take place.

Hemagglutination Inhibition Test. Certain viruses are capable of coating red blood cells and causing them to settle to the bottom of test tubes in an agglutinated pattern. If such a virus is exposed to its specific antibody before being mixed with the red cells, the virus will be unable to attach to the surface of the red cells. In this latter instance, as in control mixtures, the red cells will settle to the bottom of the test tube, forming a compact button or a doughnut-shaped mass. This test is known as the hemagglutination inhibition test, and is used to detect viral antibodies such as those associated with mumps virus.

TOXIN–ANTITOXIN REACTIONS

Bacteria are able to produce highly toxic substances to which an antibody response may develop. Bacteria such as the diphtheria and tetanus bacilli secrete exotoxins which can be demonstrated in cell-free filtrates of bacterial cultures. Gram-negative bacteria, on the other

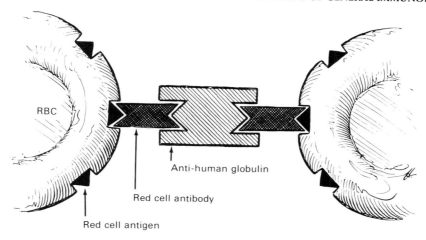

FIG. 1-22. Coombs test, showing agglutination of antibody-coated red blood cells when anti–human globulin serum is added. (Bellanti JA: Immunology, Philadelphia, WB Saunders, 1971, p 143)

hand, are associated with endotoxins, which are an integral part of the bacterial cell wall and are produced after disintegration of the bacteria. Exotoxins, in general, are more powerful antigens than endotoxins.

Roux and Yersin demonstrated in 1888 that cell-free filtrates of diphtheria cultures were toxic for guinea pigs. In 1890, von Behring and Kitasato showed that animals injected with inactivated toxins of the diphtheria and tetanus bacilli were resistant to infections with these organisms. This demonstrated that specific immunity to bacterial toxins can be produced.

Exotoxins

Exotoxins are proteins which are potent pharmacologic poisons. Diphtheria toxin interferes with protein synthesis and becomes reversibly bound to cells. All cells seem to be sensitive to diphtheria toxin, although some species, such as man, are more susceptible than others. Injection of diphtheria toxin produces local hemorrhage, vascular congestion, and necrosis. Systemic consequences of injection include pleural and pericardial effusions, renal hemorrhage, circulatory failure, and death.

After injection of diphtheria toxin into a sensitive animal, there is a latent period of 6–15 h before symptoms are first noted. In the guinea pig, diphtheria toxin becomes reversibly bound to cells in 20 min. During this in-

terval, if antitoxin is given, the guinea pig is readily saved. After 20 min, it becomes more difficult to save the animal except with large doses of antitoxin. If 2 h elapse between administration of toxin and antitoxin, the animal no longer can be saved. Thus, the toxic products of diphtheria toxin may be neutralized if antitoxin is given at a very early stage.

Toxoids

Ehrlich was the first to note that toxins treated for 3–4 weeks with formaldehyde at 37 C lose their toxicity but retain their antigenicity. He hypothesized that a toxophore group was destroyed during this treatment, while a haptophore group, responsible for antigenic properties, was preserved. Toxoid preparations, such as those of diphtheria and tetanus, are now used routinely for active immunization of children and adults.

Antitoxic Serum

A hyperimmune serum containing antibodies to a bacterial toxin may be produced in the horse and other species. These are sometimes given in emergency situations for passive protection of the unimmunized human against irreversible damage due to bacterial exotoxins. Commercial antiserums (antitoxins) are available for the toxins of diphtheria, tetanus, gas gangrene, and botulism.

Schick Test

The Schick test is a standard test for measuring a person's antitoxic immunity to diphtheria. A minute dose of diphtheria toxin is injected into the forearm, and the reaction is observed over a 1-week period. If no circulating antibodies to the toxin are present, a toxic reaction will occur locally, characterized by erythema, edema, and tenderness which begins at 24 h and reaches a maximum in 1 week. If antitoxin antibodies are present in the circulation, the toxin will be neutralized and the Schick test will be negative. A negative Schick test indicates immunity to diphtheria.

LYSIS AND CYTOTOXICITY

The end result of certain types of immunologic reactions is the immobilization or destruction of target cells. Such reactions include destruction of bacteria (bacterial lysis), destruction of red blood cells (hemolysis), or destruction of other living cells (cytolysis). The term **cytotoxicity** is frequently used to refer to the general adverse effects of immunologic reactions on intact cells. Cytotoxic effects may be produced either by the interaction of antibody with cell-bound antigens, through the fixation of complement to antigen–antibody complexes on cells, or else by the action of lymphoid T cells and their soluble mediators. In other words, two main types of immune cytotoxic mechanisms are recognized. One involves the action of humoral antibody and the complement system on target cells. In the second, cytotoxicity is mediated by immune lymphocytes and their secretions rather than by serum antibody.

A variety of assays have been developed to detect cytotoxic antibodies. These assays indicate cell damage by entry of a dye into the cell, loss of a cell's ability to adhere to a surface, or loss of cell-bound ^{51}Cr. The last method is the one most commonly used for measuring cytotoxicity.

SUGGESTED READING

Bach JF: Immunology. New York, Wiley & Sons, 1978

Barrett JT: Basic Immunology and its Medical Application. St. Louis, Mosby, 1976

Bellanti JA: Immunology. Philadelphia, WB Saunders, 1978

Bigley NJ: Immunologic Fundamentals. Chicago, Year Book Medical, 1975

Eisen HN: Immunology. Hagerstown, Harper & Row 1974

Freedman SO, Gold P (eds): Clinical Immunology. Hagerstown, Harper & Row, 1976

Fudenberg HH, Stites DP, Caldwell JL, Wells JV (eds): Basic and Clinical Immunology. Los Altos, Lange, 1976

Gell PGH, Coombs RRA (eds): Clinical Aspects of Immunology. Oxford, Blackwell, 1968

Holborow EJ, Reeves WG: Immunology in Medicine. New York, Grune & Stratton, 1977

Humphrey JH, White RG: Immunology for Students of Medicine. Philadelphia, FA Davis, 1970

Movat HZ (ed): Inflammation, Immunity and Hypersensitivity. New York, Harper & Row, 1971

Rahi AH, Garner A: Immunopathology of the Eye. Oxford, Blackwell, 1976

Roitt IM: Essential Immunology. Oxford, Blackwell, 1974

Rose NR, Friedman H (eds): Manual of Clinical Immunology. Washington DC, American Society of Microbiology, 1976

Rose NR, Milgrom F. Van Oss CJ (eds): Principles of Immunology. New York, MacMillan, 1973

Sell S: Immunology, Immunopathology, and Immunity. Hagerstown, Harper & Row, 1975

Thaler MS, Klausner RD, Cohen HJ: Medical Immunology. Philadelphia, JB Lippincott, 1977

TWO
TWO
TWO mechanisms of immune reactivity

GENERAL CONSIDERATIONS

Following the interaction between antigen and specific antibody or between antigen and sensitized lymphocytes, the effector mechanisms of immunity come into play. These mechanisms may have a beneficial effect and eliminate the antigen, or they may produce tissue damage, in which case we may say that a state of hypersensitivity exists.

Hypersensitivity responses may be categorized according to the mechanism involved in producing tissue injury. Coombs and Gell described four basic mechanisms for effecting immune responses (Fig. 2-1). A fifth mechanism, known as stimulatory hypersensitivity, has been described more recently. These responses have been designated as type I, type II, type III, type IV, and type V hypersensitivity reactions. Types I, II, III, and V involve antigen–antibody interactions. Type IV, or delayed hypersensitivity, depends on specifically sensitized T lymphocytes rather than antibodies.

ATOPIC OR ANAPHYLACTIC REACTIONS (TYPE I REACTIONS)

Type I hypersensitivity is the antigen–antibody interaction that is usually associated with allergic or atopic conditions. It occurs when an inciting allergen combines with immunoglobulin which is bound to mast cells or basophils. Vasoactive substances (*e.g.,* histamine) are released from the tissue mast cells or from baso-

phils in the peripheral blood (Fig. 2-2). These soluble mediator substances produce an effect on certain target organs. The ultimate manifestations of such an allergic reaction may be a skin rash, pulmonary obstruction, nasal and lacrimal secretion, or vascular collapse and shock.

Chronic recurrent allergic reactions such as hay fever are generally referred to as **atopic** conditions. Acute wheal-and-flare reactions and systemic shock are generally termed **anaphylactic** reactions. (In the United States, the terms **atopy** and **allergy** are synonymous. In Britain, allergy refers to all nonprotective immune reactions, including delayed hypersensitivity and immune-complex reactions.) An atopic individual is one who is prone to develop allergic reactions. The offending antigen in allergy is known as an **allergen,** and the antibody with which it reacts is known as **reagin.**

REAGINIC ANTIBODY

Reagin was the term originally applied to the antibody in serum that is detectable by the Wassermann test for syphilis. In this test, the antibody reacts with an antigen extracted from ungulate heart muscle. This antibody, however, has no relation to atopy or anaphylaxis. In current usage the term **reagin** refers to the antibody found in an allergic individual's serum. It is generally of the IgE type. Reaginic antibody can also be found in the IgG, IgA, and IgM classes of immunoglobulin; however, IgE appears to be the most important type of reagin.

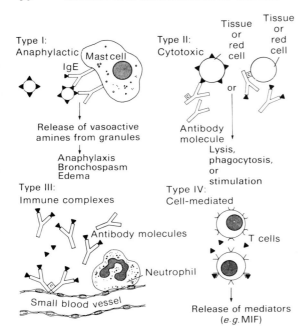

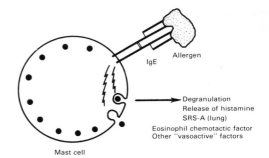

FIG. 2-2. Mechanism of antigen-mediated release of chemical mediators in type I reaction. The Fc region of the IgE antibody molecule binds to the mast cell membrane; antigen binds to the Fab portion of the antibody molecule. (Bigley NJ: Immunologic Fundamentals. (Copyright © 1975 by Year Book Med. Pub., Inc. Chicago, p 157. Used by permission.)

FIG. 2-1. Schematic illustration of the four mechanisms of immune reactivity (types I, II, III, and IV). C indicates complement; ▲, antigen; U and V, specific receptors for antigens. (Reproduced with permission from Wells JV: Immune mechanisms in Immunology. In Fudenberg HH et al: Basic and Clinical Immunology, Los Altos, Lange, 1976, p 226)

IgE has the unusual property of fixing to cells. Between 10,000 and 40,000 IgE molecules may coat a single basophil. IgE molecules attach by their Fc portions to mast cells, which are fixed tissue cells, or to basophils, which are granulocytes found in the peripheral blood. These cells become sensitized by IgE, and subsequent interaction with antigen leads to the release of soluble mediators from these cells. One antigen molecule reacts with two cell-bound IgE molecules, forming a bridge. This bridging causes a physical distortion of the antibody molecule and triggers events at the cell surface which lead to release of the mast cell products.

Reaginic activity may be transferred from a sensitized individual to a nonsensitized one. If serum from an allergic individual is injected intradermally into a normal subject, challenge with an appropriate antigen will elicit a wheal-and-flare reaction (the **Prausnitz–Kustner reaction**). This reaction results from the fixation

of the donor's IgE to the recipient's mast cells, and subsequent interaction between the cell-bound IgE and specific antigen.

Antibody which fixes to the skin of animals of the same species is known as **homocytotropic,** while antibody which fixes to the skin of a different species is known as **heterocytotropic.** These reaginic antibodies are present in very small concentrations in serum. They are heat-labile and do not fix complement.

Reaginic antibodies are most often detected by skin testing. Antigen injected directly into the skin of a sensitive individual will elicit an immediate-onset reaction. Alternatively, an allergic person's serum may be passively transferred to a normal individual and the injected site challenged with antigen. *In vitro* tests may also be used. The Schultz–Dale test relies on the release of histamine by mast cells following IgE–antigen interaction. The released histamine causes contraction of smooth muscle in guinea pig intestine or rat uterus which can be measured with a kymograph. Histamine release can also be measured photometrically after the passive coating of basophils or mast cells with reaginic antibody, and the addition of a specific antigen. The radioallergosorbent test (RAST) depends on the formation of IgE antibody–antigen complexes and the subsequent binding of radiolabeled anti-IgE to this complex. Soluble antigen is covalently bound to insoluble particles. This insoluble antigen is then added to a patient's serum, where binding will take place with specific IgE antibody. These complexes are then washed and treated with radiolabeled anti-IgE. The anti-IgE will bind to the insoluble IgE–antigen complexes and the extent of this binding can be assayed.

MEDIATOR RELEASE

Mediator substances may be released from mast cells or basophils by a nonlytic mechanism in which lysosomes attach to the inner cell membrane and extrude their contents to the outside. A second, lytic, mechanism involves the binding of complement to antigen–antibody complexes on the surfaces of mast cells. Nonlytic release appears to be the usual mechanism in atopic conditions; however, lytic release may produce anaphylactic symptoms mediated by IgG or IgM.

Among the substances released by mast cells and basophils is histamine, which increases vascular permeability, apparently by causing separation of vascular endothelial cells. In the presence of calcium ions, histamine also causes contraction of smooth muscle, producing pain and itching. Histamine activates adenyl cyclase, causing intracellular cyclic adenosine $3',5'$ monophosphate (cAMP) to accumulate in peripheral leukocytes. This results in inhibition of IgE-mediated histamine release. Another substance released by the mast cell is slow-reacting substance of anaphylaxis (SRS-A), which is responsible for the bronchial spasm seen in asthmatics. Eosinophil chemotactic factor of anaphylaxis (ECF-A) is another mediator; it attracts eosinophils to the site of an allergic reaction. Serotonin and heparin may also be released during anaphylactic reactions.

CLINICAL ENTITIES

Cutaneous Anaphylaxis

This is the typical wheal-and-flare, or urticarial, reaction which is elicited when a sensitive individual is given a scratch test or intradermal injection of an antigen. It is characterized by erythema, edema, and itching. Histologically, edema is prominent, but little

cellular infiltration is seen. The reaction is caused by the interaction of antigen and cell-bound IgE, with release of histamine and other mediators.

Systemic Anaphylaxis

This is a generalized reaction elicited by injection of an antigen into a susceptible individual. It is characterized by vascular collapse, falling temperature, smooth muscle contraction, slowed heart rate, and a decrease in serum complement levels. Death usually results from laryngeal edema and respiratory distress. Often, systemic anaphylaxis is produced by drugs such as penicillin, but bee and wasp stings may also be responsible.

Hereditary Angioedema

This is a hereditary condition associated with a deficiency of C1-esterase inhibitor or with the presence of an inactive form of the inhibitor. In this condition activation of the complement system cannot be checked. It is characterized clinically by edema of the upper respiratory tract, eyelids, lips, tongue, and trunk. The gastrointestinal system may also be involved, producing acute abdominal distress. Patients may die from asphyxiation. Attacks may be halted by injection of fresh-frozen plasma, which contains C1-esterase inhibitor. Hereditary angioedema is discussed in more detail in Chapter 4.

Urticaria

Urticaria (see also in Ch. 4) is manifested by widespread raised, erythematous, and pruritic skin lesions which occur in response to a wide variety of stimuli. These may be allergic stimuli or physical factors such as heat, cold, or sunlight.

Atopic Allergy

Atopic allergy encompasses a large range of common human allergies, including asthma, hay fever (allergic rhinitis), urticaria, and eczema. Itching, sneezing, and respiratory distress due to bronchospasm may be seen clinically. The type of reaction observed depends on the entry route of the antigen, its dose, and the individual's inherited susceptibility to atopic disease.

CELL RECEPTORS AND ALLERGIC REACTIONS

Target cells are thought to have receptors on their surfaces which can be stimulated by autonomic agonists. α-Adrenergic receptors are stimulated primarily by norepinephrine, while β-receptors are stimulated by isoproterenol (Fig. 2-3). Epinephrine stimulates both α- and β-receptors. The α-receptors can be blocked by ergot alkaloids, haloalkylamines (*e.g.,* phenoxybenzamine, dibenamine), benzodioxans, and imidazolines; β-adrenergic receptors are blocked by propranolol, practolol, dichloroisoproterenol, and pronethalol. α-Adrenergic stimulation leads to contraction of vascular and bronchial smooth muscle in the guinea pig, while β-adrenergic stimulation causes smooth muscle relaxation and decreased capillary permeability.

Cholinergic or γ-receptors are stimulated by acetylcholine and are blocked by atropine and related drugs. Their stimulation is generally associated with smooth muscle contraction and increased capillary permeability.

The release of mediators from mast cells can also be stimulated by adrenergic and cholinergic agonists. Stimulation or blockade of these receptors has an effect on the intracellular concentration of cyclic nucleotides within the target cells (Fig. 2-4). Current evidence suggests that the β-adrenergic receptor is a cell membrane enzyme, adenylate cyclase. When activated, this enzyme acts upon intracellular ATP and catalyzes the formation of cyclic AMP (cAMP) which in turn modulates the activity of cellular enzymes. Phosphodiesterase acts upon cAMP and converts it to an inactive 5′-AMP. A hormone which stimulates cell receptors can be viewed as a first messenger which activates a second messenger, cAMP. Elevated levels of cAMP induce a cell to perform its physiologic function: relaxation of smooth muscle, lipolysis of fat cells, or inhibition of mediator release by mast cells.

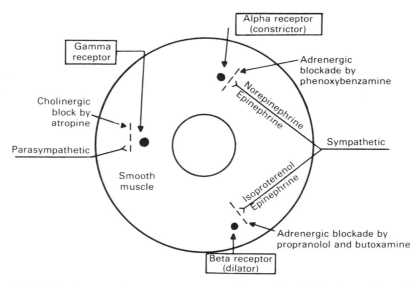

FIG. 2-3. Autonomic receptors on smooth muscle of blood vessels and bronchi. (Reed CE: The role of the autonomic nervous system in the pathogenesis of bronchial asthma: Is the normal bronchial sensitivity due to beta adrenergic blockade? In Proceedings of the Sixth Congress of the International Association of Allergology. Excerpta Medica Foundation, 1968, p 404).

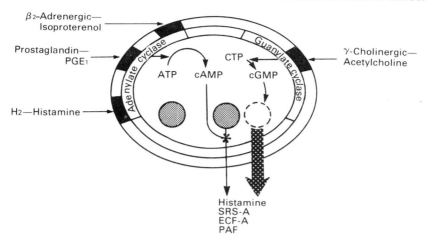

FIG. 2-4. Schematic illustration of a cell showing relationship between various receptor subunits and cAMP. (Reproduced with permission from Frick OL: Immediate hypersensitivity. In Fudenberg HH *et al*: Basic and Clinical Immunology, Los Altos, Lange, 1976, p 217)

The adenylate cyclase receptor appears to have at least three subunits, each of which can respond independently. Thus, β-adrenergic drugs, prostaglandins (PGE_1 and PGE_2), and histamine are all capable of stimulating adenylate cyclase. The β-receptor can be blocked by propranolol while the histamine receptor can be blocked by H_2-blockers such as burimamide or metiamide. The prostaglandin receptor may possibly be blocked by aspirin or indomethacin. Blockade of one or two of these receptors does not prevent a rise in cAMP upon stimulation of another, unblocked, receptor. In status asthmaticus, the β-receptor may be unresponsive to epinephrine, but, the target cells can apparently still respond to PGE_1. Corticosteroids seem to improve the ability of epinephrine to increase intracellular levels of cAMP.

It has been suggested that ATPase may act as the α-receptor. ATPase may compete with adenylate cyclase for ATP and may convert ATP directly to an inactive form, 5'-AMP, without producing the intermediary cAMP. The ultimate effect of this on the mast cell or basophil would be a lowering of cAMP levels and an increased release of soluble mediators.

cAMP is metabolized to inactive 5'-AMP by phosphodiesterase. This enzyme can be inhibited by the methylxanthines, including theo-phylline, theobromine, and caffeine. By preventing the metabolism of cAMP, the methylxanthines increase intracellular levels of cAMP and prevent mediator release by mast cells. This mechanism may be the basis for the effect of theophylline in allergic asthma. Epinephrine, which increases cAMP levels by receptor stimulation, has a synergistic effect with theophylline in asthma.

The γ-receptor on target cells is thought to be guanylate cyclase. It is stimulated by acetylcholine and inhibited by atropine. Stimulation of guanylate cyclase converts guanosine triphosphate (GTP) to cyclic GMP (cGMP). Elevated levels of intracellular cGMP have the opposite effect of cAMP, causing an increase in the release of mediators from mast cells and contraction of bronchial smooth muscle. cGMP is metabolized by phosphodiesterase and converted to inactive 5'-GMP. Guanyl phosphodiesterase, however, is only one-tenth as susceptible to methylxanthines as is adenyl phosphodiesterase. Therefore, the methylxanthines have a preferential effect on the cAMP system.

Obviously, the interactions between hormones and target cells are quite complex. An overall homeostatic balance is thought to exist between the β-adrenergic sympathetic system and the cholinergic parasympathetic system.

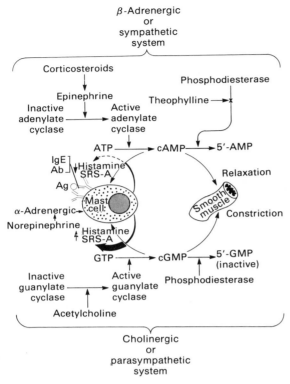

FIG. 2-5. The balance theory of sympathetic and parasympathetic regulation. (Reproduced with permission from Frick OL: Immediate hypersensitivity. In Fudenberg HH *et al:* (eds) Basic and Clinical Immunology. Los Altos, Lange, 1976, p 220)

This balance theory is illustrated for asthma in Figure 2-5. Selective stimulation and inhibition of the cAMP and cGMP pathways by drugs may have great importance in the treatment of a variety of allergic conditions.

TREATMENT OF ALLERGIC DISEASE

A variety of methods of treatment are available which inhibit the chain of events in allergic disease. A most effective therapy is avoidance of contact with the offending allergen, a method which is not always feasible. As discussed in the following paragraphs, immunotherapy may be useful in the treatment of certain allergic conditions through mechanisms of hyposensitization, desensitization, tolerance, or nonspecific IgE formation. If cAMP can be increased by stimulation of β-adrenergic receptors, the release of mast cell mediators can be decreased and atopic symptoms diminished. Drugs such as cromolyn interfere with the release of mediators after allergen has combined with sensitized mast cells. This drug appears to stabilize lysosomal membranes and in some way prevents the release of amines from mast cells. The effects of mediators such as histamine can be blocked in certain instances with drugs such as antihistamines. Thus, the chain of events in allergic reactions may be broken at various places. The discovery of new drugs and the clarification of the biochemical events involved will surely lead to further control of the allergic reaction.

Immunotherapy

Immunotherapy of atopic disease involves an attempt to alleviate the allergic symptoms by giving injections of specific allergens in increasingly higher doses. The mechanism of this type of therapy is unclear. At least four possibilities exist to account for the effects of immunotherapy (Fig. 2-6). First, hyposensitization therapy is accompanied by the production of blocking antibody. This precipitating IgG antibody is nonreaginic but reacts with the same antigen as reaginic antibody. A competitive inhibition occurs, with blocking antibody and reagin competing for the same allergen. Blocking antibody can be demonstrated *in vitro*, where it prevents the release of mediators from sensitized mast cells when a specific allergen is added.

A second explanation for the beneficial effects of immunotherapy is that it causes desensitization. In this process IgE antibody is consumed by repeated small doses of allergen. The IgE antibody becomes tied up to such an extent that it is not available to attach to reactive tissue sites. A third mechanism proposes that individuals produce decreased amounts of IgE antibody upon repeated exposure to an allergen. This decrease in IgE antibody production is a form of immune tolerance. A fourth proposed mechanism by which specific immunotherapy may work is through the production of nonspecific IgE, which may combine with the effector-cell surface receptors and block the attachment of allergen-specific IgE antibody. Thus, the binding sites of

Hyposensitization:

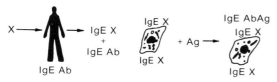

Desensitization:

Tolerance:

Non-antigen-specific IgE:

FIG. 2-6. Proposed mechanisms of immunotherapy in atopic diseases. The possible mechanisms include 1) hyposensitization with production of IgG blocking antibody, 2) desensitization, with consumption of IgE antibody by repeated small doses of allergen, and 3) tolerance, with a decrease in IgE antibody production following repeated small doses of antigen. A fourth possible mechanism involves the production of nonspecific IgE which might block effector cell receptors. (Sell S: Immunology, Immunopathology and Immunity, Hagerstown, Harper & Row, 1975, p 171)

mast cells become saturated with nonspecific IgE, and this prevents the sensitization of the mast cells by allergen-specific IgE.

CYTOTOXIC HYPERSENSITIVITY (TYPE II REACTIONS)

Type II hypersensitivity reactions are considered to be cytotoxic or cytolytic in nature. They may involve the combination of IgG or IgM antibody with cell-membrane antigens, or the attachment of a free antigen or hapten to a cell followed by antibody and complement interaction. The attachment of antigen and antibody to a cell may lead to cell lysis. In cytotoxic reactions, the antigen–antibody interaction may cause target cell destruction by three different mechanisms; 1) cell lysis or inactivation through the participation of complement, 2) phagocytosis of target cells with or without the participation of complement, and 3) inactivation or lysis of target cells in the presence of lymphoid effector cells (**cell-dependent cytotoxicity**).

COMPLEMENT-DEPENDENT CELL LYSIS

Blood elements, kidney, skin, or other tissues may all serve as target organs for complement-dependent antibody-mediated cell lysis.

Blood Elements

The most familiar example of a type II cytotoxic reaction is the transfusion reaction that occurs when a recipient's circulating antibody contacts erythrocytes from an incompatible donor. The individual with type A blood has antibodies against erythrocytes of type B. If this individual accidentally receives type B blood, the anti-B antibodies interact with the B erythrocyte antigen, causing the cells to agglutinate and lyse. Ultimately, the damaged cells are destroyed by the spleen. Antibodies to platelets may be produced in such entities as idiopathic thrombocytopenic purpura. Alternatively, antiplatelet antibodies may be produced by the administration of the drugs apronalide (Sedormid) and quinidine, leading to a drug-induced thrombocytopenia. Antibodies to drugs may also adsorb to granulocytes, leading to granulocytopenia. In diseases in which autoantibodies are produced, such as sytemic lupus erythematosus, serum antibodies specific for lymphocytes may be found.

Kidney

Cytotoxic antibodies may be produced against almost any tissue. However, clinically speaking, the kidney is one of the most important organs to be involved in this type of reaction. Deposition of antibodies directed against the glomerular basement membrane occurs in

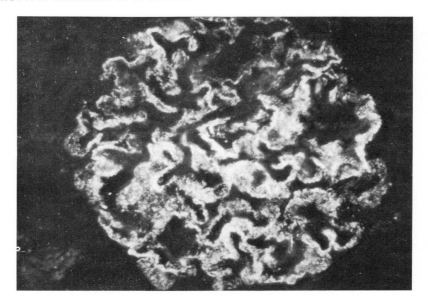

FIG. 2-7. Direct immunofluorescent staining of a renal glomerulus with fluorescein-labeled anti-IgG in patient with membranous glomerulonephritis. x940. (Courtesy of Dr. C. Biava)

three types of disease. Patients who received renal transplants when this procedure was first developed were treated with antilymphocyte serum. This material contained antibodies to lymphocyte membrane antigens, which apparently cross reacted with glomerular basement membrane antigens. Although this antibody could be demonstrated by immunofluorescence along the glomerular basement membrane, its role in producing renal disease was probably masked by the more significant process of graft rejection.

In membranous glomerulonephritis, IgG antibodies are deposited along the glomerular basement membrane in a linear pattern (Fig. 2-7). Linear deposition of glomerular basement membrane antibodies may also be demonstrated in polyarteritis nodosa, scleroderma, systemic lupus erythematosus, diabetic glomerulonephritis, malignant hypertension, and toxemia of pregnancy. These diseases may be the result of immune complex deposition in blood vessels and antibodies to glomerular basement membrane. Antibodies to glomerular basement membrane may simply be secondary to renal damage.

A number of other tissues may be target organs for type II hypersensitivity reactions. In cicatricial pemphigoid, circulating antibody may be deposited along the basement membrane at the dermal–epidermal junction. Other tissues, including muscle, thyroid, heart, and brain, have also been involved in type II cytotoxic reactions in various experimental and clinical situations.

Antibody and Complement in Cytotoxicity

As discussed earlier in this chapter, following antigenic stimulation, B lymphocytes transform to plasma cells and produce antibody. This antibody can attach to the cell-bound antigen which stimulated its production. During immune lysis, specific antibody becomes fixed in this way to membrane-bound antigens. The antigens may be part of the surface membrane or may become secondarily attached to the cell. Antibodies such as IgG or IgM attach to a cell at specific combining sites. Complement proteins will then combine with the antigen–antibody complex and can generate damage through phospholipase activity. If complement is activated in this way, cytotoxicity may occur. The target cell becomes rounded, the nucleus and cytoplasmic granules become more prominent, swelling of the cell and rupture of the cytoplasmic membrane occur, and a ghost cell is left. Such effects may be observed *in vitro*. C8 is the major cytolytic component in the complement system; however, its activity is enhanced by C9.

Through the enzymatic phospholipase action, 100-Å holes are generated in the cell membrane, and the cellular contents are allowed to escape. The functional holes which are produced in the cell membrane allow the free exchange of potassium and sodium ions between the injured cell and the surrounding medium. Osmotic pressure within the cell increases and water enters, leading to swelling and osmotic lysis. Electron microscopy reveals damage to the mitochondria, endoplasmic reticulum, and cytoplasmic matrix. Lysosomal rupture may occur as well. For this mechanism to occur, it is necessary that the immunoglobulin involved be capable of activating the complement system. Such activity is restricted to IgM and IgG antibody, except for the IgG4 subclass.

Another mechanism of immune destruction of target cells is **opsonic adherence.** Cells coated with antibody may be rendered more susceptible to phagocytosis by macrophages. Antibodies may alter the smooth surface of bacteria, making the surface more sticky and making it easier for phagocytes to ingest the microorganism. These antibodies are referred to as **opsonins.** Components of the complement system may also adhere to the cell surface and act as additional opsonizing factors.

Cytotoxic antibodies are found in the serum of patients with malignant melanoma and may play a role in preventing tumor metastasis. Cytotoxic antibodies directed against thyroid tissue are found in patients with autoimmune thyroiditis. It should be pointed out that not all antibodies directed against cell surface antigens are harmful. In fact, some may even be protective to the target cell, and prevent cytotoxic reactions.

IMMUNE-COMPLEX REACTIONS (TYPE III REACTIONS)

Immune-complex reactions occur following the deposition of antigen–antibody complexes in tissues, causing fixation of complement and consequent inflammatory cell responses. This type of reaction is recognized as being important in a variety of clinical entities.

ARTHUS REACTION

The Arthus reaction results from the deposition of antigen–antibody complexes in small blood vessels, leading to a vasculitis and local tissue inflammation. The reaction begins 1–2 hours after immune-complex deposition, reaching a maximum at 3–6 hours, and disappearing after 10–12 hours. Histologically, neutrophils are the hallmark of the Arthus reaction. These are replaced by mononuclear cells and eosinophils at later stages. The reaction may be produced by injecting antigen locally into animals or individuals who have precipitating antibodies in their circulation, or by injecting antibody locally when antigen is present in the circulation. A necrotizing vasculitis ensues, owing to deposition of the antigen–antibody complexes in vessel walls. The immune complexes fix complement and attract neutrophils, which in turn release lysosomal enzymes. The neutrophils are capable of rapidly phagocytizing and degrading antigen–antibody complexes. If neutrophils are prevented from reaching the site of deposition, as by the use of nitrogen mustard or antineutrophil antiserum, the typical Arthus lesion does not develop.

SERUM SICKNESS

Serum sickness is a systemic disease (see Ch. 9) produced mainly by immune-complex deposition. It is usually caused by injection of a foreign serum such as horse serum antitoxin. The injected protein serves as an immediate immunogen and persists in tissues long enough to act as an eliciting antigen for a type III reaction. Thus, the acute manifestations of serum sickness are due to IgE-mediated (type I) damage and the chronic symptoms are associated with immune-complex deposition.

The pathogenesis of serum sickness is indicated in Figure 2-8. During the first phase, the serum level of antigen falls rapidly as the antigen equilibrates through the body. Further decline in the level of antigen is associated with nonimmune protein catabolism. During the

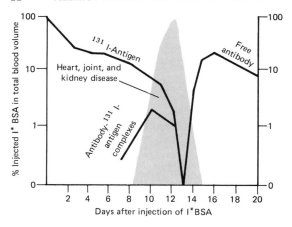

FIG. 2-8. Role of antigen–antibody complex in disease. Serum sickness is characterized by elimination of antigen and formation of antigen–antibody complexes. Lesions of heart, joints, and kidneys develop as antigen–antibody complexes are deposited and complement levels in serum decrease. Free antibody subsequently appears in the circulation. **I*BSA** = ^{131}I-labeled bovine serum albumin. (Dixon FJ: Harvey Lect., 58: 21-52, 1963)

next phase, the level of antigen declines because of the formation of immune complexes (immune elimination). The first immune complexes formed are small because relatively little antibody is available. As antibody is produced in greater amounts, larger immune complexes are formed. These react with complement, the level of which drops abruptly at this stage. Acute inflammatory lesions are produced at the site of the immune-complex localization. The immune complexes eventually become large enough that they are removed from the circulation by the reticulo-endothelial system. Following this removal, free antibody may be detected in the circulation.

The deposition of the immune complexes in tissues is influenced by properties of the affected tissues. Thus, the renal glomeruli are frequent sites for immune-complex deposition owing to their rich blood supply, the filtering capacity of glomeruli, and the phagocytic activity of mesangial cells. The size of the immune complexes also influences whether they will be deposited. Only complexes of 19S or larger will be trapped in vessel walls. Finally, the release of the vasoactive substances during

immune elimination—*e.g.,* the release of histamine and serotonin from platelets—may increase vascular permeability and facilitate the deposition of immune complexes.

FACTORS INFLUENCING IMMUNE-COMPLEX DISORDERS

Some of the diseases felt to be mediated by immune complexes are listed in Table 2-1. The development of immune-complex disease

TABLE 2-1. EXAMPLES OF HUMAN DISEASES ASSOCIATED WITH IMMUNE COMPLEXES IN PLASMA AND DEPOSITED IN TISSUES

Microbial infections
  Bacterial and spirochetal
    Acute poststreptococcal glomerulonephritis
    Syphilis
    Mycoplasmal pneumonia
    Subacute bacterial endocarditis
    Shunt nephritis (*Staphylococcus albus*)
    Lepromatous leprosy
  Viral
    Chronic HB$_s$Ag infections
    HB$_s$Ag in polyarteritis nodosa
    Guillain–Barré syndrome
    Infectious mononucleosis glomerulonephritis
Parasitic infections
  Malarial nephrotic syndrome
  Tropical splenomegaly syndrome
  Leishmaniasis
  Trypanosomiasis
  Schistosomiasis
Disseminated malignancy
  Solid tumors
    Carcinoma of lung
    Carcinoma of breast
    Carcinoma of colon
    Malignant melanoma
  Leukemia
    Acute lymphoblastic leukemia
    Chronic lymphocytic leukemia
  Lymphoma: Hodgkin's disease
Autoimmune disorders
  Systemic lupus erythematosus
  Hashimoto's thyroiditis
  Rheumatoid arthritis
Miscellaneous
  Essential mixed cryoglobulinemia
  Celiac disease
  Dermatitis herpetiformis
  Crohn's disease
  Ulcerative colitis
  Henoch–Schönlein nephritis
  Hepatic cirrhosis
  Sickle cell anemia
Drug reactions
  Serum sickness
  Penicillamine nephropathy

(Wells JV: In Fudenberg HH *et al* (eds): Basic and Clinical Immunology. Los Altos, Lange, 1976, p. 233)

depends on a variety of factors. Certain species of animals appear to be more susceptible to their development. Genetic factors within a species also seem to influence the development of immune-complex disease. Human diseases associated with immune-complex deposition, such as rheumatoid arthritis, have a higher incidence in certain families.

Almost any antigen which elicits an antibody response may induce immune-complex deposition. This includes heterologous proteins, drugs, bacteria, and viruses. IgG and IgM antibody are the classes of immunoglobulins generally involved in the formation of immune complexes. Both precipitating and nonprecipitating antibodies may form immune complexes. These complexes are known to bind to platelet membranes and can lead to the release of vasoactive amines. Binding of immune complexes to neutrophils can also occur and will lead to the release of lysosomal enzymes from these cells.

DELAYED HYPERSENSITIVITY (TYPE IV REACTIONS)

Delayed hypersensitivity, a form of cell-mediated immunity, differs from humoral immunity in that delayed hypersensitivity reactions are mediated by sensitized T lymphocytes rather than by humoral antibody. The term **delayed hypersensitivity** was coined by Hans Zinsser, who noted the indurated, erythematous skin reactions which occurred in response to bacterial antigens. A delay of several hours occurs between the time of challenge and the onset of a visible reaction. The reaction develops slowly, reaching maximum intensity at 24–72 hours. Antibody-mediated reactions, on the other hand, develop immediately after challenge and last for hours rather than days. Over the years, the tuberculin reaction has become the most familiar delayed hypersensitivity reaction; however, similar reactions were shown to develop in response to a variety of immunologic stimuli. These include reactions to various microorganisms, such as viruses, and to contact allergens, protein antigens, grafts, and tumors.

In 1942, Landsteiner and Chase showed that delayed hypersensitivity reactions could be transferred to unimmunized hosts by lymphoid cells, but not by serum (see Passive Transfer). Thus, these cellular reactions could be differentiated from other forms of hypersensitivity which could be passively transferred by antibody-containing serum. Freund, in 1956, showed that the injection of antigens in oil emulsions containing tubercle bacilli greatly enhanced the development of delayed hypersensitivity.

Recently, it has been shown that T cells from the thymus-dependent areas of lymphoid tissue are the most prominent cells in delayed hypersensitivity reactions. As discussed in Chapter 1, these cells originate from bone marrow stem cell precursors and are in some way processed by the thymus. They reside within the thymus, in the paracortical regions of lymph nodes, and in thymus-dependent areas of the spleen. T cells have been shown to elaborate a number of soluble mediators known as lymphokines (discussed subsequently). These can be assayed *in vitro*, and may be responsible for certain *in vivo* phenomena observed in delayed hypersensitivity reactions. In addition, other cells besides lymphocytes are involved in delayed hypersensitivity reactions. These include neutrophils, macrophages, and basophilic leukocytes.

INDUCTION OF DELAYED HYPERSENSITIVITY

As in other forms of hypersensitivity, introduction of an antigen does not always elicit a cell-mediated immune response. Such factors as the type of antigen, the route of administration, and the use of adjuvants may influence the development of a response and the type of response observed. Protein antigens, when incorporated in mycobacterial adjuvants and given by the intradermal route, may lead to the development of delayed hypersensitivity, while the same antigen given repeatedly in large intramuscular doses may favor the development of antibody. An even larger dose of the same antigen may result in the state of complete nonreactivity known as immune tolerance. It should also be noted that a single injection of an antigen may elicit an early delayed hypersensitivity response and a subsequent antibody response.

EXPRESSION OF DELAYED HYPERSENSITIVITY

When a skin test antigen is applied to any sensitive animal, reactions generally appear within 4–6 hours and reach a maximum at 18–24 hours. The time course of delayed reactions in humans is prolonged, with reactions reaching a maximum at about 48 hours. Erythema and induration are characteristic features of delayed skin reactions; severe reactions may show a central pallor. If specific antibody is also present, an Arthus or anaphylactic reaction may precede the delayed skin reaction.

Delayed hypersensitivity is most often studied by eliciting skin reactions in the guinea pig. In man, delayed skin reactions are frequently elicited by a very small test dose, one containing microgram quantities of antigen. In the mouse, delayed hypersensitivity is best elicited by injection of antigen into the foot pad or application of antigen to the ear.

Although delayed hypersensitivity is usually investigated by skin testing, generalized reactions may be elicited when antigenic challenge is administered systemically to sensitized animals. These generalized reactions consist of fever and disappearance of mononuclear cells from the circulation.

Delayed hypersensitivity skin reactions are characterized histologically by the perivascular infiltration of mononuclear cells. Although specifically sensitized T lymphocytes are important in the development of delayed hypersensitivity, only about 5% of the lymphocytes found at a skin test site are indeed antigen-specific. Radioactive labeling has shown that most of the cells which accumulate are nonspecific, unsensitized mononuclear cells. The distribution of the mononuclear infiltrates within the skin may vary, depending upon the species being tested. In the rat, lymphocytes are found deep in the dermis, whereas in man and guinea pigs a more superficial infiltrate is observed. A delayed skin reaction differs histologically from an ordinary inflammatory lesion, which shows an initial neutrophil response followed by a chronic mononuclear response. Neutrophils may participate in delayed reactions to a certain extent. They are particularly prevalent if the skin test antigen is contaminated with irritant substances such as endotoxin. Neutrophils may also appear if tissue necrosis occurs, or if antigen–antibody responses are being elicited.

Other changes observed in delayed hypersensitivity skin reactions include dilated lymphatic channels, activation of the endothelial cells of blood vessels, and activation of fixed tissue histiocytes.

Delayed hypersensitivity skin reactions are associated with increased permeability of the local vasculature. This increased permeability is accompanied by exudation of fluid and plasma proteins. In addition, extensive fibrin deposition may be observed. These deposits bind tissue water and probably contribute to the induration which is characteristic of delayed hypersensitivity reactions.

Cutaneous Basophil Hypersensitivity

A form of delayed hypersensitivity reaction, known as cutaneous basophil hypersensitivity when it occurs in the skin, has recently been recognized. Raffel and Newel termed these reactions "Jones–Mote reactions" because they were similar to reactions induced by Jones and Mote in humans by giving repeated injections of heterologous serum. Dvorak has found that basophil-rich reactions are frequently seen in delayed hypersensitivity skin reactions to protein antigens and antigen–antibody complexes, in contact sensitivity, in viral hypersensitivity, and in graft and tumor rejection.

Cutaneous basophil hypersensitivity (CBH) reactions are best elicited 5–10 days after sensitization. With certain antigens, such as vaccinia virus and contact allergens, CBH may be elicited for many weeks after sensitization. CBH reactions are erythematous and usually lack induration.

Microscopically, CBH reactions are characterized by perivascular infiltrates of mononuclear cells, as are other delayed hypersensitivity reactions. In addition, large infiltrates of basophilic leukocytes are typically seen. Basophils may comprise 30%–60% of the

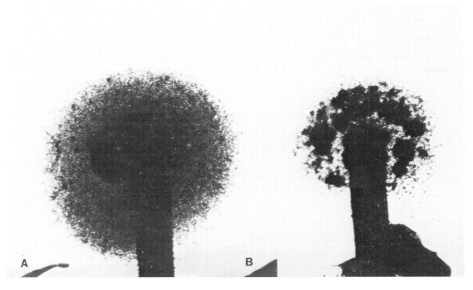

FIG. 2-9. Migration inhibition factor (MIF) assay. A. Control with normal migration of guinea pig peritoneal macrophages. B. Inhibition in the presence of specific antigen. (Courtesy of Dr. G. Senyk)

papillary dermal infiltrate and a smaller fraction of the deep dermal infiltrate. In allergic contact dermatitis in man, basophils account for 10%–15% of the total dermal and epidermal inflammatory cells. (It should be remembered that basophils normally account for only 0.5% of circulating leukocytes in man and guinea pigs.)

Like other types of delayed hypersensitivity reactions, CBH reactions depend on the interaction of sensitized T lymphocytes with antigen. Basophils, although present in large numbers and having the capability of binding heterotropic antibody, do not appear to possess immunologic specificity in these reactions. It has not been possible to transfer CBH reactions passively using basophils from sensitized donors.

The function of basophils remains obscure. It is well known that these cells contain vasoactive substances such as histamine and heparin. CBH reactions, however, show little morphologic evidence of a histamine effect and little alteration of vascular permeability. There is a well-known inverse correlation between the number of mast cells and the number of basophils in a particular species. While basophils are readily found in man and guinea pigs, rats and mice possess fewer basophils and proportionately more mast cells.

IN VITRO CORRELATES OF DELAYED HYPERSENSITIVITY

In recent years, it has been shown that sensitized T lymphocytes, when cultured in vitro with specific antigen, undergo certain morphologic changes and also release a variety of mediator substances known as lymphokines.

Lymphokines

Lymphokines are substances which are secreted by sensitized T lymphocytes in the presence of specific antigen. Lymphokines influence the behavior of other cells involved in the inflammatory response. While these mediators may or may not play a role in vivo, studying them may lead to a better understanding of delayed hypersensitivity mechanisms.

1) Assay of **migration inhibition factor (MIF)** has become one of the most popular in vitro tests for delayed hypersensitivity (Fig. 2-9). Rich and Lewis first recognized that the mi-

gration of sensitized lymphoid cells was inhibited in the presence of specific antigen. George and Vaughn demonstrated the migration of peritoneal macrophages from capillary tubes and the inhibition of this migration in the presence of specific antigen. David and his coworkers, and Bloom and Bennett, working independently, showed that only small numbers of lymphocytes were required for antigen-induced inhibition of macrophage migration. It was subsequently recognized that a glycoprotein, which became known as MIF, was responsible for the inhibitory effect.

2) **Macrophage aggregation factor (MAF),** a lymphokine discovered by Nelson and Boyden in 1963, causes macrophages to aggregate and adhere to the mesothelial lining of the peritoneal cavity. This results in the disappearance of mononuclear cells from peritoneal exudates. 3) Sensitized lymphocytes, when cultured in the presence of specific antigen, elaborate a variety of **chemotactic factors,** which attract certain types of white blood cells. So far, chemotactic factors have been demonstrated for neutrophils, monocytes, lymphocytes, eosinophils, and basophils. 4) **Lymphocyte mitogenic factor** increases the incorporation of tritiated thymidine into cultured lymphocytes. It may affect unsensitized cells and thereby amplify the activation of lymphocytes.

5) **Skin reactive factor** induces an indurated, erythematous skin lesion when injected intradermally into normal guinea pigs. It produces a visible reaction 3 hours after injection which is characterized by infiltration of mononuclear cells and later by neutrophils. 6) **Lymphotoxin (LT)** is cytopathic for a number of mammalian cell cultures. It is presently felt that sensitized lymphocytes need not come into direct contact with target cells in order to express LT activity. 7) **Macrophage activation** is a process that is thought to be induced by a lymphokine: animals with cellular immunity acquired during an infection have macrophages with increased bactericidal properties.

8) **Interferon** is a substance elaborated by lymphocytes and other types of mammalian cells. It protects other reinfected cells from viral infection. Interferon is not virucidal itself, nor is it specific for the virus which produced

it. Its mechanism of action is thought to involve the binding of a translation-inhibiting protein to host cell ribosomes. This prevents the translation of viral RNA but not host cell RNA and therefore interferes with viral replication. **Lymph node permeability factor** is a lymphokine which causes increased vascular permeability, lymphocyte emigration, and deposition of fibrinoid material.

Obviously, the physiologic actions of lymphokines would be helpful in explaining some of the events which occur during cell-mediated immunity. These mediator substances may stimulate the production of lymphocytes; attract macrophages, monocytes, and basophils; kill bacteria and viruses; and increase the blood flow and permeability of local vessels. It should be emphasized that correlation between *in vitro* events and those which occur *in vivo* is speculative. Furthermore, it is not known whether a single lymphocyte may produce several lymphokines, or under which circumstances a given lymphokine will be produced. It is known, however, that histologic responses differ depending on the type of antigen involved and the mode of sensitization. Perhaps the lymphokines which are elaborated depend on the antigenic stimulus and the type of mediator most suited for its neutralization.

ANTIBODY FORMATION IN DELAYED HYPERSENSITIVITY

The role of antibody in cell-mediated immune responses is complex and not completely understood. Antibody molecules may participate in a variety of reactions that are generally considered to be in the realm of cellular immunity. Thus, antibody may be detected in certain forms of graft rejection and in resistance to many viral and bacterial infections. Possibly some cooperation between humoral and cellular immunity exists in situations where both mechanisms are present. While some investigators have claimed a major role for humoral antibody in delayed hypersensitivity reactions, there is no conclusive evidence to support this concept. One source of confusion seems to be the hypersensitivity reactions which have both a humoral and a cellular component. In hypersensitivity reactions which are purely delayed in type, such as hypersensitivity to contact allergens and to antigen–antibody complexes prepared in antibody excess cellular hypersensitivity exists and antibody is not detectable even by the most sensitive methods.

It is possible that cell-bound antibody plays a role in delayed hypersensitivity and may account for the immunologic specificity of these reactions. B cells have been shown to bind antigen and both B and T cells contain antibody on their surfaces.

HAPTENS AND DELAYED HYPERSENSITIVITY

If antibody-mediated hypersensitivity is induced by a simple chemical, or hapten conjugated to a carrier protein, the host develops antibody which is specific for the hapten moiety. Delayed reactivity, however, develops against the hapten and a portion of the carrier protein adjacent to the hapten linkage. Thus, delayed hypersensitivity reactions are said to have **carrier specificity.** It would seem that the lymphocyte receptor responsible for delayed hypersensitivity is larger than that responsible for antibody production. An exception is seen in sensitization to arsanilic acid, which can elicit delayed hypersensitivity with hapten specificity only. This may be attributable to some physical or chemical property of this particular hapten.

PASSIVE TRANSFER

In their classic studies, Landsteiner and Chase demonstrated that delayed hypersensitivity reactions could be transferred from sensitized to normal animals by lymphoid cells. This differentiated delayed reactions from antibody-dependent reactions, which were transferred by immune serum. Delayed hypersensitivity reactions can be elicited for only a few days in noninbred animals. After this time, the donor cells undergo rejection by the recipient. In man, however, Lawrence has shown that delayed hypersensitivity reactions can be elicited for long periods (1–2 years) after the passive transfer of lymphoid cells. He also demon-

strated that delayed hypersensitivity could be transferred to nonsensitive individuals with an extract of lymphocytes known as **transfer factor.** This transferred state of immunity is highly specific; that is, the individual acquires cellular immunity only to the antigen used for sensitizing the donor.

Transfer factor can be produced by osmotic lysis or by freezing and thawing of circulating cells. It has a molecular weight of less than 10,000 and is not in itself immunogenic. It may represent an RNA nucleotide–peptide complex which is informational or provides some part of a receptor for antigen. On the other hand, Uhr has suggested that transfer factor is a special form of immunogen capable of stimulating an immune response in a very short period of time. Further study of transfer factor may yield important information about the molecular events involved in cellular immunity, and may also reveal possibilities for the treatment of diseases with an immune basis.

SUPPRESSION OF CELLULAR IMMUNITY

As discussed in Chapter 1, immune tolerance is a state of relative immunologic suppression, in which the individual responds poorly or not at all to an immunologic stimulus.

While tolerance produces specific suppression of an immune response, a variety of other substances induce a nonspecific suppression of the host's immune response. These include antimetabolite drugs, corticosteroids, antilymphocyte serum, and ionizing radiation. Heparin and warfarin also suppress cellular immunity, perhaps by interfering with the clotting mechanism. Thymectomy, when performed early in life, will specifically suppress T cell responses.

BIOLOGIC SIGNIFICANCE OF CELLULAR IMMUNITY

The practical significance of cellular immunity is an important consideration. Besides causing clinical delayed hypersensitivity reactions such as contact allergy, cellular immunity is responsible for protection against certain microbial infections, for mediating allograft rejection, and for surveillance of neoplasia.

Cellular Immunity in Bacterial Infections

Since the time of Robert Koch, it has been recognized that a heightened reactivity occurs when an infectious organism is reintroduced into a previously infected animal. Thus, in a tuberculous animal, skin testing with mycobacteria results in an anamnestic reaction consisting of intense local inflammation and induration.

During a cellular immune response, macrophages, like T cells, are activated and their phagocytic properties are enhanced. Macrophages, however, do not have immunologic specificity; that is, activated macrophages will dispose of unrelated bacteria as well as those responsible for their activation. However, macrophage activation develops at the same time as delayed skin reactivity and reappears anamnestically following rechallenge. Other evidence supporting the close association between cellular immunity and delayed hypersensitivity reactions comes from the study of children who have congenitally defective delayed hypersensitivity. These children have impaired resistance to bacterial infections whether or not their serum concentration of immunoglobulins is normal.

Transplant Rejection

The survival of a tissue transplant depends on the degree of foreignness between donor and recipient. Thus, autografts, in which the same individual is both donor and recipient, and isografts, grafts between identical twins, will survive indefinitely, while allografts, transplants between other individuals of the same species, are ordinarily rejected. The rapidity of rejection is directly related to the genetic disparity between the donor and host. More specifically, rejection is related to the differences in histocompatibility genes which determine cell surface isoantigens in the donor and host (see Histocompatibility Antigens, Ch. 1, and Transplantation Immunology, Ch. 11).

It is recognized that antibodies to foreign tissues are formed during graft rejection. Antibodies are not, however, felt to be important in the usual type of rejection of allografts. Rather, extensive evidence indicates that cellular immune mechanisms are associated with allograft rejection.

Microscopically, allograft rejection, like other delayed hypersensitivity reactions, produces perivascular infiltrates of mononuclear cells. In addition, neutrophils may be found, and recently it has been shown that large numbers of basophils may be present. Possibly, the vasoactive contents of basophils may in some way contribute to graft destruction by a vascular mechanism.

The rejection of second or subsequent allografts is accelerated and is at least partially dependent on circulating antibodies. This includes the hyperacute rejection of renal allografts, in which microvascular occlusion by fibrin is mediated by antibodies with specificity for the graft.

Immune Surveillance

The possibility that a response similar to allograft rejection is active in protection of the host against neoplasia was first suggested by Louis Thomas in 1959. This concept has been furthered by Burnet, who pointed out that there must be some host mechanism for detecting and eliminating potentially dangerous mutant cells. It was subsequently recognized that tumors possess antigens which do not appear on normal host cells (see Tumor Antigens, Ch. 1 and Ch. 12). Furthermore, the host mounts an immune reaction against these so-called tumor-specific transplantation antigens (TSTAs). Some of these TSTAs, which are present on many spontaneously arising tumors, share specificity with antigens present in normal fetal tissues but undetectable in adults.

As in allograft rejection, cellular immune mechanisms seem to be of greater importance than antibody in immune suveillance. Thus, lymphocytes from a patient with neuroblastoma can inhibit neuroblastoma tumor cells when cultured *in vitro*. On the other hand, the patient's serum may enhance the growth of the tumor. This latter effect, known as **enhancement,** may in fact be due to antibody.

Other evidence in favor of cellular immunity in immunologic surveillance comes from patients with immunodeficiency syndromes such as the Wiskott–Aldrich syndrome, in which there is a progressive deficiency of cell-mediated immunity and an extreme susceptibility to lymphoid malignancies. Additionally, patients with renal allografts who are maintained on immunosuppressive therapy also show an increased risk of malignancy.

If the concept of immune surveillance against neoplasia is accepted, it follows that many tumors would be destroyed before becoming clinically significant. Thus, Beckwith and Perrin found the incidence of neuroblastoma to be 40 times higher in infant autopsies than was found clinically. Furthermore, adrenal calcifications were observed in older children, a finding which may represent a destroyed tumor.

It should be pointed out that immunologic surveillance is somewhat theoretic at the present time. Many tumors produced experimentally are considered too weak to immunize a host, and those that do immunize may do so too late to be effective or may stimulate the wrong type of response. Still, a great deal of evidence favors the surveillance hypothesis as a mechanism for prevention of life threatening neoplasia.

Immune Cells in Cytotoxic Reactions

Cytotoxic reactions can be mediated by sensitized T lymphocytes. This type of cell-mediated immunity is important in certain microbial infections, contact allergy, autoimmune disease, and transplant and tumor immunity. Cell-mediated immunity does not require the participation of antibody or complement. Cell-mediated cytotoxicity is specific, however, and may occur by one of two proposed mechanisms: 1) activated lymphocytes may be directly responsible for target cell damage, or 2) soluble mediators produced by activated lymphocytes could mediate cytotoxicity.

The specificity of cytotoxic reactions indicates that sensitized lymphocytes will only attack target cells, while "bystander" cells in the reaction mixture will remain unharmed. Electron microscopic and cinematographic studies indicate that lymphocytes may attach to target cells by means of an organelle or tail known as a uropod. This association between lymphocyte and target cell seems to be transient, and may involve the release or injection of some cytotoxic substance into the target cell. This might explain why only specific target cells are killed and why no substantial amounts of cytotoxic factors are detectable in the medium.

STIMULATORY HYPERSENSITIVITY (TYPE V REACTIONS)

Under certain circumstances, antibody may stimulate target cells to overproduce their normal products. These target cells presumably have surface receptors which transmit a signal to the interior of the cell upon stimulation. This mechanism may be similar to the adenylate cyclase–cAMP pathway.

Long-acting thyroid stimulator (LATS) is an IgG autoantibody that is probably directed against antigen or the thyroid cell surface. When LATS binds to thyroid cells, it stimu-

TABLE 2-2. SUMMARY OF THE FOUR MAIN TYPES OF DIRECT CYTOTOXICITY

Type	Activating agents	Effector cells	Specificity Effector cells	Target cells
1. Allograft-induced	Alloantigens	T cells	Specific	Specific
2. Tumor antigen-induced	Cell membrane antigens (including tumor-specific antigens)	T cells and "armed" macrophages	Specific	Specific ↓ Nonspecific
3. Mitogen-induced	Phytohemagglutinins (PHA) Soluble antigens	T cells (?) B cells	Nonspecific (PHA) Specific (antigens)	Nonspecific
4. Antibody-dependent	7S antibody specifically bound to cell membrane antigens	K cells and macrophages	Nonspecific	Specific, antibody-dependent

(Wells JV: In Fudenberg HH *et al* (eds): Basic and Clinical Immunology. Los Altos, Lange, 1976, p. 237)

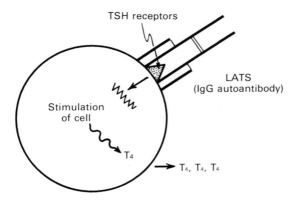

FIG. 2-10. Proposed mechanism for antibody-mediated stimulatory (type V) hypersensitivity. Long-acting thyroid stimulator (LATS) binds to or near thyroid-stimulating hormone (TSH) receptor on thyroid cell, causing constant production of T_4 hormone. (Bigley NJ: Immunologic Fundamentals Copyright © 1975 by Year Book Med. Pub., Inc. p 171. Used by permission.)

lates a constant production of T_4 hormone (Fig. 2-10). LATS has an effect similar to that of thyroid-stimulating hormone (TSH); however, LATS is not under the control of the thyroid–pituitary axis.

Other examples of stimulatory hypersensitivity may include the induction of pinocytosis by antimacrophage serum, stimulation of lymphocyte surface immunoglobulin by antigen or antibody, and transformation of lymphocytes by antilymphocyte serum.

HUMORAL AMPLIFICATION SYSTEMS

While most of the mechanisms which mediate tissue damage are studied as isolated systems, it should be recognized that in the body these different mechanisms may interact with one another. Thus, type II and type III reactions

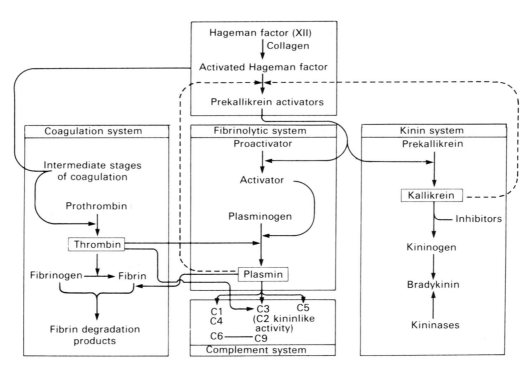

FIG. 2-11. Schematic diagram demonstrating multiple relationships between the coagulation, fibrinolytic, complement, and kinin systems. (Reproduced with permission from Wells JV: Immune mechanisms in tissue damage. In Fudenberg *et al* (eds): Basic and Clinical Immunology, Los Altos, Lange, 1976, p 239).

may both be observed in response to a viral infection. Other bodily systems such as the complement and coagulation systems may be brought into play and may influence the final outcome of the immunologic reaction (Fig. 2-11).

The complement system involves the complex interaction of at least 11 separate serum proteins, as was described in Chapter 1. Certain products of the complement system such as C3a and C5a can serve as anaphylatoxins and can cause the release of histamine and other substances from mast cells, leading to edema, smooth muscle contraction, and increased capillary permeability. C3a, C5a, and the trimolecular complex C567 are chemotactic for neutrophils. Thus, neutrophils and products of mast cell secretion may contribute to the reaction observed when antigen and antibody interact in the presence of complement. Plasmin, a fibrinolytic enzyme, can directly attack C1, C3, and C5. The proteolytic enzyme thrombin, which converts fibrinogen to fibrin, can attack C3, and a fragment of C2 which has kininlike activity can cause contraction of smooth muscle and increase vascular permeability.

The coagulation system can also be activated as a result of an immunologic reaction. Hageman factor can be activated by damaged blood vessel endothelium or by exposure to collagen. The clotting system is also activated in delayed hypersensitivity reactions in which extensive fibrin deposition can be demonstrated. The water-retaining property of polymerized fibrin seems to account for the induration seen in classic delayed hypersensitivity skin reactions.

The kinin or kallikrein system is activated by coagulation factor XII, which leads to the formation of bradykinin. This substance produces smooth muscle contraction, increased vascular permeability, and arterial dilation. The formation of bradykinin can be inhibited by C1-esterase inhibitor, a factor which is absent in patients with hereditary angioedema; increased activity of the kinin system may occur in this disease. The fibrinolysin system can also amplify and modify immunologic reactions. The proteolytic enzyme plasmin (fibrinolysin) can digest fibrin, fibrinogen, various other clotting factors, C1 inactivator, and complement components C1, C3, and C5.

These four humoral amplification systems (complement, coagulation, kinin, and fibrinolysin) are closely interrelated, and serve to amplify and control the immune response. They produce effects on hemostasis and tissue repair which are important features of hypersensitivity reactions.

SUGGESTED READING

Bellanti JA: Immunology. Philadelphia, WB Saunders, 1978

Bigley NJ: Immunologic Fundamentals. Chicago, Year Book Medical, 1975

Eisen HN: Immunology. Hagerstown, Harper & Row, 1974

Freedman SO, Gold P (eds): Clinical Immunology. Hagerstown, Harper & Row, 1976

Fudenberg HH, Stites DP, Caldwell JL, Wells JV (eds): Basic and Clinical Immunology. Los Altos, Lange, 1976

Gell PGH, Coombs RRA (eds): Clinical Aspects of Immunology. Oxford, Blackwell, 1968

Humphrey JH, White RG: Immunology for Students of Medicine. Philadelphia, FA Davis, 1970

Movat HZ (ed): Inflammation, Immunity and Hypersensitivity. New York, Harper & Row, 1971

Rahi AH, Garner A: Immunopathology of the Eye. Oxford, Blackwell, 1976

Roitt IM: Essential Immunology. Oxford, Blackwell, 1974

Rose NR, Friedman H (eds): Manual of Clinical Immunology. Washington DC, American Society for Microbiology, 1976

Rose NR, Milgrom F, Van Oss CJ (eds): Principles of Immunology. New York, MacMillan, 1973

Sell S: Immunology, Immunopathology, and Immunity. Hagerstown, Harper & Row, 1975

THREE
THREE
THREE
the ocular immune response

The eye resists foreign invaders through a variety of specific and nonspecific defense mechanisms. Like other parts of the body, the eye is constantly exposed to a flood of microorganisms but is capable of warding off most of these with little or no alteration of its structure or function. Much of the eye's natural resistance depends on anatomic and physiologic properties of its external structures—the lids, tears, conjunctiva, and cornea (30a,b). Once a foreign substance (such as a bacterium) has entered the eye, the defense mechanisms are far less effective than at the eye's outer surface, and destructive effects are more likely to occur. In this chapter, we will consider the specific and nonspecific defense mechanisms which characterize the different ocular tissues. We will be concerned not only with the way the eye responds under normal circumstances, but also with the immunologic responses of the eye when it is exposed to various infectious agents and antigenic stimuli.

LIDS

The eyelids have the obvious function of protecting the eye from trauma by the blink mechanism and by screening out small particles through the action of the cilia. In addition, the lids keep the eye lubricated with tears and help to sweep foreign substances from the eye and into the tear drainage. The skin of the eyelids possesses the same antimicrobial properties that skin has elsewhere in the body. In addition the lids possess a number of glands whose secretions contribute to the tear film and also contain numerous antimicrobial substances.

TEARS

The tear film consists of three layers: 1) An outer oily layer, composed of phospholipids, is produced by the meibomian glands. This layer retards evaporation of the tear film and aids in spreading the tears over the surface of the cornea. 2) The middle layer of the tear film is composed of aqueous secretions from the lacrimal and accessory lacrimal glands of Krause and Wolfring. This layer, which contains lysozyme and immunoglobulins, is deficient in Sjögren's syndrome. 3) The innermost layer of the tear film is a thin, mucoid layer which is derived mainly from the goblet cells of the conjunctiva. The mucoid layer facilitates spreading of the aqueous layer over the surface of the eye. We have become more aware of mucoid deficiencies in recent years, particularly in cases of cicatricial pemphigoid and in the Stevens–Johnson syndrome.

LYSOZYME

The tears contain both antibody and lysozyme (22). Lysozyme is a cationic, low-molecular-weight enzyme which reduces the local concentration of susceptible bacteria by attacking the mucopeptides of their cell walls. Although most gram-positive bacteria are affected by lysozyme, *Staphylococcus aureus* is not, since the lysozyme-susceptible site on this organism's cell wall is blocked structurally from lysozyme attack.

Tear lysozyme is thought to be produced by the lacrimal gland and is present in a much higher concentration in tears than in serum (53). Tear lysozyme concentration is elevated during the morning and reduced during the hours of sleep (53). Lactoferrin, another major tear protein, has bacteriostatic properties, presumably due to its ability to make certain metals unavailable for microorganisms (14).

IMMUNOGLOBULINS

All of the major immunoglobulin classes except IgD have been detected in human tears. IgA is the major immunoglobulin in tears and, as in other external secretions, it is the 11S, dimeric variety containing secretory piece which predominates (11,18,57,70,86). IgG is usually detectable in only small amounts, while IgM is only rarely detectable (18). IgD has not been detected in any study of tears. IgE is detectable by radioimmunoassay (12,70), and this immunoglobulin may be increased in patients suffering from allergic disorders of the external eye (12).

Tear immunoglobulin appears to be produced by plasma cells within the lacrimal gland, while secretory component is produced within the acinar epithelial cells of the gland (29). Various studies have shown that the level of IgA in tears varies from 7 to 85 mg/100 ml and IgG concentrations range from trace amounts to 14 mg/100 ml. In the inflamed eye, tear immunoglobulins are generally increased and resemble more closely the distribution of the immunoglobulins in serum. This is probably due to a transudation of serum proteins into the tears (70). The exact mechanism by which secretory IgA works is not known. Its clearest role is in bacterial disease, where in some way it prevents attachment of bacteria to mucosal cells (22). No specific immunoglobulin changes can presently be correlated with specific disease entities other than an increase in IgE in some allergic conditions (18,70).

Complement is detectable in human tears,

and both C3 (11) and C4 (18) have been quantitated. The relationship of complement to specific ocular diseases requires further study.

CONJUNCTIVA

NORMAL STRUCTURE AND FUNCTION

The normal conjunctiva forms a natural barrier to invasion by exogenous substances. Inflammatory cells present from the time of birth have been studied in several animal species (71) and the quantity of leukocytes appears to increase with age and antigenic exposure. The normal human conjunctiva contains an extraordinary number of infiltrative, inflammatory cells, among which lymphocytes, plasma cells, and neutrophils are found. Fixed-tissue mast cells are also found in great numbers in the conjunctiva, as in other vascularized tissues (3). No doubt many of the inflammatory cells normally present in the conjunctiva are engaged in phagocytosis and in processing antigen for its elimination and for the individual's immunologic memory. The epithelial cells of the conjunctiva may also participate in phagocytosis (124). Epithelial phagocytosis has been shown to be active in conjunctival infection with *Listeria* and *Chlamydia*. Both epithelial cells and leukocytes possess lysosomes containing acid hydrolases which have a strong antimicrobial effect.

The normal palpebral conjunctiva varies a great deal in its surface morphology from a satin-smooth appearance to a uniform or nonuniform papillary appearance (43). Papillae represent collections of nonspecific inflammatory cells and tissue elements which are bound closely to the tarsal plate or the limbus. Follicles may also be seen in the normal conjunctiva, especially in the lower fornix. These are not related to disease and are especially common in childhood. Conjunctival follicles represent tightly packed collections of lymphocytes in various stages of development. Lymphoid aggregates containing mature and immature lymphocytes are found just below the epithelium in the conjunctiva of adult rabbits after 10 weeks of age (9).

The conjunctiva is endowed with several other nonspecific protective mechanisms.

Constant epithelial turnover and a cool temperature due to tear evaporation may serve a protective function. In addition, certain unknown factors make the conjunctiva usually resistant to certain viruses (such as those which cause the common cold), yet highly susceptible to the gonococcus and the agent of inclusion conjunctivitis. (In contrast, the nasal mucosa is highly susceptible to cold viruses yet resistant to the gonococcus.) The prominent vascularity of the conjunctiva and the frequently observed dilation of its vessels suggests that the exchange of substances across the vessel walls is a fundamental response of the conjunctiva to noxious substances.

PATHOLOGIC RESPONSES

The conjunctiva can undergo a variety of morphologic changes in response to microorganisms, toxins, and various antigens. The type of response depends largely on the nature of the stimulus. Hyperemia occurs in response to physical stimuli such as wind, sun, or smoke, or in response to allergens, toxins, and infectious agents. A brilliant red appearance suggests a bacterial conjunctivitis, while a milky appearance suggests an allergic conjunctivitis. Tearing often accompanies hyperemia and may be increased by transudation across the vessel walls. Exudation is seen in all types of acute conjunctivitis. A purulent exudate is characteristic of bacterial conjunctivitis, while a stringy exudate is more often seen in allergic conjunctivitis. Drooping of the upper eyelid (**pseudoptosis**) may be due to increased weight of the lid from cellular infiltration and edema. **Chemosis,** or edema of the conjunctiva, is often associated with an acute allergic response and several other types of conjunctivitis.

Papillary hypertrophy occurs when inflammatory cells accumulate within the conjunctiva, causing it to heap up in mounds that are bound to the tarsal plate by strong connective tissue fibrils. A tuft of vessels forms in the substance of the **papilla** and branches over it like the spokes of an umbrella. When the papillae are small, the conjunctiva frequently has a smooth, velvety appearance, as in bacterial conjunctivitis. In allergic conditions, such as

vernal and atopic keratoconjunctivitis, the papillae of the upper tarsus may be large, flat-topped, polygonal, and milky in appearance. These giant papillae may also form at the limbus, where they appear as gelatinous excrescences. **Follicles** are characteristic of viral and chlamydial infections and also of toxic conjunctivitis due to the application of certain topical medications. When they are located on the upper palpebral conjunctiva or at the limbus, they are strongly suggestive of chlamydial disease. Those located in the lower fornix or at the lateral margins of the upper tarsus have limited diagnostic value. The follicle is rounded, whitish gray in color, and avascular, although small vessels may encircle it (109).

Pseudomembranes and **membranes** result from a coagulation process on the surface of the conjunctiva. A true membrane involves the entire epithelium, and when it is removed a raw bleeding surface remains. A pseudomembrane is a coagulum on the surface of the epithelium, and when it is removed the epithelium remains intact and bleeding does not occur. Both membranes and pseudomembranes accompany various types of bacterial conjunctivitis, erythema multiforme major (Stevens-Johnson syndrome), and chemical burns. Neutrophils are abundantly present in smears taken from such cases.

Granulomas appear on the conjunctiva in response to various infectious agents or in the form of a chalazion (lipogranuloma). A grossly visible preauricular node may accompany such a granulomatous response.

Conjunctival scrapings are often helpful in determining the etiology of an inflammatory response (63,104). A predominantly neutrophilic reaction is characteristic of fungal infections and all but two bacterial infections (*Branhamella catarrhalis* and *Moraxella*). Several diseases of unknown etiology also produce a neutrophil response, including erythema multiforme and Reiter's syndrome. An eosinophil response is characteristic of allergic inflammation, such as vernal conjunctivitis, hay fever, and drug-related allergies. Mast cells are also characteristically seen in conjunctival smears from patients with vernal conjunctivitis. Mononuclear cells predominate in conjunctival scrapings from viral conjunctivitis, while neutrophils are usually seen in response to chlamydial infections.

HUMORAL IMMUNE RESPONSES

All five immunoglobulins are routinely found in the human conjunctiva (2). Most are present in the subepithelial tissue and almost none are found in the epithelium. Immunoglobulin-producing plasma cells are not routinely identified in the perilimbal conjunctiva with the use of immunofluorescent techniques (4). Immediate hypersensitivity reactions have been studied in the guinea pig conjunctiva following systemic sensitization with normal rabbit serum (25). Topical conjunctival challenge produces edema, hyperemia, and infiltration by a large number of eosinophils and neutrophils. Both IgE and IgG homocytotropic antibody can be demonstrated in serum and when these are passively transferred to normal guinea pigs, conjunctival hypersensitivity can be demonstrated by topical challenge (25). Antihistamines, cromolyn (disodium cromoglycate), and steroids do not modify the clinical signs, but they do inhibit the neutrophil and eosinophil response (24).

CELLULAR IMMUNE RESPONSES

Cellular immune responses have not been well studied in the conjunctiva and it is often stated that these responses can only be elicited on mucous membranes with great difficulty. We have recently studied a model of contact sensitivity in the guinea pig conjunctiva in which a nontoxic hapten, oxazolone, elicits a delayed-onset reaction 5–7 days after topical cutaneous sensitization (31). The conjunctival response contains predominantly mononuclear cells but a large number of eosinophils is also seen. A reaction which is widely believed to represent delayed hypersensitivity in the conjunctiva is the **phlyctenule,** a transient nodular lesion seen in response to a variety of microbial agents. Both B and T lymphocytes have been identified in the human conjunctiva and lacrimal gland taken from patients with phlyctenular conjunctivitis and Sjögren's syndrome (10). B cells are generally found in higher

numbers but are more concentrated in the central follicles, while T cells are found mainly in peripheral follicles and scattered throughout the tissue.

CORNEA

NORMAL STRUCTURE AND FUNCTION

The cornea has long been a favorite site for immunologic study. Because of its transparency and convenient location, a mild inflammatory response or ingrowth of new blood vessels can be easily monitored. It also provides a window through which direct observations of the inner eye can be made. The cornea has the unique property of being avascular except at the corneoscleral limbus. Lymphatic drainage is also lacking, except when new blood vessels have grown into a previously normal cornea. The avascularity of the cornea and the lack of lymphatic channels has given rise to the concept that the cornea is a "privileged site." This feature is dramatically demonstrated in corneal transplantation, where allografts may survive indefinitely instead of being rejected as they could be in other anatomic sites. Antigens and other substances which enter the cornea from the blood stream must enter from the limbus and diffuse into the cornea. This seems to prevent large molecules, such as IgM, from entering the central cornea (4). Conversely, substances injected into the central cornea enter the circulation through the limbal vessels but do not drain through lymphatic channels. Cellular elements can also enter the cornea through the limbal blood vessels, and many types of corneal inflammation are accompanied by a great outpouring of cells from these vessels into the cornea (32).

Antigen may diffuse from the cornea to the anterior chamber, although Descemet's membrane probably inhibits this diffusion. The relative importance of this route is presently unknown.

Mast cells are found at the limbus in most animal species (32,56), in association with the limbal blood vessels. The function of these cells is not known although it has been suggested that they may regulate the tone or other functions of the limbal vessels.

PATHOLOGIC RESPONSES

Epithelial Keratitis

Epithelial keratitis commonly accompanies blepharoconjunctivitis, particularly the type associated with staphylococcal infection. It is also commonly seen after long-term administration of certain topical drugs (idoxuridine, gentamicin) to the eye. This type of superficial keratitis is usually a toxic rather than an immunologic alteration of the cornea. A nontoxic epithelial keratitis is seen in a variety of clinical entities such as corneal exposure and dry eye syndromes. This type of keratitis can usually be distinguished from the toxic variety on the basis of the clinical course and the distribution of the corneal lesions.

There may be an immunologic cause for some forms of superficial epithelial keratitis, for example, the keratitis which occurs in the early stages of a viral keratoconjunctivitis such as epidemic keratoconjunctivitis (EKC). Recently we have demonstrated epithelial keratitis secondary to contact sensitivity in the guinea pig, using oxazolone, a chemical which is not ordinarily toxic to the cornea (31).

Trantas' Dots

Trantas' dots are white, chalky deposits found at the limbus, and are seen in patients with atopic and vernal conjunctivitis (see Fig. 7-6 in Ch. 7). They are composed of large numbers of eosinophils, and are transient, their presence usually correlating with the activity of the allergic disease.

Marginal Infiltrates

Marginal or catarrhal corneal infiltrates form near the limbus and are usually associated with bacterial infections, particularly those due to staphylococci. They begin beneath the epithelium but may ulcerate later in their course. A clear interval is present between the infiltrate and the adjacent limbal blood vessels. The lesions last 4–14 days and heal without treatment. They are most commonly seen at the 10, 2, 4, and 8 o'clock positions, possibly because of contact between the cornea and the staphylococcus-infected lids. They are usually considered to be the result of an antibody-mediated reaction to bacterial antigens or exotoxins, the most frequent being those of *Staphylococcus aureus.* The characteristic location and appearance of catarrhal infiltrates probably depends on the optimal concentration of antigen and antibody being present 1 or 2 mm inside the limbal blood vessels. The lucid interval may be due to removal of antigen or leukocytes by the blood vessels in this area. Marginal catarrhal lesions are occasionally associated with acute catarrhal conjunctivitis due to *Haemophilus aegyptius,* or with chronic conjunctivitis caused by *Moraxella lacunata,* β-hemolytic streptococci, or coliform organisms (105).

Wessely Rings

These ring-shaped infiltrates form in the corneal stroma and are concentric with the limbus. Wessely originally described the phenomenon following intracorneal injection of horse serum (118). Similar rings have been observed in experimentally produced Arthus reactions in the cornea (38), and in association with infectious corneal ulcers (66). Although these rings are generally referred to as immune rings, their pathogenesis is often obscure. Generally, corneal rings are considered to be due to an antigen–antibody interaction in the cornea, presumably resulting from outwardly diffusing antigen meeting and reacting with antibody diffusing inward from the limbus. This may be viewed as similar to the Ouchterlony double-diffusion test for antigen–antibody interaction with the cornea acting as a gel. The reactants meet to form a line of precipitation, and an inflammatory response forms along the line of precipitation. Corneal rings can be produced experimentally by the injection of endotoxin into the rabbit cornea (73,74). An infiltration of neutrophils and components of the alternate complement pathway are found when these rings are studied by histopathologic techniques (73). It may be that corneal rings associated with gram-negative and other corneal infections are due to endotoxin rather than to antigen-antibody complexes.

Stromal Infiltration

Stromal infiltration of the cornea results from an influx of inflammatory cells due to several pathogenetic mechanisms. Those which are immunologic in nature may be the result of either humoral or cell-mediated immune reactions. Whatever the etiology, neutrophils are the most prominent cellular component of most types of corneal inflammation. The cornea seems to have the ability to attract neutrophils even when the same reaction at another anatomic site has different cellular constituents (32).

Subepithelial Opacities

Subepithelial corneal opacities are common in viral infections, especially EKC. The etiology of these infiltrates is unknown but they are widely believed to represent sites of viral antigen deposition to which inflammatory cells have been attracted (65). Corticosteroids will cause these infiltrates to disappear but when steroids are withdrawn the infiltrates generally reappear. This may be due to the ability of steroids to eliminate inflammatory cells but not antigen–antibody complexes.

Phlyctenules

Phlyctenules are small nodular lesions which occur for the first time at the limbus but may subsequently occur on the conjunctiva or cornea. Toward the end of their 10- to 14-day course they typically ulcerate and leave a pathognomonic limbus-based triangular scar and sometimes a vascular pannus. They are most commonly associated with staphylococcal infections or tuberculosis, but have also been seen after infections with *Candida albicans, Coccidioides immitis,* the agent of lymphogranuloma venereum, and certain nematodes (106). They are thought to be due to a delayed hypersensitivity mechanism, and indeed it has been demonstrated that phlyctenules can be produced experimentally by topical challenge in animals made hypersensitive to tuberculin (117) and staphylococci (35).

Vascularization

Ingrowth of blood vessels into the corneal stroma is seen in a wide variety of conditions and the pathogenesis of this process has been the subject of intensive study. Two schools of thought arose to explain vasculogenesis in the cornea. One theory proposed that vascularization is always preceded by corneal edema and that the compactness of the normal corneal tissue prevents vascularization (19). A second hypothesis proposed that certain vasostimulating factors were produced by corneal tissue (16). Most recent investigators feel that the compactness of the corneal stroma is not a major factor in inhibiting corneal vascularization since many clinical situations in which corneal edema persists are not associated with vessel ingrowth. Recent interest has centered around the relationship between inflammation and corneal vascularization (55,64). It has been shown that in every model of corneal vascularization studied, except possibly one associated with neoplastic cells implanted in the cornea (40), a leukocytic infiltrate always precedes corneal vascularization (64). Recently, neutrophils and a heat-labile fraction isolated from them have been implicated as more specific factors responsible for inducing corneal vascularization (34). The infiltration of leukocytes and subsequent vascular ingrowth can be inhibited by treatment with corticosteroids (64) or by a protease inhibitor found in cartilage, aorta (42), and vitreous (13).

Keratic Precipitates

Collections of inflammatory cells are deposited on the endothelial surface of the cornea in a number of anterior-segment inflammatory conditions. The cells are presumably derived from iris vessels and are considered to be an indication of iris inflammation. Keratic precipitates often accompany deep corneal inflammation such as herpetic keratitis, in which case they are invariably located directly behind the area of corneal involvement. More severe types of corneal infiltration, such as bacterial corneal ulcers, elicit a much greater outpouring of inflammatory cells with diffuse keratic precipitates and frequently with the formation of a hypopyon. An early sign of graft rejection is the appearance of keratic precipitates at the margin of the graft closest to the limbal blood vessels. These cells are presumably cytotoxic lymphocytes which are derived from the limbal vessels (78).

HUMORAL IMMUNE RESPONSES

Except for IgM, all immunoglobulins and albumin can routinely be demonstrated in the cornea by direct immunofluorescence (4). Most of the immunoglobulin is concentrated in the stroma. Larger molecules, including IgM, may sometimes be found in the corneas of older individuals presumably due to an increased permeability of the limbal blood vessels with increasing age (116).

It is now well recognized that antigen–antibody reactions can take place in the cornea and lead to inflammation. The Wessely phenomenon, in which an antigen–antibody precipitate develops in the cornea, can be produced by challenging actively or passively sensitized animals with intracorneal injections of protein antigens (39,80). At one time it was believed that the cornea could not support a typical Arthus reaction, since this phenomenon requires damage to blood vessels by antigen–antibody complexes and inflammatory components (81). Furthermore, because of the avascularity of the cornea and its presumed exemption from Arthus-type reactions, it was believed that corneal clouding after antigenic challenge must be due to a delayed hypersensitivity mechanism (83). Indeed, the corneal response was often employed as a means of differentiating Arthus-type from delayed hypersensitivity responses. More recently, several investigators have shown that in fact the cornea can support antigen–antibody reactions and that damage can result to corneal collagen fibrils even in the absence of corneal vascularization (39,80). Thus, to use the cornea as a site for the differentiation of immediate and

delayed hypersensitivity reactions would seem to be invalid (39).

A number of investigators have looked at the corneal immune response following injection of protein antigens into the corneas of rabbits and guinea pigs (26,76,97,100,103). Following injection of a large dose of antigen, a biphasic reaction occurs in the rabbit cornea (26,76). During the early phase (3–5 days), transient corneal clouding occurs and lymphocytes and immature plasma cells accumulate at the limbus. This early phase is believed to be a manifestation of delayed hypersensitivity since 1) typical delayed-type skin reactions can be elicited during this phase, 2) the corneal reaction can be transferred with lymphoid cells but not with serum, and 3) circulating antibody is not detectable at this early time interval (76). At a later stage (7–14 days), a typical Wessely phenomenon occurs. This reaction is characterized by precipitation of immune complexes in the cornea, Arthus-type skin reactivity, circulating antibody, and infiltration of the cornea by large numbers of plasma cells. During this late phase, antibody-producing cells can be demonstrated in the homolateral preauricular and cervical lymph nodes, the cornea, and the uveal tract (97,100). No appreciable number of antibody-producing cells are found in the spleen or in the contralateral lymph nodes. Thus, a state of local hypersensitivity can be induced in the cornea which depends primarily on the immunologic activity of the local tissues.

The antibody response which follows intracorneal injection of protein antigens can be inhibited in a variety of ways, *e.g.*, by corticosteroids (99) and systemically administered mercaptopurine (Purinethol) (27,90), but locally administered antilymphocyte serum (101), fenoprofen (102), and local irradiation (85) do not interfere with antibody production.

CELLULAR IMMUNE RESPONSES

Delayed hypersensitivity reactions in the cornea have been investigated experimentally by a number of workers (17,32,54,76,84,98). Injection of a protein antigen into the cornea of a sensitized animal results in a delayed-onset

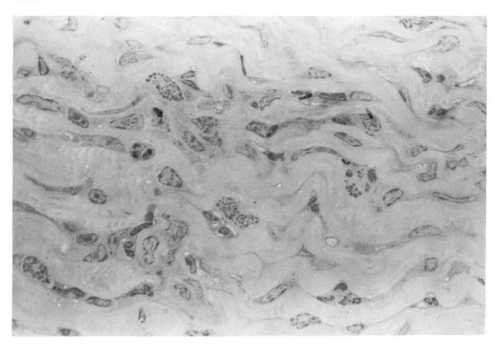

FIG. 3-1. Basophils infiltrating central cornea of guinea pig in cutaneous basophil hypersensitivity reaction induced with ovalbumin in incomplete Freund's adjuvant. (Giemsa, ×630)

clouding of the cornea with subsequent vascularization. The cellular reaction is centered around the limbus but gradually involves the central corneal stroma. As in other types of immunologic responses, the character of the cellular infiltrate depends on the method of sensitization, the nature of the antigen, the type of animal used, and whether or not complete Freund's adjuvant is used in sensitization (32). In guinea pigs immunized with protein antigens in incomplete Freund's adjuvant (without mycobacteria), the corneal reaction contains large numbers of mononuclear cells, numerous basophils in the central cornea (Fig. 3-1), and eosinophils at the limbus (32). If the same antigens are administered in complete Freund's adjuvant (with mycobacteria), the infiltrates are much more cellular and contain mainly neutrophils at 24 hours after challenge, and mononuclear cells at 48 hours. Such reactions bear a similarity to cutaneous basophil hypersensitivity in the skin (Fig. 3-2) and classic delayed hypersensitivity reactions elicited by intradermal injections (23). Fibrin deposi-

tion occurs in classic delayed hypersensitivity reactions both in the skin and in the eye. Large numbers of histiocytes, activated lymphoid elements, and inflammation of the conjunctival epithelium are also seen in the early phases of these reactions (54). A similar histologic picture can be induced in the guinea pig cornea by the injection of lymphokines produced by antigen-stimulated lymphocytes or by mixed cultures of allogeneic lymphocytes (17).

As noted previously, a single injection of a protein antigen into the cornea of a rabbit produces a biphasic reponse (26,76). The early phase of this response (3–5 days) is characterized by sudden diffuse corneal clouding and a dilation of limbal blood vessels. This response is usually considered to represent a delayed hypersensitivity reaction characterized histologically by the presence of lymphocytes and immature plasma cells (26). Antibodies are not detectable at this early stage; however, delayed skin reactions can be elicited and passively transferred to unimmunized guinea pigs (76), and production of migration inhibition factor

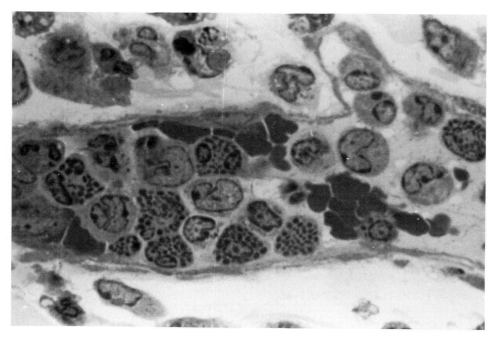

FIG. 3-2. Cutaneous basophil hypersensitivity reaction in guinea pig skin after sensitization with ovalbumin in incomplete Freund's adjuvant. (Giemsa, ×794)

(MIF) can be detected in draining lymph node cells (98). Delayed hypersensitivity reactions in the cornea, as in the skin, are best elicited at early phases after sensitization and are later supplanted by reactions mediated by humoral mechanisms, sometimes in combination with a delayed hypersensitivity component.

ANTERIOR CHAMBER

The anterior chamber provides a transparent site for examination of immunologic events in the eye, and it has long been considered an immunologically privileged site. This latter attribute, which allows tissue grafts to survive for prolonged periods of time, has often been attributed to the lack of lymphatic drainage from the anterior chamber (1). Although tissues grafted into the anterior chamber of the eye do have a prolonged survival, most investigators agree that such allografts are ultimately rejected (30, 72).

The reason for the prolongation of graft survival has been the subject of considerable in-

terest. Lack of graft recognition by the host's immune system is not the reason for delayed rejection, since an anterior chamber graft becomes rapidly vascularized by iris vessels (30) and can sensitize the host within 7 days of implantation (111). Thus, blockade of the afferent, or sensitizing, arc of the immune response does not explain this phenomenon. Kaplan and his associates (59-61) have concluded that the prolonged survival of grafts in the anterior chamber results from presentation of the antigen to the host's immune system by the vascular route and processing of the antigen by the spleen rather than by regional lymph nodes. They suggest that this initial encounter of antigen with the spleen results in the diversion of what would otherwise be a cell-mediated, tissue-destructive response. Instead, a protective response occurs, due possibly to the production of enhancing antibodies or the generation of suppressor T lymphocytes by the spleen. Whatever the mechanism, it seems to require the presence of an intact and functioning spleen and the continued presence of antigen within the eye over at least a 4-day interval following injection (62). Vessella and associates (111) have also proposed that the delay in rejection could be related either to the development of blocking factors in serum or to the recruitment of suppressor T cells.

UVEAL TRACT

NORMAL STRUCTURE AND FUNCTION

The uvea undoubtedly has certain special features which make it a frequent target of immunologic reactions. Like other tissues, the uveal tract contains fibroblasts, histiocytes, and mast cells. Considerable elastic tissue is found in Bruch's membrane of the choroid and in the choroidal stroma. Many similarities between ocular and joint tissues have been pointed out (52), both in chemical composition and in physical characteristics. These similarities might explain the participation of both of these tissues in certain types of uveitis syndromes. The homogeneous ground substance of the choroid contains large amounts of elas-

tic and collagen material, especially around blood vessels and in the intercapillary and subcapillary regions (51). Mast cells, plasma cells, lymphocytes, and phagocytes may be found in the interstitial tissue of the uveal tract. Many melanocytes and fibroblasts occupy the choroidal stroma in addition to the large number of blood vessels. Bruch's membrane, which separates the choriocapillaries from the retinal pigment epithelium, is unusually porous allowing nutrients to traverse it and waste products to be removed. Because of its composition, Druch's membrane is subject to all the diseases which affect elastic and collagenous tissues, and these alterations can in turn affect the uveal blood vessels (51). The outer choroid contains larger blood vessels, nerve plexuses, ganglion cells, arterioles, small arteries, venules, melanocytes, macrophages, and mast cells.

The choroid is very rich in mast cells (see Fig. 3-3) and in fact contains far more mast cells than any other tissues studied by Smelser and Silver (96). More mast cells are found in

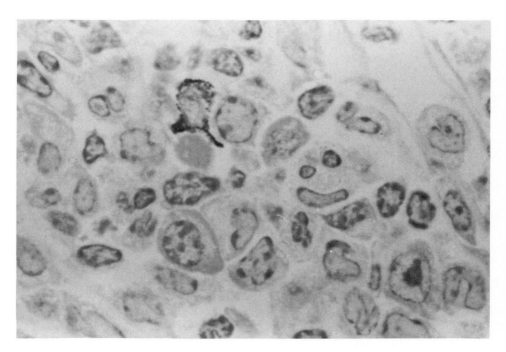

FIG. 3-3. Classic delayed hypersensitivity reaction in guinea pig uveal tract after sensitization with ovalbumin in complete Freund's adjuvant. Note mast cell (small dark granules) surrounded by immature lymphocytes, plasma cells, and eosinophils. (Giemsa, ×794)

the posterior uvea than near the ora serrata, yet the normal rabbit iris is devoid of mast cells. The relation between mast cells, uveal function, and the production of disease is unclear, but these cells are known to contain numerous vasoactive substances which could possibly be released during recurrent uveal inflammation. Two types of mast cells have been identified in the uveal tract (51). One is a spindle-shaped cell with large granules and the other is a more rounded cell containing less distinct granules.

The vitreous overlies the uveal tract and by virtue of its relative anatomic isolation from the blood can act as a depot from which antigen diffuses out very slowly. There appear to be two main routes of exit from the vitreous. One is forward toward the iris, ciliary body, and aqueous humor; the other potential site of antigen escape is around the retinal vessels, especially in the area of the optic nerve.

The iris stroma contains only minimal amounts of IgG and no IgM. The choroid, on the other hand, contains large amounts of IgG and all other immunoglobulins (4).

PATHOLOGIC RESPONSES

It is believed that the uveal tract can support each of the four classic types of immunologic reactions described by Gell and Coombs (36): 1) anaphylactoid reactions, 2) cytotoxic reactions, 3) immune-complex reactions, and 4) cell-mediated immunity (75,92). Since human uveitis is only rarely studied at the microscopic level, extensive work has been done using various animal models of immunologically induced uveitis. The clinical and histopathologic features in these models vary considerably, since the type of histopathologic response depends on a number of factors: 1) the chemical nature of the antigen, 2) its dosage, 3) the route of injection, 4) the use of adjuvants, 5) the species of animal, and 6) the site, time, and dosage of the challenge injection. In addition, methods of tissue preparation, including fixation and staining techniques, will influence the accuracy with which different cell types can be identified by light microscopy. Since many of these factors have been extremely variable, it is not surprising that the results of experimental studies make comparisons difficult.

A number of early studies were concerned with distinguishing granulomatous and nongranulomatous uveitis (122, 123). Granulomatous uveitis was felt to be caused by direct infection with a nonpyogenic infectious agent such as the tubercle bacillus. Nongranulomatous uveitis was assumed to be a sterile reaction resulting from an allergic, or less often a toxic or physical, insult. Microscopically, granulomatous reactions resemble the tuberculin reaction and were considered to be mainly a manifestation of delayed hypersensitivity (122). Nongranulomatous reactions consist of nonspecific inflammatory cell infiltration and were considered to be allergic, toxic, or physical in origin (123). The use of histologic terminology to distinguish clinically recognizable conditions has often been criticized and many ophthalmologists prefer to classify uveitis according to other criteria.

Several methods of immunization have been used in creating models of experimental uveitis. The most popular involve 1) the introduction of a small amount of a bland protein antigen into the vitreous of a rabbit or guinea pig eye, 2) systemic immunization with a protein antigen followed by intravitreal challenge with the same antigen, and 3) immunization of an animal with uveal tissue or its components.

HUMORAL IMMUNE RESPONSES

Anaphylactoid Reactions

Despite the impressive numbers of mast cells in the uveal tract, patients with anaphylactoid reactions in the uveal tract are thought to be encountered only rarely. One such patient was described who had recurrent iridocyclitis and macular edema in association with exacerbations of hay fever (82). Experimentally, ocular anaphylaxis has been studied only occasionally. By perfusion of the head of a hypersensitive dog with dilute solutions of antigen, the pupils can be made to contract in a striking manner (120). The rabbit uvea has been passively sensitized with antibodies to ovalbumin, and a few hours later Evans blue dye has been injected intravenously followed by an immediate intravitreal injection of a small amount of purified ovalbumin. An almost immediate hyperemia of the iris develops, followed by a markedly bluish tint because of the presence of the blue dye in the aqueous of the challenged eye (92). Passive reverse ocular anaphylaxis can be induced by injecting antibody into the vitreous and, some hours later, injecting a mixture of antigen and Evans blue dye intravenously. The same picture of hyperemia and a blue aqueous results.

Anaphylactoid reactions are characterized histologically by the presence of a large number of neutrophils in the anterior chamber and around the ciliary body; the posterior uvea does not seem to participate in the reaction (67). An interesting model of type I hypersensitivity has recently been developed by injecting *Ascaris suum* larvae into the vitreous of guinea pigs and demonstrating an IgE antibody response in the aqueous humor (21). A brisk IgE response also follows a secondary intravitreal injection of larvae into animals immunized systemically with *A. suum.*

Cytotoxic Reactions

Immunization of laboratory animals with uveal tissue and uveal or retinal antigens has been carried out for many years with the hope of developing an animal model for endogenous uveitis or sympathetic ophthalmia. Elschnig was the first to show complement-fixing antibodies to uveal tissue in experimental animals immunized with uveal tissue (28). He also demonstrated the presence of an organ-specific antigen (one found in the uvea of many species) in the uveal tract. Woods demonstrated positive intradermal skin tests in uveitis patients (121), and Hallett *et al* (50) showed complement-fixing antibodies, using bovine uveal antigen in a group of uveitis patients. Precipitating hemagglutinating antibodies directed against uveal antigens have been reported by others (69). Collins (20) produced a type of uveitis histologically similar to sympathetic ophthalmia by immunizing guinea pigs with homologous uveal tissue in complete Freund's adjuvant. Aronson (5, 6), using a similar model, produced a uveitis in which a large number of plasma cells infiltrated the uvea

and in which humoral antibodies and positive skin tests could be demonstrated. Two uveal antigens were demonstrated in these studies: one found in higher concentrations in pigmented tissues and the other found in higher concentrations in albino uvea. It was also demonstrated that almost any long-standing uveitis was characterized by the presence of antiuveal precipitating antibodies in the circulation (8). Furthermore, experimental uveitis can be passively transferred to unimmunized guinea pigs with cells from immunized donors (7).

Within the last several years, attempts have been made to identify the specific antigenic components of uvea or retina which induce immunologic inflammation. Wacker and his colleagues (58, 112, 113) localized and purified a soluble antigen which surrounded retinal photoreceptor cells and which produced a uveitis when administered to guinea pigs in small amounts. A recent study has shown that immunization of rabbits with rod outer segments induces complement-fixing antibodies which seem to have a protective rather than a pathogenic effect (108). Purified antigens have also been isolated from the uveal tract (15) and these may cross react with antigens in stromal collagen.

Despite the extensive work in this field of autoallergic disease of the eye, it remains unclear whether experimentally produced uveitis bears any meaningful relationship to human uveitis. Although there are clear indications that pigment-bearing cells are specifically attacked in both sympathetic ophthalmia and the related Vogt–Koyanagi–Harada syndrome (75), the mechanism underlying this form of attack has not been fully elucidated. It should be kept in mind that when uveal antibodies are demonstrated, they may be more the consequence of inflammation than the cause.

Immume-Complex Reactions

Arthus reactions are undoubtedly one of the most important factors in the production of uveal inflammation (75). Antigen–antibody complexes may play a role in the occlusive vasculitis of Behçet's disease (89), in the periarterial exudates seen in toxoplasma retinochoroiditis, and in a variety of rheumatic conditions which affect the eye.

Arthus reactions have been produced experimentally in the eyes of rabbits and guinea pigs (94, 114). These reactions can be induced by injection of a protein antigen into the vitreous followed by injection of homologous antibody intravenously, or in a reverse fashion by intravitreal injection of antibody followed by intravenous injection of antigen. The typical Arthus reaction is characterized by an acute fibrinous hemorrhagic uveitis which reaches its peak in less than 24 h and subsides rapidly. Microscopically, passive Arthus reactions are characterized by diffuse polymorphonuclear leukocytic infiltration of the uveal tract and cornea and and a smaller mononuclear cell component (94). In the active Arthus reaction, animals are actively sensitized with a systemic injection of protein antigen prior to intravitreal challenge. These reactions contain neutrophils and mononuclear cells but are less intense than the passive Arthus reactions (94). The active Arthus reaction is probably a more complex response than the passive Arthus reaction and may contain an element of delayed hypersensitivity. In the passive Arthus reaction, at 24 hours, there is severe chemosis, intense iridocyclitis, proteinaceous exudate, and cells and fibrin within the anterior chamber (92). Recently, prostaglandins have been found in the aqueous humor, the anterior uvea, and the choroid of rabbits primed for uveal Arthus reactions (79).

Antibody Formation in the Eye

All tissues capable of sustaining chronic inflammatory responses, including the eye, are capable of producing antibody (119). Thus, the eye can act as a lymph node does under certain circumstances and may form antibody in an efficient manner. If an antigen is injected into the vitreous, a spontaneous uveitis will develop in about 1 week which will slowly resolve over the following week to 10 days (125). If the animal is challenged with the same antigen 6 months to a year later, the eye will again become inflamed even if the antigenic challenge is given intravenously (91). The primary response to the initial injection of antigen de-

pends on immunologically component cells which originate outside the eye but are drawn to the eye where a depot of antigen persists. In contrast, the cells responsible for the secondary uveitis produced by subsequent antigenic challenge are already present in the eye, having been seeded there by previous inflammation of the uveal tract (91). (Large numbers of immunologically uncommitted cells are also recruited from outside the eye and participate in the secondary inflammation.) This seeding of the eye with antigen-specific cells may be an important factor in the pathogenesis of certain types of recurrent uveitis in humans. Although the eye may act in a manner similar to a regional lymph node, upon rechallenge the formation of IgG is higher and the formation of IgM lower than in other organized lymphoid tissues (87).

Progressive Immunization

As noted in the previous paragraph, a single injection of protein antigen into the vitreous of the rabbit produces a clinically apparent uveitis after a latent period of 6–8 days (125). The intraocular reaction is primarily mononuclear and usually nongranulomatous. Severe inflammation can produce a retinal detachment, degeneration of photoreceptors, preretinal membrane formation, fixed retinal folds, vitreous degeneration, and gliosis of the retina and optic disc. The spontaneous inflammatory reaction has been compared to the progressive immunization reaction of Gell and Hinde (37), an evolving immunologic reaction produced after repeated injections of antigen into the skin. It appears to represent an early delayed hypersensitivity response followed by a superimposed antibody response. The initial ocular inflammation, which occurs prior to the detection of circulating antibody, may be the result of a delayed hypersensitivity mechanism (93). In similar studies, mast cells have been shown to disappear during the acute phase of inflammation and to reappear as the rection subsides (68). They may also accumulate in the iris, a tissue which normally lacks significant numbers of mast cells (95).

Hall has shown that cells from the uveal tract and draining lymph node produce antibody to intravitreally injected antigen and that circulating antibody appears 7 days after such an injection (44, 46). She feels that antibody found in the aqueous and vitreous during later phases of the antibody response is produced by cells of the uveal tract rather than by cells in draining lymph nodes (46). The uveal antibody response can be suppressed by cyclophosphamide (45) and can be either enhanced or suppressed by concanavalin A (49), depending on the time and route of injection of this mitogen.

An interesting sidelight of these experiments is the demonstration of nonspecific enhancement of the secondary response (47, 48, 88). If rabbits are injected intravitreally with one antigen and challenged several months later in the opposite eye with an intravitreal injection of an unrelated antigen, the second eye responds by producing high levels of antibody to the antigen injected into the first eye. It has been suggested that a lymphokine produced during the immune response to the second antigen stimulates cells in the uveal tract to produce antibody to the first antigen.

CELLULAR IMMUNE RESPONSES

Delayed hypersensitivity responses are thought to play an important role in many types of uveitis, including sympathetic ophthalmia, Vogt–Koyanagi–Harada syndrome, and sarcoid uveitis (75). Additionally, compromised cellular immunity may be of significance in the pathogenesis of certain infectious types of uveitis, including those associated with toxoplasmosis, tuberculosis, leprosy, and herpes simplex infection. Cell-mediated hypersensitivity has been demonstrated to uveal and to retinal antigens using in vitro techniques in patients with various forms of uveitis (77), and this may indicate that these antigens play a role in inciting certain types of uveal inflammation.

Experimentally, delayed hypersensitivity reactions have been studied extensively in the uveal tract by injecting animals with protein antigens (33, 94), lymphokines (17), or mycobacterial adjuvants (115). Delayed hypersensitivity reactions begin approximately 4 hours after intraocular challenge and reach a peak between 24 and 48 hours. The iris becomes markedly hyperemic and the anterior chamber contains a proteinaceous exudate, cells, and fibrin (94). Microscopically, the uvea becomes massively infiltrated by mononuclear cells (Fig. 3-3) and a smaller number of neutrophils, and there may be involvement of the cornea, sclera, and retina. Recently, we have shown (33) that eosinophils are a prominent component of delayed hypersensitivity reactions in the uveal tract, accounting for approximately 50% of the total inflammatory cells when mycobacterial adjuvants are not used, and up to 30% when such adjuvants are employed (Fig. 3-4). These reactions differ markedly from delayed-onset reactions elicited simultaneously in the skin, which are composed mainly of basophils and mononuclear cells. The character of the inflammatory response depends greatly on the procedure used in sensitization and especially on whether or not mycobacterial adjuvants are used. The reason for the abundance of eosinophils in delayed hypersensitivity reactions of the uveal tract is not known, but these cells are thought to play a role in controlling allergic reactions by inactivating products of basophil and mast cell secretion (41).

An interesting form of ocular lesion is produced by immunization of rats with mycobacterial adjuvants (115). These animals develop an iridocyclitis, conjunctivitis, episcleritis, and keratitis. Ocular tissues become infiltrated with mononuclear cells and neutrophils, representing what may be a unique type of delayed hypersensitivity in which direct ocular challenge is not necessary. Another interesting model of uveitis mediated by T lymphocytes is induced in the mouse by the intraocular injection of lymphocytic choriomeningitis (LCM) virus (107). This type of uveitis is mediated not directly by virus but rather by T lymphocytes directed against viral-infected uveal tissue.

LENS

The crystalline lens is a unique tissue immunologically because of its anatomic isolation from the rest of the body at an early stage of embryonic development. Lens antigens are out

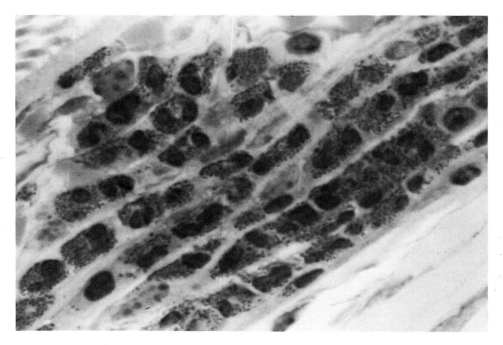

FIG. 3-4. Delayed hypersensitivity reaction in guinea pig uveal tract after sensitization with ovalbumin in incomplete Freund's adjuvant. Note large number of eosinophils infiltrating the choroid. (Giemsa, ×794)

of contact with the immune system during the development of "self" recognition. Exposure to lens antigens at a later stage could therefore result in an immunologic response to a tissue which is considered foreign. Thus, the clinical condition known as endophthalmitis phaco-anaphylactica may be the result of autosensitization to one's own lens antigens (110). A more detailed discussion of the immunologic properties of the lens takes place in Chapter 7.

REFERENCES

1. Adler FH: Physiology of the Eye, 4th ed. St Louis, Mosby, 1965, p 96
2. Allansmith MR, Hutchison D: Immunoglobulins in the conjunctiva. Immunology 12:225, 1967
3. Allansmith MR, Korb DR, Greiner JV et al: Giant papillary conjunctivitis in contract lens wearers. Am J Ophthalmol 83:697, 1977
4. Allansmith MR, Whitney CR, McClellan BH, Newman LP: Immunoglobulins in the human eye. Location, type, and amount. Arch Ophthalmol 89:36, 1973
5. Aronson SB: Hypersensitivity reactions in the uveal tract caused by uveal antigen-antibody reactions. In Maumenee AE, Silverstein AM: Immunopathology of Uveitis. Baltimore, Williams & Wilkins, 1964, pp 182–191
6. Aronson SB: The homoimmune uveitises in the guinea pig. Ann NY Acad Sci 124:365, 1965
7. Aronson SB, McMaster PRB: Passive transfer of experimental allergic uveitis. Arch Ophthalmol 86:557, 1971
8. Aronson SB, Yamamoto E, Goodner EK, O'Connor GR: The occurrence of an autoantiuveal antibody in human uveitis. Arch Ophthalmol 72:621, 1964
9. Axelrod AJ, Chandler JW: Morphologic characteristics of conjunctival-associated lymphoid tissue in the rabbit. Invest Ophthalmol Vis Sci [Suppl] 17:182, 1978
10. Belfort R Jr, Mendes NF: T and B lymphocytes in the human conjunctiva and lacrimal gland. Invest Ophthalmol Vis Sci [Suppl] 17:182, 1978
11. Bluestone R, Easty DL, Goldberg LS et al: Lacrimal immunoglobulins and complement quantified by counter-immunoelectrophoresis. Br J Ophthalmol 59:279, 1975
12. Brauninger GE, Centifanto YM: Immunoglobulin E in human tears. Am J Ophthalmol 72:558, 1971

13. Brem S, Preis I, Langer R et al: Inhibition of neovascularization by an extract derived from vitreous. Am J Ophthalmol 84:323, 1977

14. Broekhuyse RM: Tear lactoferrin: a bacteriostatic and complexing protein. Invest Ophthalmol 13:550, 1974

15. Broekhuyse RM, van der Eerden JJJM: Ocular antigens VI: immunogenic determinants in ocular and non-ocular tissues related to uveal pigment granules. An immunofluorescent and immunodiffusion study. Exp Eye Res 19:353, 1974

16. Campbell FW, Michaelson IC: Blood-vessel formation in the cornea. Br J Ophthalmol 33:248, 1949

17. Chandler JW, Heise ER, Weisner RS: Induction of delayed-type sensitivity-like reactions in the eye by the injection of lymphokines. Invest Ophthalmol 12:400, 1973

18. Chandler JW, Leder R, Kaufman HE, Caldwell JR: Quantitative determinations of complement components in tears and aqueous humor. Invest Ophthalmol 13:151, 1974

19. Cogan DG: Vascularization of the cornea. Its experimental induction by small lesions and a new theory of its pathogenesis. Arch Ophthalmol 41:406, 1949

20. Collins RC: Experimental studies on sympathetic ophthalmia 32:1687, 1949

21. Donnelly JJ, Rockey JH, Soulsby EJL: Intraocular IgE antibody induced in guinea pigs with *Ascaris suum* larvae. Invest Ophthalmol Vis Sci 16:976, 1977

22. Drutz DJ, Mills J: Immunity and infection. In Fudenberg HH, Stites DP, Caldwell JL, Wells JV (eds): Basic and Clinical Immunology. Los Altos, Lange, 1978

23. Dvorak HF, Dvorak AM, Simpson BA et al: Cutaneous basophil hypersensitivity. II. A light and electron microscopic description. J Exp Med 132:558, 1970

24. Dwyer R StC, Darougar S, Jones BR: Immediate hypersensitivity in the guinea pig conjunctiva. II. Effect of treatment with antihistamines, steroids and disodium cromoglycate. Mod Probl Ophthalmol 16:186, 1976

25. Dwyer R StC, Turk JL, Darougar S: Immediate hypersensitivity in the guinea pig conjunctiva. I. Characterisation of the IgE and IgG antibodies involved. Int Arch Allergy Appl Immunol 46:910, 1974

26. Elliott JH, Flax MH, Leibowitz HMI: The limbal cellular infiltrate in experimental corneal hypersensitivity. I. Morphologic studies after primary sensitization. Arch Ophthalmol 76:104, 1966

27. Ellis PP, Sellyei LF Jr, Kurland LR: Modification of corneal immune response. II. Effects of 6–mercaptopurine. Am J Ophthalmol 61:709, 1966

28. Elschnig A: Studien zur sympathischen Ophthalmie. II. Die antigene Wirkung des Augenpigmentes. Graefes Arch Ophthalmol 76:509, 1910

29. Franklin RM, Kenyon KR, Tomasi TB Jr: Immunohistologic studies of human lacrimal gland: localization of immunoglobulins, secretory component and lactoferrin. J Immunol 110:984, 1973

30. Franklin RM, Prendergast RA: Primary rejection of skin allografts in the anterior chamber of the rabbit eye. J Immunol 104:463, 1970

30a. Friedlaender MH: Ocular allergy and immunology. J. Allergy Clin Immunol 63:51, 1979

30b. Friedlaender MH, Allansmith MR: Ocular allergy. Ann Ophthalmol 7:1171, 1975

31. Friedlaender MH, Cyr R: Contact sensitivity in the guinea pig eye. Invest Ophthalmol Vis Sci 18 (Suppl): 95, 1979

32. Friedlaender MH, Dvorak HF: Morphology of delayed type hypersensitivity reactions in the guinea pig cornea. J Immunol 118:1558, 1977

33. Friedlaender MH, Howes EL Jr, Hall JM et al: Histopathology of delayed hypersensitivity reactions in the guinea pig uveal tract. Invest Ophthalmol Vis Sci 17:327, 1978

34. Fromer CH, Klintworth GK: An evaluation of the role of leukocytes in the pathogenesis of experimentally induced corneal vascularization. III. Studies related to the vasoproliferative capability of polymorphonuclear leukocytes and lymphocytes. Am J Pathol 82:157, 1976

35. Funaishi S: Experimentelle untersuchungen über die Aetiologie der phlyctanularäten Augenentzundungen. Klin Monatsbl Augenheilkd 71: 141, 1923

36. Gell PGH, Coombs RRA: Clinical Aspects of Immunology. Oxford, Blackwell, 1968, pp 583–594

37. Gell PGH, Hinde IT: Observations on the histology of the Arthus reaction and its relation to other known types of skin hypersensitivity. Int Arch Allergy 5:23, 1954

38. Germuth FG, Maumenee AE, Pratt-Johnson J et al: Observations on the site and mechanism of antigen-antibody interaction in anaphylactic hypersensitivity. Am J Ophthalmol 46:282, 1958

39. Germuth FG Jr, Maumenee AE, Senterfit LB, Pollack AD: Immunohistologic studies on antigen-antibody reactions in the avascular cornea. I. Reactions in rabbits actively sensitized to foreign protein. J Exp Med 115:919, 1962

40. Gimbrone MA Jr, Cotran RS, Leapman SB et al: Tumor growth and neovascularization in an experimental model using the rabbit cornea. J Natl Cancer Inst 52:413, 1974

41. Goetzl EJ, Wasserman SI, Austen KF: Eosinophil polymorphonuclear leukocyte function in immediate hypersensitivity. Arch Pathol 99:1, 1975

42. Goren SB, Eisenstein R, Choromokos E: The

inhibition of corneal vascularization in rabbits. Am J Ophthalmol 84:305, 1977

43. Greiner JV, Covington HI, Allansmith MR: Surface morphology of the human upper tarsal conjunctiva. Am J Ophthalmol 83:892, 1977

44. Hall JM: Specificity of antibody formation after intravitreal immunization with bovine gamma globulin and ovalbumin. I. Primary response. Invest Ophthalmol 10:775, 1971

45. Hall JM, Ohno S, Pribnow JF: The effect of cyclophosphamide on an ocular immune response. I. Primary response. Clin Exp Immunol 30:309, 1977

46. Hall JM, Pribnow JF: Responses of the reticuloendothelial system of the rabbit to intraocular injections of foreign protein. Cell Immunol 5:419, 1972

47. Hall JM, Pribnow JF: Specificity of antibody formation after intra-vitreal immunization with bovine gamma globulin and ovalbumin. Cell Immunol 11:64, 1974

48. Hall JM, Pribnow JF: Nonspecific stimulation of a secondary ocular antibody response. Invest Ophthalmol 15:863, 1976

49. Hall JM, Pribnow JF: Effect of concanavalin A on ocular immune responses. J Reticuloendothel Soc 21:163, 1977

50. Hallett JW, Wolkowicz MI, Leopold IH et al: Autoimmune complement fixation test in endogenous uveitis. Arch Ophthalmol 68: 168, 1962

51. Hogan MJ: Ultrastructure of the choroid. Its role in the pathogenesis of chorioretinal diseases. Trans Pac Coast Otoophthalmol Soc 42:61, 1961

52. Hogan MJ: Similarities of ocular, joint and other tissues: anatomic and histochemical observations. In Maumenee AE, Silverstein AM (eds): Immunopathology of Uveitis. Baltimore, Williams & Wilkins, 1964, pp 39–59

53. Horwitz BL, Christensen GR, Ritzmann SR: Diurnal profiles of tear lysozyme and gamma A globulin. Ann Ophthalmol 10:75, 1978

54. Howes EL Jr: Cellular hypersensitivity in the cornea. An analysis of the limbus and limbal cellular infiltration by light and electron microscopy. Arch Ophthalmol 83:475, 1970

55. Inomata H, Smelser GK, Polack FM: Corneal vascularization in experimental uveitis and graft rejection. An electron microscopic study. Invest Ophthalmol 10:840, 1971

56. Iwamoto T, Smelser GK: Electron microscope studies on the mast cells and blood and lymphatic capillaries of the human corneal limbus. Invest Ophthalmol 4:815, 1965

57. Josephson AS, Weiner RS: Studies of the proteins of lacrimal secretions. J Immunol 100:1080, 1968

58. Kalsow CM, Wacker WB: Localization of a uveitogenic soluble retinal antigen in the normal guinea pig eye by an indirect fluorescent antibody technique. Int Arch Allergy 44:11, 1973

59. Kaplan HJ, Streilein JW: Do immunologically privileged sites require a functioning spleen? Nature 251:553, 1974

60. Kaplan HJ, Streilein JW; Analysis of immunologic privilege within the anterior chamber of the eye. Transplant Proc 9:1193, 1977

61. Kaplan HJ, Streilein JW: Immune response to immunization via the anterior chamber of the eye. I. F_1 lymphocyte-induced immune deviation. J Immunol 118:809, 1977

62. Kaplan HJ, Streilein JW: Immune response to immunization via the anterior chamber of the eye. II. An analysis of F_1 lymphocyte-induced immune deviation. J Immunol 120:689, 1978

63. Kimura SJ, Thygeson P: The cytology of external ocular disease. Am J Ophthalmol 39:137, 1955

64. Klintworth GK: The contribution of morphology to our understanding of the pathogenesis of experimentally produced corneal vascularization. Invest Ophthalmol Vis Sci 16:281, 1977

65. Knopf HLS, Hierholzer JC; Clinical and immunological responses in patients with viral keratoconjunctivitis. Am J Ophthalmol 80:661, 1975

66. Laibson PR: Cornea and sclera. Arch Ophthalmol 88:554, 1972

67. Lanzieri M: Passive uveal anaphylaxis in guinea pigs. J Immunol 95:651, 1965

68. Larsen G: Experimental uveitis. A histopathologic study with special reference to the mast cell. Acta Ophthalmol (Kbh) 39:1, 1961

69. Luntz MH: Immune reaction to autologous lens proteins induced in guinea pigs. JAMA 186:33, 1963

70. McClellan BH, Whitney CR, Newman LP, Allansmith MR: Immunoglobulins in tears. Am J Ophthalmol 76:89, 1973

71. McMaster PRB, Aronson SB, Bedford MJ: Mechanisms of the host response in the eye. IV. The anterior eye in germ-free animals. Arch Ophthalmol 77:392, 1967

72. Medawar PB: Immunity to homologous graft skin. III. The fate of skin homografts transplanted to the brain, to subcutaneous tissue, and to the anterior chamber of the eye. Br J Exp Pathol 29:58, 1948

73. Mondino BJ, Rabin BS, Kessler E et al: Corneal rings with Gram-negative bacteria. Arch Ophthalmol 95:2222, 1977

74. Morawiecki J: Prazipitationserscheinungen in der lebenden Hornhaut bei Antigen-Antikorperreaktionen. Ophthalmologica 132:236, 1956

75. O'Connor GR: Uveitis of immunologic origin: clinical syndromes. Trans Pac Coast Otoophthalmol Soc 57:213, 1976

76. Parks JJ, Leibowitz HMI, Maumenee AE: A transient stage of suspected delayed sensitiv-

ity during the early induction of immediate corneal sensitivity. J Exp Med 115:867, 1962

77. Perkins ES: Recent advances in the study of uveitis. Br J Ophthalmol 58:462, 1974

78. Polack FM, Kanai A: Electron microscopic studies of graft endothelium in corneal graft rejection. Am J Ophthalmol 73:711, 1972

79. Rahi AHS, Bhattacherjee P, Misra R: Release of prostaglandins in experimental immune-complex endophthalmitis and phacoallergic uveitis. Br J Ophthalmol 62:105, 1978

80. Rahi AHS, Tripathi RC: Anatomy of passive Arthus reaction in the cornea. A preliminary communication. Mod Probl Ophthalmol 16:155, 1976

81. Rich AR, Follis RH: Studies on the site of sensitivity in the Arthus phenomenon. Johns Hopkins Med J 66:106, 1940

82. Ruedemann AD: Ocular manifestations of allergy. In Thomas JW (ed): Allergy in Clinical Practice. Philadelphia, Lippincott, 1961, pp 256–274

83. Salvin SB, Gregg MB: The specificity of allergic reactions. IV. The cornea. Proc Soc Exp Biol Med 107:478, 1961

84. Schlossman S, Stetson CA: Vascularization of the cornea during delayed hypersensitivity reactions. J Immunol 79:208, 1957

85. Sellyei LF Jr, Ellis PP: Modification of corneal immune response. I. Effects of irradiation. Am J Ophthalmol 61:702, 1966

86. Sen DK, Sarin GS, Mani K, Saha K: Immunoglobulin in tears of normal Indian people. Br J Ophthalmol 60:302, 1976

87. Shimada K. Silverstein AM: Local antibody formation within the eye: a study of immunoglobulin class and antibody specificity. Invest Ophthalmol 14:573, 1975

88. Shimada K, Silverstein AM: Induction of booster antibody formation without specific antigenic drive. Cell Immunol 18:484, 1975

89. Shimada K, Yaoita H, Shikano D: Chemotactic activity in the aqueous humor of patients with Behçet's disease. Jpn J Ophthalmol 16:94, 1972

90. Shulka BR, Gupta NC, Ahuja OP: Corneal immune response. Indian J Ophthalmol 20:84, 1972

91. Silverstein AM: Ectopic antibody formation in the eye: pathologic implications. In Maumenee AE, Silverstein AM (eds): Immunopathology of Uveitis. Baltimore, Williams & Wilkins, 1964, pp 83–97

92. Silverstein AM: Uveal hypersensitivity reactions to protein antigens. In Maumenee AE, Silverstein AM, (eds): Immunopathology of Uveitis. Baltimore, Williams & Wilkins, 1964, pp 209–217

93. Silverstein AM, Welter S, Zimmerman LE: A progressive immunization reaction in the actively sensitized rabbit eye. J Immunol 86:312, 1961

94. Silverstein AM, Zimmerman LE: Immuno-

genic endophthalmitis produced in the guinea pig by different pathogenetic mechanisms. Am J Ophthalmol 48:435, 1959

95. Smelser GK: The mast cell in experimental uveitis. In Maumenee AE, Silverstein AM (eds): Immunopathology of Uveitis. Baltimore, Williams & Wilkins, 1964, pp 252–255

96. Smelser GK, Silver S: The distribution of mast cells in the normal eye: a method of study. Exp Eye Res 2:134, 1963

97. Smolin G, Hall J: Afferent arc of the corneal immunologic reaction. II. Local and systemic response to bovine γ-globulin. Arch Ophthalmol 90:231, 1973

98. Smolin G, Hall J, Cignetti F: The afferent arc of the corneal immunologic reaction: migration inhibitory factor. Invest Ophthalmol 12:152, 1973

99. Smolin G, Hall JM, Okumoto M, Ohno S: High doses of subconjunctival corticosteroid and antibody-forming cells in the eye and draining lymph nodes. Arch Ophthalmol 95: 1631, 1977

100. Smolin G, Hall J, Stein M: The afferent arc of the corneal immunologic reaction. I. Local response to bovine gamma globulin. Can J Ophthalmol 7:336, 1972

101. Smolin G, Okumoto M, Meyer RF, Hall JM: Effect of local antilymphocyte serum on antibody forming cells. Can J Ophthalmol 12:54, 1977

102. Smolin G, Okumoto M, Ohno S, Hall JM: Failure of fenoprofen to affect the corneal immunologic reaction. Ann Ophthalmol 10:351, 1978

103. Thompson R, Gallardo E, Khorazo D: Precipitins in the ocular tissues of rabbits generally and locally immunized with crystalline egg albumin. Am J Ophthalmol 19:852, 1936

104. Thygeson P: The cytology of conjunctival exudates. Am J Ophthalmol 29:1499, 1946

105. Thygeson P: Marginal corneal infiltrates and ulcer. Arch Ophthalmol 39:432, 1948

106. Thygeson P: Observations on nontuberculous phlyctenular keratoconjunctivitis. Trans Am Acad Ophthalmol Otolargyngol 58:128, 1954

107. Ticho U, Silverstein AM, Cole GA: Immunopathogenesis of LCM virus-induced uveitis: the role of T lymphocytes. Invest Ophthalmol 13:229, 1974

108. Tilgner S, Stelzner A, Dietze U et al: Experimentelle allergische chorioretinitis. Graefes Arch Ophthalmol 204:113, 1977

109. Vaughan D, Asbury T: General Ophthalmology. Los Altos, Lange, 1978

110. Verhoeff FH, Lemoine AN: Endophthalmitis phacoanaphylactica. Trans Int Congr Ophthalmol 1:234, 1922

111. Vessella RL, Raju S, Cockrell JV, Grogan, JB: Host response to allogeneic implants in the anterior chamber of the rat eye. Invest Ophthalmol Vis Sci 17:140, 1978

112. Wacker WB, Donoso LA, Kalsow CM et al:

Experimental allergic uveitis. Isolation, characterization and localization of a soluble uveitopathogenic antigen from bovine retina. J Immunol 119:1949, 1977

113. Wacker WB, Lipton MM: The role of two retina antigens in production of experimental allergic uveitis and its suppression by mycobacteria. Int Arch Allergy 41:370, 1971

114. Waksman BH, Bullington SJ: A quantitative study of the passive Arthus reaction in the rabbit eye. J Immunol 76:441, 1956

115. Waksman BH, Bullington SJ: Studies of arthritis and other lesions induced in rats by injection of mycobacterial adjuvant. III. Lesions of the eye. Arch Ophthalmol 64:751, 1960

116. Walton KW: Studies on the pathogenesis of corneal arcus formation. I. The human corneal arcus and its relation to atherosclerosis as studied by immunofluorescence. J Pathol 111:263, 1973

117. Weekers L: L'exanthème de la conjonctivite phylecténulaire envisagé comme une toxituberculide. Arch Ophthalmol 29:294, 1909

118. Wessely K: Ueber anaphylaktische Erscheinungen an der Hornhaut. München Med Wochenschr 58:1713, 1911

119. Witmer R: Antibody formation in the rabbit eye studied with fluorescein-labeled antibody. Arch Ophthalmol 53:811, 1955

120. Woods AC: Ocular anaphylaxis. I. The reaction to perfusion with specific antigen. Arch Ophthalmol 45:557, 1916

121. Woods AC: Sympathetic ophthalmia: use of uveal pigment in diagnosis and treatment. Trans Ophthalmol Soc UK 45:208, 1925

122. Woods AC: Endogenous Uveitis, 2nd ed. Baltimore, Williams & Wilkins, 1956

123. Woods AC, Friedenwald JS, Wood RM: The histopathology of the acute and chronic ocular hypersensitive reactions in the experimental rabbit. Am J Ophthalmol 40:631, 1955

124. Zimianski MC, Dawson CR, Togni B: Epithelial cell phagocytosis of *Listeria monocytogenes* in the conjunctiva. Invest Ophthalmol 13:623, 1974

125. Zimmerman LE, Silverstein AM: Experimental ocular hypersensitivity. Histopathologic changes observed in rabbits receiving a single injection of antigen into the vitreous. Am J Ophthalmol 48:447, 1959

FOUR
FOUR
FOUR

diseases affecting the eye and the skin

The skin of the eyelids is susceptible to the same types of hypersensitivity disorders and infections which involve the skin of other parts of the body. Because of anatomic factors, the lids are especially prone to show evidence of inflammation. The eyelid skin is thinner than any other skin of the body and is frequently subjected to trauma, allergens, and toxic substances. The loose subcutaneous tissues allow accumulation of fluid, which becomes walled off from the surrounding structures by the orbital septum, creating prominent periorbital edema.

Many of the significant advances in the field of immunology have been made through the study of cutaneous responses. The first observation of the phenomenon we now know as cutaneous delayed hypersensitivity was made by Jenner in 1798 (56). Subcutaneous tests to detect tuberculin sensitivity were performed during the 1880s by Robert Koch. Blackley, during the 1860s, demonstrated immediate urticarial skin reactions to inhalant allergens. In 1912, dinitrochlorobenzene (DNCB) sensitivity was first reported in industrial workers (11). This chemical and related haptens have been studied extensively in order to define the mechanisms of sensitization and tolerance. In 1921, Prausnitz and Kustner demonstrated the passive transfer of skin sensitivity in humans (85). The skin-sensitizing antibody responsible for this phenomenon is now known to be IgE (52, 57).

During the early 1940s Landsteiner and Chase demonstrated that contact allergy and tuberculin skin reactivity could be transferred passively by means of blood lymphocytes from sensitized donors (19, 67). This established the dependency of delayed hypersensitivity reactions on lymphocytes rather than on serum factors. In 1956, Lawrence achieved the same results with an extract of sensitized lymphocytes known as transfer factor (68).

The clinical use of corticosteroids and other immunosuppressive agents has been associated with an increase in cutaneous infections. In patients receiving immunosuppressives, the incidence of herpes zoster, herpes simplex, and candida infections has greatly increased (65). The incidence of cutaneous malignancies has also increased during the era of immunosuppression (45, 65).

The skin has served as an important site for the study of immunologic mechanisms in health and disease states. Unlike the case with most other organs, rections are easily observable on the skin and can often be biopsied. Exciting developments have taken place in cutaneous immunology during the past 40 years. Antibodies to skin components have now been demonstrated in pemphigus vulgaris, pemphigoid, and dermatitis herpetiformis. A number of other disease states with a possible immunologic mechanism are currently under investigation also, including erythema multiforme, psoriasis, and chronic urticaria. Undoubtedly, the study of cutaneous disease and the use of the skin for experimental studies will continue to advance the science of immunology in future years.

ATOPIC DERMATITIS

Atopic dermatitis is one of the eczematous skin eruptions. It often occurs in childhood, but may be seen in adolescents and adults as well. The incidence in children under 5 years of age is estimated at 3%. Frequently, patients with atopic dermatitis have a history of respiratory allergy or allergic reactions to certain foods. Although immunologic abnormalities have been noted in atopic dermatitis, this condition also seems to represent an abnormal reactivity of the skin to various stimuli. This abnormal skin reactivity may be genetically determined and it is considered by some to represent a metabolic or biochemical defect. Although patients with atopic dermatitis undergo extensive allergic testing, frequently it is impossible to find a relationship between this condition and a known allergen.

Immunopathology

There has been much interest in the abnormal and paradoxic skin responses observed in atopic dermatitis patients (122). A response known as **white dermographism** occurs in response to stroking the skin with a blunt instrument. Normally one would expect to see erythema and wheal formation, but in patients with atopic dermatitis, the erythema is often replaced by a white line surrounded by an area of blanching. This response is not specific for atopic dermatitis and may be observed in other skin conditions. The **delayed blanch phenomenon** occurs after the injection of acetylcholine or methacholine into the skin of atopic dermatitis patients. In normal individuals, vasodilation and erythema are observed. In atopic dermatitis patients, however, a white, spreading reaction appears 5–30 min after the injection and persists for up to 60 min. The blanching of atopy was originally thought to be due to paradoxic vasoconstriction (72). However, it is now believed that vasodilation does occur but that erythema is obscured by an outpouring of edema fluid into the skin

(25). It is this exudation of serum from capillaries which is the unique feature in atopic persons. Patients with atopic dermatitis also have decreased levels of circulating plasma norepinephrine, but higher concentrations than normal in affected areas of skin (102). Some believe that atopic patients have a tendency to bind large concentrations of norepinephrine to the skin. These patients also have cold hands and demonstrate pallor of the ears, nose, and perioral regions.

Serum IgE concentrations are generally elevated in patients with atopic dermatitis (106). Upon remission of the clinical manifestations of the disease, IgE concentrations may decline markedly (58). Higher IgG and lower serum complement levels have been noted in some cases, but these may be the result of the chronic skin infections which are often present in atopic dermatitis patients. In most cases, serum levels of IgA, IgM, and IgD are normal. Despite the elevation of serum IgE, most atopic patients have normal numbers of peripheral blood lymphocytes bearing IgE and other immunoglobulins. An increase in the number of lymphocytes with complement receptors may be found.

Recently, evidence has been presented which indicates that a deficiency of cellular immunity exists in patients with atopic dermatitis. Cutaneous delayed hypersensitivity responses to ubiquitous antigens, including candida and streptokinase–streptodornase (SKSD), may be poor (75). This form of delayed cutaneous anergy is most marked in children with severe dermatitis. Such patients may also fail to become sensitized to topical application of dinitrochlorobenzene (DNCB). Furthermore, the mean percentages of T cells in the peripheral blood of eczema patients may be lower than in normal controls, and the T lymphocyte response to low concentrations of the mitogen phytohemagglutinin may be significantly depressed (91). Other abnormalities in atopic patients include an increase in the peripheral eosinophil count and in the absolute number of B lymphocytes (91). Perhaps because of a defect in cellular immunity, atopic patients have an increased susceptibility to viral and fungal infections (73, 117).

A further association with deficiencies in

cellular immunity is suggested by certain well-studied immunodeficiency syndromes. Patients with the Wiskott–Aldrich syndrome, ataxia–telangiectasia, and sex-linked hypogammaglobulinemia all have a form of eczema which is indistinguishable from atopic dermatitis.

Since T lymphocytes are important regulators of IgE synthesis and other types of antibody production, it has been postulated that a disorder of T regulator cells is responsible for the failure to terminate IgE antibody responses to certain antigens in atopic dermatitis. IgE binds to mast cells in the skin, initiating the release of histamine and other chemical mediators during antigenic stimulation. The overly reactive skin of atopic patients may respond excessively to the effects of histamine and other chemical mediators.

Histologically, atopic dermatitis lesions show intraepithelial vesicles, vascular dilatation in the dermis, and perivascular infiltration by inflammatory cells. Hyperkeratosis and acanthosis are present in chronic lesions. Lysosomes have been demonstrated in the stratum granulosum of atopic skin by electron microscopy, suggesting a possible autodigestive component in the pathogenesis of this disease.

Clinical Features

General. The skin lesions of atopic dermatitis (Fig. 4-1) vary with age. In infants (2–24 months), the lesions are exudative, vesicular, and crusted. The affected areas are most commonly the forehead, cheeks, and extensor surfaces of the extremities. In severe cases, a generalized eruption over the entire body may occur. In later childhood (2–12 years), the skin becomes lichenified and pigmented, and lesions are confined to the flexor surfaces with a predilection for the popliteal regions. The wrists, ankles, buttocks, and neck may also be involved. In adolescents and adults, dry, thickened, and lichenified lesions affect mainly the flexor surfaces. The face, neck, hands, and feet may also be involved. Vitiligo or spotty hyperpigmentation of the skin may be seen in association with chronic atopic dermatitis.

Ocular Findings. The skin of the eyelids may be involved, with erythematous and exudative lesions. In later stages, scaling and crusting may occur. Secondary staphylococcal blepharitis requiring treatment may also occur. Atopic keratoconjunctivitis may be observed in patients with atopic eczema (Fig. 4-2). Clinically, there may be hyperemia, chemosis, and filamentous discharge. Less commonly, giant papillary hypertrophy ("cobblestones") may be observed on the palpebral conjunctiva; in contrast to vernal conjunctivitis, the lower tarsus is more frequently involved in atopics (103). Trantas' dots (see Fig. 7-6), which con-

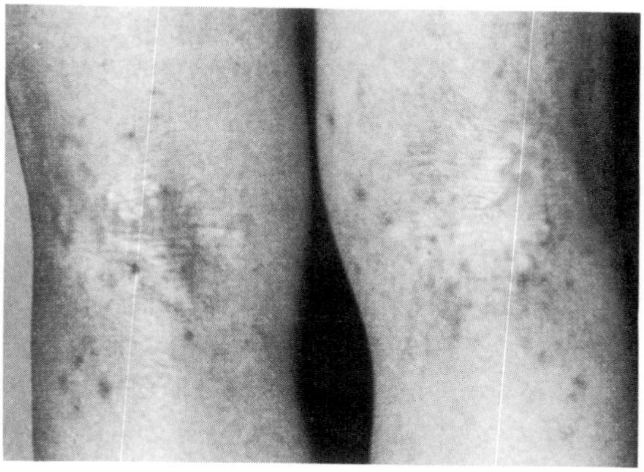

FIG. 4-1. Skin lesions in atopic dermatitis. (Korting GW: The Skin and Eye. Engl. ed. 1973, Georg Thieme Verlag, Stuttgart, Germany)

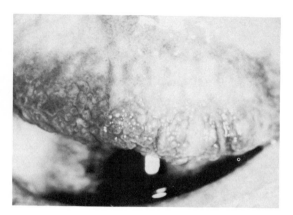

FIG. 4-2. Atopic keratoconjunctivitis with papillary response of the upper palpebral conjunctiva. (Courtesy Dr. H. B. Ostler)

sist of localized deposits of eosinophils, can occur at the limbus. Linear or stellate scarring may be present on the palpebral conjunctiva. In vernal conjunctivitis, no scarring is seen. According to Thygeson, papillary hypertrophy of the lower palpebral conjunctiva is so unusual in vernal conjunctivitis that it helps to differentiate this condition from atopic conjunctivitis. Vernal conjunctivitis will frequently become arrested by age 18. It is not uncommon to see atopic conjunctivitis in older patients. Occasionally, shrinkage of the fornices is noted in atopic keratoconjunctivitis.

Punctate staining of the cornea may be present and, if the disease is severe, scarring and vascularization of the cornea may occur. Keratoconus is sometimes associated with atopic dermatitis: it is said to occur in 25% of the cases. Copeman reviewed 100 patients with keratoconus and found that 32 had some form of eczema (24). The incidence of atopic eczema in the general population is about 3% compared with an incidence of 16% in this group of keratoconus patients. Karseras and Ruben also found a strong association between keratoconus and atopic conditions (63). It has been suggested that local irritation of the eyelids due to eczema or hay fever may lead to excessive eye rubbing. This, coupled with a congenitally thinned and weakened cornea, may be associated with the development of keratoconus.

Atopic cataracts (Fig. 4–3) have been described as a complication of atopic dermatitis (10). Their incidence has been estimated at 8%–10%. They are seen mainly in the severe chronic forms of the disease, especially in children and young adults. Atopic cataracts usually appear at least 10 years after the onset of skin involvement. Once the cataract is detected, however, it may evolve rapidly into complete opacification within 6 months. These cataracts are frequently bilateral and involvement may be symmetric. Occasionally, however, a unilateral cataract is seen. Classically, atopic cataracts have a shieldlike opacification affecting the anterior cortex. Frequently, the cataract begins as a posterior subcapsular opacity. Histologically, a localized degeneration and proliferation of the subcapsular epithelium is seen. Degeneration of the adjacent

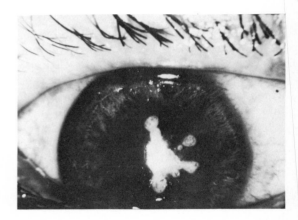

FIG. 4-3. Anterior shieldlike cataract of atopic dermatitis. (Courtesy Dr. H. B. Ostler)

cortex may occur and may lead to widespread opacification of the lens.

Spontaneous retinal detachment is said to be more common in patients with atopic dermatitis than in the general population (51). Whether this is associated with continued rubbing of the eyes or with degenerative vitreous changes is uncertain.

Differential Diagnosis

It may be difficult to distinguish atopic dermatitis from seborrheic dermatitis, especially during infancy. Infants with cradle cap or exudative eczema of the scalp may develop typical atopic dermatitis in later years. The differentiation between atopic and seborrheic dermatitis is easier during later childhood and adulthood. The skin lesions of phenylketonuria and Letterer–Siwe disease may be indistinguishable from atopic dermatitis in infancy. Other types of infantile atopic dermatitis such as Leiner's disease (erythroderma desquamativum) and Ritter's disease (dermatitis exfoliativa neonatorum) occur during the first few weeks of life and are quite similar to atopic dermatitis. Neurodermatitis, localized neurodermatitis, and contact dermatitis may also simulate atopic dermatitis. As mentioned earlier, an atopic dermatitis may be a feature of immunodeficiency syndromes including the Wiskott–Aldrich syndrome, ataxia–telangiectasia, and sex-linked agammaglobulinemia. The differentiation of vernal conjunctivitis from the conjunctivitis of atopic dermatitis is discussed under Ocular Findings.

Treatment

The skin of atopic dermatitis patients is easily irritated and therefore they should take care to avoid nonspecific irritants such as harsh soaps and detergents, too frequent bathing, excessive sweating, chapping in cold weather, irritating fabrics such as wool and nylon, scratching, and emotional stress (61).

Topical steroids may be used for the skin lesions. A fluorinated corticosteroid such as triamcinolone or betamethasone in a water-soluble base may be applied three times a day to localized skin lesions. For exudative lesions, wet saline dressings may be applied several times a day. For thick and lichenified lesions, 1% crude coal tar in Lassar's paste or cold cream may be effective. Coal tar derivatives, however, can sensitize the skin to strong sunlight. Antihistamines, such as hydroxyzine 5–25 mg, may be given as often as four times a day to help control itching. If the skin lesions are widespread and not controlled by topical therapy, oral corticosteroids may be added. As little as 5–10 mg prednisone a day combined with a full regimen of topical treatment may keep a patient relatively free of dermatitis. For acute involvement of large areas of skin, a high dose of prednisone may be given and tapered slowly until skin lesions improve. Long-term use of corticosteroids should be avoided, especially in children because of the tendency of these drugs to suppress growth. Patients with active atopic dermatitis should not be vaccinated for smallpox because of the danger of their developing generalized vaccinia.

In atopic keratoconjunctivitis, if an inciting antigen can be identified it should be eliminated. Topical corticosteroids may be used for short periods of time; however, their long-term usage should be avoided. Some recent success has been obtained with the use of 2–4% cromolyn eye drops. This medication stabilizes mast cells and prevents the release of their mediators.

Surgery of atopic cataracts should not be undertaken lightly. Several investigators have reported complications such as severe hemor-rhage, retinal detachment, iridocyclitis, and corneal edema. A relatively high incidence of pre- and postoperative retinal detachment has also been reported (22, 51). In patients with keratoconus associated with atopic eczema, penetrating keratoplasty may be carried out with a high degree of success.

CONTACT DERMATITIS

Contact dermatitis is probably the most common immunologic disease encountered by dermatologists. It results from the exposure of the skin to a wide variety of substances commonly found in the environment, including drugs, dyes, plant resins, preservatives, cosmetics, and metals. There are two varieties of contact dermatitis: 1) irritant, the more common form, and 2) allergic. **Irritant contact dermatitis** is caused by excessive moisture or by acids, alkalis, resins, or chemicals capable of injuring any person's skin if persistent contact is allowed. Allergy or hypersensitivity plays no role in irritant contact dermatitis. **Allergic contact dermatitis,** unlike the irritant variety, only occurs in sensitized individuals and involves the mechanism of cell-mediated immunity. In allergic contact dermatitis, an individual becomes sensitized to a given chemical or other sensitizing substance, and upon reexposure to the same chemical an erythematous delayed skin reaction is elicited.

Immunopathology

Irritant dermatitis is provoked by substances with primary irritant properties or by frequent defatting of the skin caused by excessive moisture. With continued defatting of the skin or repeated irritant exposure, edema, erythema, vesiculation, and scaling of the skin develop. The damaged or inflamed eczematous skin, while inflamed, has a higher risk of developing a true allergic contact dermatitis. Removal of the irritant or curtailment of the practice leading to skin inflammation will allow the irritant dermatitis to resolve.

In allergic contact dermatitis, the sensitizing substances are generally haptens of small molecular weight which bind to dermal proteins, forming complete antigens. The haptens do not significantly alter the configuration of these carrier proteins. Upon initial application of a contact sensitizer, most of the applied chemical is rapidly removed by the blood stream. Whether sensitization occurs in the draining lymph node, at a peripheral skin site, or elsewhere, is not actually known. Initial exposure, however, does result in the production of specifically sensitized T lymphocytes capable of responding to the antigen when reexposure occurs. A second application of the sensitizing substance therefore leads to an inflammatory response and an accumulation of mononuclear cells and other inflammatory cells characteristic of cell-mediated responses. In the guinea pig, contact sensitivity can be transferred to unsensitized guinea pigs with mononuclear white blood cells or with lymph node cells. This was first demonstrated in the classic experiments of Landsteiner and Chase in 1942 (67). The chemical substances which mediate these erythematous reactions may be the lymphokines which are produced by sensitized lymphocytes on exposure to a specific antigen. The role of prostaglandins in allergic contact dermatitis has also been studied with interest. Prostaglandin E is capable of inducing delayed-onset inflammation and a dusky erythema of the skin lasting for up to 10 h.

It should be emphasized that allergic contact dermatitis lesions do not depend on humoral antibody and are not absent in individuals with deficiencies of the humoral immune system. Patients with deficiencies of cell-mediated immunity, however, do have absent or diminished contact sensitivity. This group of patients includes individuals with certain malignancies, sarcoidosis, and certain immunodeficiency states such as the Wiskott–Aldrich syndrome.

Histologically, lesions of contact dermatitis are characterized by mononuclear cell infiltration of the dermis. During the acute phases, the epidermis shows edema or spongiosis followed by intraepidermal vesiculation. During chronic stages, irregular epidermal thickening and hyperkeratosis may be seen. Recently, it has been shown by Dvorak (32, 33) that contact dermatitis lesions in guinea pigs and in humans contain large infiltrations of basophilic leukocytes.

Clinical Features

Contact dermatitis lesions are characterized by erythema, exudation, edema, and vesiculation during the acute phase. During the chronic phase, scaling, eczematization, crusting, and lichenification predominate (Fig. 4-4). The site of the skin lesion is often a clue to the diagnosis: lesions appear in localized areas which have been exposed to offending substances. Areas of exposure, including the hands, face, neck, and legs, may be affected. Lesions of irritant dermatitis and allergic contact dermatitis may look the same; however, irritant lesions generally occur 1–2 h after contact, whereas lesions of allergic contact dermatitis develop over a 48-h period following exposure.

The eye is a frequent site of involvement in contact dermatitis (30). Drugs including neomycin sulfate, atropine and its derivatives, chloramphenicol, penicillin, and related compounds may all act as sensitizers. Antazoline, an ophthalmic antihistamine solution, is also a potential sensitizer. Besides the skin lesions of contact dermatitis, contact sensitizers may produce a conjunctivitis characterized usually by a papillary response, pronounced vasodilatation, chemosis, and watery discharge. An erythematous blepharitis may also occur, and in very severe cases a keratitis may develop that is typified by small yellow necrotic opacities just inside the limbus. Primary irritant conjunctivitis can produce similar findings. The fine epithelial punctate keratitis produced by chronic use of gentamicin, topical anesthet-

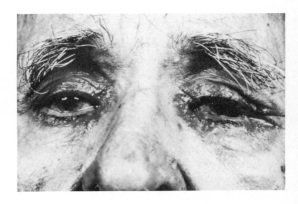

FIG. 4-4. Contact allergy caused by neomycin. (Courtesy Dr. R. S. Weinberg)

ics, echothiophate (phospholine iodide), phenylephrine, and epinephrine are well known to the ophthalmologist. Recently, Mathias and his co-workers (74a) have reported a convincing case of contact dermatitis and conjunctivitis associated with the use of tetracaine and two unusual allergens, echothiophate iodide and phenylephrine hydrochloride.

Rubbing the eyes after handling soaps, detergents, or chemicals may provoke a contact dermatitis rection. Allergic reactions to cosmetics affect primarily the eyebrows and upper lids because of the method of application. Mascara, eyebrow pencil, and face creams all may act as allergens. Nail polish can cause sensitization around the eye by accidental touching of the area. Lip gloss and eye gloss cosmetics contain lanolin fractions which may also act as sensitizers.

Parabens are used in a great many lotions, creams, and cosmetics because they are excellent antimicrobial agents which prevent spoilage from bacterial and fungal growth. Paraben allergy was first reported in 1966 (99) and is now thought to be one of the leading causes of contact dermatitis. Nickel sulfate is a common sensitizer found in jewelry and undergarments. Chromates, which are used in costume jewelry, leather products, bleaches, industrial chemicals, fabrics, and automobile products, are common offenders. p-Phenylenediamine is widely used in hair dyes, clothing, and shoes. It contains a benzamine nucleus and may cross react with a variety of therapeutic agents including sulfonamides, benzocaine, and hydrochlorothiazide.

Diagnosis

A diagnosis of allergic contact sensitivity is made by patch testing. The suspected allergen is applied to the skin and covered with a patch for 48 h. Sometimes a true allergic response will not be maximal until 72 h after application. An erythematous reaction, delayed in onset, indicates a positive test and should raise a strong suspicion of previous sensitization. It should be realized that substances with primary irritant properties may also produce a positive response within a few hours of application. This is one pitfall of patch testing; however, these primary irritant reactions can

be avoided by using low doses of testing substances.

At times, it may be hard to identify the actual allergen, and in these situations detailed detective work may be necessary.

Treatment

The basis of treatment in contact dermatitis is the removal of the allergen or irritant from the patient's environment. Often this is difficult because of economic or occupational factors. If continued exposure to an allergen is necessary, well-designed clothing may offer suitable protection. Medications containing neomycin, sulfonamides, or other common sensitizers should be avoided in sensitive patients.

In acute skin lesions, cool saline compresses should be applied. Topical fluorinated corticosteroid lotions such as triamcinolone or betamethasone may be used. In chronic lesions, steroid lotions or ointments are also of use. The only form of contact dermatitis which may require a systemic corticosteroid is widespread, severe poison ivy dermatitis (35). A 10 to 14-day course of prednisone may be used in this situation since it may lessen the intensity of the disease as well as the loss of time from work or school. Desensitization treatment by the oral and parenteral routes has been tried with poison ivy; however, the efficacy of this mode of therapy is still in dispute. For the conjunctivitis or keratoconjunctivitis that is associated with drugs which are primary irritant substances or contact allergens, the best treatment is withdrawal of the drug and substitution of an appropriate, nonirritating medication.

URTICARIA

Urticaria is a cutaneous eruption having multiple pathogenic mechanisms which may be immunologic or nonimmunologic. Its prevalence in the general population is high and is estimated to be between 10% and 25%. No specific cause can be found in 70% of patients with chronic urticaria (42). In others, psychogenic, allergic, and physical factors may play a role; these are discussed in more detail under Clinical Features. An etiologic classification of urticaria is listed in Table 4-1.

TABLE 4-1. CAUSES OF CHRONIC URTICARIAL LESIONS

Idiopathic (90% of cases)
Drugs
    Immunologic drug reactions
    Nonimmunologic release of chemical mediators
Food additives and preservatives
Food allergens
Infection
    Parasitic (*e.g.,* ascariasis, hookworms, strongyloidiasis, filariasis, echinococcosis, schistosomiasis)
    Viral (*e.g.,* Coxsackie virus, infectious mononucleosis, viral hepatitis)
    Bacterial?
Contactants (penetrants)
Psychogenic factors
Urticaria pigmentosa
Genetic abnormalities (*e.g.,* hereditary urticaria, deafness and amyloidosis)
Systemic diseases (*e.g.,* collagen vascular disorders, Hodgkin's disease, malignancy, amyloidosis)
Physical allergy
    Light (solar) urticaria
        Idiopathic
        Secondary to abnormality of protoporphyrin IX metabolism
    Heat urticaria
        Generalized (cholinergic)
        Localized
    Cold urticaria
        Acquired essential
        Acquired, secondary to cryoglobulinemia, cryofibrinogenemia or cold hemolysin syndrome
        Familial
    Urticaria due to trauma
        Dermographism
        Pressure urticaria

(Freedman SO: Clinical Immunology of the Skin. In Freedman SO, Gold P (eds): Clinical Immunology, 2nd ed. Hagerstown, Harper & Row, 1976, p 212)

The skin lesions of urticaria are sharply circumscribed elevated areas of edema. If the swelling is extensive, and involves the subcutaneous tissues, the term angioedema is used. Urticaria may be divided into acute and chronic forms. Acute urticaria is often associated with immunologic mechanisms. Chronic urticaria, which lasts more than 8 weeks, frequently has no identifiable cause. At times, emotional or allergic factors may be implicated.

Immunopathology

The immunologic mechanisms involved in urticaria are not well understood. The clinical signs of urticaria may be simulated by injection of histamine into the skin. This results in localized vasodilation, increased vascular permeability, and itching. Plasma histamine levels, however, are not elevated in urticaria, except for cold urticaria. This may be due to the rapid uptake of histamine by various tissues (6). Cell-bound IgE is not increased in patients with urticaria. Serum IgE levels may be elevated but are often within normal limits (41). Occasionally, depressed levels of IgG, IgA, and IgM are seen in children with chronic urticaria and chronic infections (18).

Urticaria may occur during serum sickness or in response to a drug allergy such as allergy to penicillin. Most of the commonly seen immunologic causes of urticaria are related to infection, foods, and drugs.

In urticaria not involving IgE antibody, cytotoxic mechanisms and immune (antigen–antibody) complexes often play a role. Type II (cytotoxic) hypersensitivity is the mechanism involved in hemolytic transfusion reactions, in which IgG or IgM antibodies react with erythrocyte antigens and induce cell lysis. Activation of the complement system and production of the anaphylatoxins C3a and C5a may lead to histamine release from mast cells. Serum sickness and cryoglobulinemia are both frequently accompanied by urticaria. Cold urticaria may be passively transferred to normal recipients with cold-precipitable IgG. While this is normally attributed to aggregated IgG or mixed IgG–IgM cryoglobulins and activation of the complement system, it is possible that homocytotropic IgG antibodies may also play a role. In human serum sickness, IgE (reaginic) antibodies are thought to mediate the urticarial lesions while antigen–antibody complexes appear to be responsible for the lesions of the heart, kidneys, and joints.

While histamine has been considered the principal mediator in urticaria, its duration of action is considered too short to account for all the observed clinical manifestations. Other substances which may be important in mediating urticarial reactions include slow reacting substance of anaphylaxis (SRS-A), bradykinin, and the prostaglandins. The actual role of these mediators in urticaria has yet to be established.

Histologically, urticarial lesions are infiltrated by neutrophils and eosinophils. Dermal edema and vasodilation are prominent features of these reactions. Electron microscopic studies have also revealed a reduction in the density of mast cell granules in lesions of chronic urticaria.

Clinical Features

General. Typical urticarial lesions are characterized by erythema and wheal formation. They vary in color, size, and shape (Fig. 4-5). They are frequently transient and may be associated with intense itching.

The etiologic factors in urticaria are multiple. In general, the urticarias are classified as immunologic and nonimmunologic. Immunologic causes include hypersensitivity responses to infections, foods, and drugs. These responses may be mediated by any one of the four types of hypersensitivity reactions. Nonimmunologic causes of urticaria include physical and emotional factors, histamine-releasing drugs, and cholinergic stimuli.

Drugs commonly associated with urticaria include aspirin, tetracycline, acetazolamide and other sulfonamide derivatives, penicillin, polymyxin, and opium alkaloids such as morphine, codeine, and meperidine. Berries, shellfish, nuts, and eggs are some of the common dietary causes of urticaria. Infections with parasites, viruses (including infectious mononucleosis and hepatitis), and occasionally bacteria have been implicated in urticaria. Pollens and contact sensitizers are also known to produce urticaria and can be tested for easily. Psychogenic factors are felt to play a role in approximately 20% of urticaria cases; however, the pathophysiology is completely unknown. Urticaria may be seen during the course of certain systemic diseases. These include collagen vascular diseases (particularly systemic lupus erythematosus), Hodgkin's disease, other lymphomas, carcinomas, and amyloidosis.

Urticaria may also be induced by certain physical agents, including light, heat, cold, and trauma (100). Light urticaria occurs on areas of the skin that have been exposed to sunlight. Heat urticaria may be produced by emotional stress or physical exertion as well as by outside heat. It may be related to an increase in body temperature and excitation of the autonomic nervous system. Cold urticaria is one of the more common forms of physical allergy. It

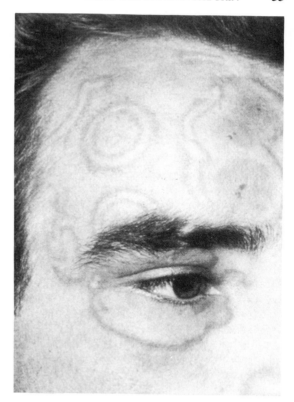

FIG. 4-5. Urticaria. (Korting GW: The Skin and Eye. Engl. ed. 1973, Georg Thieme Verlag, Stuttgart, Germany)

may be due to an antibody mechanism, since in some cases the sensitivity to cold can be passively transferred by serum to normal skin. The nature of the antigen, however, is unknown. It is felt that skin protein may be altered by cold in such a way as to make it antigenic. Skin trauma or pressure on the skin are physical factors that are also capable of inducing urticaria in susceptible individuals.

Ocular Findings. Generalized urticaria may involve the face and frequently affects the periorbital region. The loose connective tissue around the eyes may be markedly affected and the patient's eye may be completely closed from the edema. Chemosis may be seen if the edema is extensive. In cases of hereditary angioedema, exophthalmos may be present owing to periorbital edema. Optic nerve edema has also been described. Urticarial edema of the eyelids should be differentiated from edema due to myxedema, renal and cardiac diseases, trauma, and contact allergy. Unilateral edema of the eyelids can also be caused by osteomyelitis involving the maxilla. Finally, parasitic diseases including schistosomiasis and filariasis may occasionally cause periorbital swelling.

Diagnosis and Treatment

A specific etiologic agent may sometimes be identified in urticaria. In food allergy, the suspected food may be elminated from the diet for several weeks and subsequently tried again to determine its relation to the urticaria (71). Drug allergy requires a careful history and elimination of the suspected drug. A diagnosis of cold urticaria can be made by applying an ice cube to the forearm for 5 min and watching for the appearance of an urticarial lesion as the skin rewarms. Cholinergic urticaria, the type associated with exercise, emotional stress, and overheating, may be elicited by an injection of methacholine, which produces a skin lesion at the injection site. If a specific etiologic agent is identified it should be avoided. Avoiding excessive exposures of light, trauma, and sudden changes in temperature may help in the treatment of urticaria due to physical allergy. Sunscreen lotions have also been effective. When urticaria is associated with infections it appears to be self-limited.

Most patients obtain some relief of acute or chronic urticarial lesions with one of the antihistamines. Hydroxyzine is one of the most effective anti-whealing agents and suppresses histamine-induced pruritus. Cyproheptadine or diphenhydramine may be beneficial as well. Systemic corticosteroids are unpredictable and have little value for the treatment of urticaria. Aqueous epinephrine, may be given subcutaneously for temporary relief of acute urticaria. Topical antipruritic medications such as calamine lotion may have some value.

HEREDITARY ANGIOEDEMA

This interesting condition is characterized by repeated attacks of subepithelial edema involving the skin, respiratory tract, and gastrointestinal tract. Urticaria does not occur in this condition, although the skin lesions may be well demarcated. Although hereditary angioedema was recognized in 1888 (79), it was only recently discovered that a biochemical abnormality in the complement system exists in this entity (4, 28, 94).

Immunopathology

Patients with hereditary angioedema have an inherited deficiency of C1-esterase inhibitor, and α_2-globulin which inhibits activation of the first component of complement. The deficiency leads to uncontrolled activation of the complement pathway and generation of a kininlike substance. This results in repeated episodes of angioedema involving the skin and the respiratory and gastrointestinal tracts. Death may result from pharyngeal or laryngeal edema and asphyxiation. About 85% of patients' kindreds have markedly deficient or absent C1-esterase inhibitor. In the remaining 15%, the inhibitor is present in normal amounts but it is functionally inactive.

C1-esterase inhibitor acts at two stages in the activation of C1. It chiefly inhibits C1s; however, it also may inhibit C1r (36). C1-esterase inhibitor has many other physiologic functions: it is known to inhibit the kinin system, plasma thromboplastin antecedent (coagulation factor XI), plasmin, and activated Hageman factor. These other functions may contribute to the role of C1-esterase inhibitor in the manifestations of hereditary angioedema.

Clinical Features

Hereditary angioedema is inherited as an autosomal dominant trait. It has its onset in early adolescence and becomes less severe after the age of 35. It is unrelated to other allergic disorders. It is characterized clinically by recurrent episodes of edema involving the extremities, face, and airway and by recurrent abdominal pain. In many instances, a clearly identifiable traumatic event may precede the onset of edema. The edema is nonpitting, and not associated with pain or pruritus. Often, emotional upset may provoke attacks of edema. The frequency of episodes of edema is variable, with intervals between attacks ranging from a few weeks to several years.

The periorbital region may be involved (Fig. 4-6), and exophthalmos and optic nerve edema have been described. Chemosis involving the conjunctiva and spreading to the cornea has also been noted.

Diagnosis

The history in patients with hereditary angioedema is quite informative (77), since the unusual features of recurrent edema involving the extremities, face, and airway, accompanied by recurrent abdominal pain, are characteristic. In addition, there is often a strong family history of hereditary angioedema. The serum C4 level will be decreased in this condition and its measurement constitutes the best screening procedure for hereditary angioedema. Confirmation of the diagnosis can be made by assaying C1-esterase inhibitor activity by radioimmunodiffusion. In the 15% of cases with normal levels of C1-esterase inhibitor, a functional assay must be done.

Treatment

Long-term prophylaxis of attacks may be achieved by the use of antifibrinolytic agents and androgens. ε-Aminocaproic acid (EACA) suppresses attacks but has some associated toxicity (37). This drug may act by inhibiting plasmin activation and the resulting activation of C1. Short-term prophylaxis may be obtained with transfusions of fresh-frozen plasma which contains normal levels of C1-esterase inhibitor. Specific therapy for acute attacks is not available, and supportive care including prevention of airway obstruction is required.

PSORIASIS

Psoriasis is a chronic skin disease characterized by epidermal hyperplasia and an accelerated rate of epidermal turnover that result in scaling erythematous skin lesions. The disease is sometimes associated with an inflammatory arthritis. Although psoriasis is inherited as a

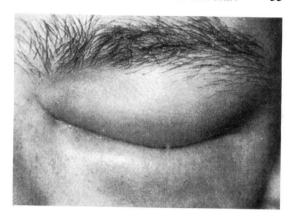

FIG. 4-6. Angioneurotic edema. (Korting GW: The Skin and Eye. Engl. ed. 1973, Georg Thieme Verlag, Stuttgart, Germany)

simple autosomal dominant trait with incomplete penetrance, environmental as well as genetic factors are important in the disease. Ocular findings including lid lesions, conjunctival changes, and corneal vascularization are said to occur in 10% of affected patients. These complications are twice as frequent in males as in females and may be the only manifestation of the disease (62).

Immunopathology

Histologically, the skin lesions of psoriasis are characterized by epidermal thickening, acanthosis, and elongated dermal papillae. There may be increased mitotic activity of the epidermis as well as hyperkeratosis and a diminished stratum granulosum. An inflammatory infiltrate consisting of mononuclear cells in the superficial corium, or neutrophils in the epidermis, may be seen.

Psoriatic patients have a three- to fourfold increase in the incidence of histocompatibility antigens HLA-B13 and B-17 (95, 118). A decreased IgM level is present in one-third of patients, especially in those with a concurrent arthritis (38). Recent studies (60) have shown an increase in serum IgG, IgA, and IgE, and an increase in salivary IgA levels, in some patients with psoriasis. Anti-IgG antibodies have been found in 45% of patients with psoriasis (44), a fact that suggests the possibility of an autoimmune disorder in this disease. Cell-mediated immunity may also be affected in patients with psoriasis, since it is difficult to induce hypersensitivity to chemical agents such as dinitrochlorobenzene in psoriatic patients, even in those not receiving immunosuppressive drugs (34). In addition, the lymphocytes of psoriatic patients show a diminished response to the mitogen phytohemagglutinin (69).

Clinical Features

General. Cutaneous lesions have three basic elements: 1) Affected areas are elevated above the surface of the surrounding, uninvolved, skin. 2) Scales cover the lesions as a result of accelerated epidermal proliferation. 3) The lesions are erythematous. Skin lesions vary in size and in configuration from drop-shaped papules to large plaques. Elbows and knees are the areas most frequently involved. The turnover time of epidermis is 3–4 days, rather than the normal 28 days. Arthritis may accompany the psoriasis in some cases.

Ocular Findings. Ocular symptoms (Fig. 4-7) may be minimal or pronounced. The lashes may be covered with scales, and the lid margins may be erythematous and crusted. A squamous blepharitis may occur, and may lead to an inflammatory ectropion with trichiasis. Aside from the lid changes, the most common ocular finding in psoriasis patients is nonspecific conjunctivitis, which may be catarrhal or purulent. Occasionally, symblepharon, xerosis, and trichiasis may follow the healing phase (108).

Nodular excrescences of piled-up epithelium may occur at the limbus. These may be surrounded by smaller stromal opacities. The surface of the nodules may be eroded. The bulbar conjunctiva adjacent to the nodule may be injected, producing an overall appearance at first glance of phlyctenular keratoconjunctivitis or acne rosacea keratitis. The epithelial nodules are produced by hyperkeratosis and may result from the initial subepithelial disease.

Corneal changes may be seen and are usually confined to the lower half of the cornea or to the periphery (62). The lower half of the cornea may show focal subepithelial infiltrates with or without epithelial erosion. Superficial and deep stromal opacities may be seen axially. These stromal opacities are usually permanent, but the epithelial opacities

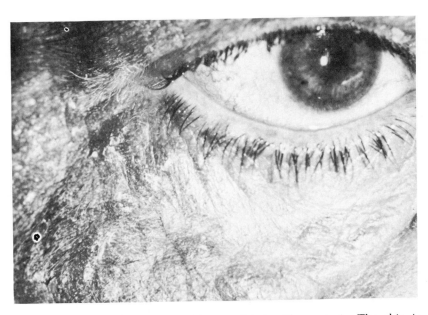

FIG. 4-7. Nonspecific conjunctivitis associated with psoriasis. The skin is scaly and erythematous. (Courtesy Dr. H. B. Ostler)

may come and go in parallel with the activity of the skin disease. Episcleritis has been reported; however, it is rare and its occurrence may be coincidental.

Psoriatic Arthritis. An inflammatory polyarthritis may develop in about 7% of psoriasis patients. Three patterns of arthritis are known to occur (89). In one series of 168 patients with psoriatic arthritis, 78% had an arthritis that was indistinguishable from rheumatoid arthritis, 17% had distal-joint arthritis most often affecting the distal interphalangeal joints of the fingers, and 5% had severe peripheral joint involvement accompanied by a deforming arthritis of the spine that was similar to ankylosing spondylitis. Patients with this latter type of deforming arthritis frequently develop a uveitis: it occurs in about one-quarter of the males in this category. Uveitis is also seen in men with the distal form of arthritis and in 4% of men and 9% of women with the rheumatoidlike arthritis.

Diagnosis

Laboratory studies are not generally helpful in the diagnosis of psoriasis. Uric acid levels may be elevated, probably owing to an increased nucleic acid degradation associated with accelerated epidermal proliferation. About 16% of patients with the rheumatoid type of psoriatic arthritis will have a positive test for rheumatoid factor; however, in general psoriatic arthritis is characterized by a negative sheep cell agglutinin test.

Treatment

Ultraviolet radiation, especially from natural sunlight, has been of value in the treatment of psoriasis for centuries. Wood and coal tars are frequently used and may produce beneficial effects by inhibition of cell replication. The combined use of tar preparations and ultraviolet light are popular in the treatment of chronic cases (113). Adrenal corticosteroids are the most prevalently used medications today in psoriasis. Their effect is enhanced when they are applied under occlusive dressings. Systemic corticosteroids will often yield prompt

benefit in psoriasis, but the well-known complications of these medications must be kept in mind. Cancer chemotherapeutic drugs have recently been employed in the treatment of psoriasis. Methotrexate, a folic acid antagonist, is the most widely used (5, 112). Methotrexate diminishes DNA synthesis by competitive inhibition of folic acid reductase. Therefore, cell replication is inhibited. This medication must be given systemically since topical application is not effective. As small a dose as possible should be used and toxicity must be evaluated. Other drugs which interfere with nucleic acid synthesis have also been used. Clofazimine (Lamprene), a phenazine derivative, has been used, but has been found to produce fine, brownish lines in the superficial layers of the cornea (115).

Treatment of the ocular findings is symptomatic. Good hygiene should be practiced. Topical corticosteroids may be used when necessary. The uveitis accompanying psoriatic arthritis requires monitoring for increased intraocular pressure, cataract formation, and the development of synechiae. Short-acting dilating agents may be used if there is a tendency to form synechiae.

TOXIC EPIDERMAL NECROLYSIS (RITTER'S DISEASE, LYELL'S DISEASE)

Toxic epidermal necrolysis (TEN) is an acute bullous eruption of the skin and mucous membranes. Two different etiologies are thought to exist. In infants and in children under the age of 10, the most common etiology is staphylococcal infection (Ritter's disease). The staphylococcus organism produces a toxin that has a specific effect on the stratum granulosum of the skin, which leads to separation and a generalized peeling of the epidermis. The mucous membranes of the mouth, tongue, trachea, and gastrointestinal tract may also show necrotic changes. Because of the chracteristic burnlike changes in the skin, cases produced by the coagulase-positive *Staphylococcus aureus* are termed **staphylococcal scaled skin syndrome (SSSS).**

In an older group of patients with similar clinical findings, the disease is felt to be drug-related. The drugs most commonly implicated are penicillin, phenytoin, sulfonamides, phenolphthalein, and phenylbutazone. The mortality in this group may be as high as 40%.

Ocular involvement may occur in toxic epidermal necrolysis. A mucopurulent or pseudomembranous conjunctivitis is the most common finding. Symblepharon formation, eyelid changes, and corneal complications may develop in severe cases.

Immunopathology

The childhood form of TEN appears to be associated with a toxin produced by *Staphylococcus aureus* known as exfoliatin. This is a protein with a molecular weight of 10,000–50,000 which has a specific effect on the stratum granulosum of the skin. Its mode of action, however, is still unknown. Exfoliatin production is controlled by plasmids. These are extrachromosomal DNA elements which replicate independently of bacterial chromosomes (64).

The pathogenesis of drug-related cases of TEN is unknown. An autoimmune mechanism in which the drug responsible for the condition acts as a hapten and leads to formation of antibodies against epidermis has been proposed (74). Complement and immunoglobulins have been demonstrated by immuno-fluorescence within the epidermis in one-fourth of the patients with this condition (50). Several investigators have observed a rise in γ- and α_2-globulins in these patients. Stein and Turk (104) have reported a decrease in IgA and IgM during the acute phase of the disease. A rise in α_1- antitrypsin, ceruloplasmin, β_{1C}-globulin, and IgG have also been noted (50). Finding a deficiency of the prealbumin protein on immunoelectrophoresis was felt by Husz *et al.* (50) to be characteristic of severe disease and possibly to signal a fatal outcome.

Clinical Features

General. Three stages of the disease are recognized. Initially, a prodromal stage occurs, characterized by erythema around the mouth and eyes. There may be general malaise and the skin may be tender or painful. Large flaccid bullae develop, and spread in a centrifugal fashion. With pressure on the skin, the epidermis will separate from the underlying dermis (**Nikolsky's sign**). This helps to distinguish the disease from Stevens–Johnson syndrome, in which the bullae are subepidermal in location, tense, and nonmobile.

During the exfoliative phase, exudation and crusting occur around the mouth and eyes (Figure 4-8). The epidermis may be peeled off like the skin of a ripe peach. Often large sheets

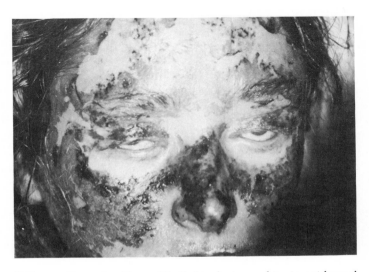

FIG. 4-8. Extensive "burn-like" skin lesions of toxic epidermal necrolysis. (Courtesy Dr. H. B. Ostler)

of epidermis are peeled off, simulating gloves and stockings. As the exfoliative stage resolves, a final desquamative stage occurs. The exposed, glazed areas of skin become duller while the areas of skin not exfoliated throw off powdery scales. Later, only the skin of the palms and soles continues to desquamate. Generally, since only the epidermis is involved, no permanent scarring occurs. Scarring only occurs if the epidermal disease is severe enough to involve the underlying structures (80). The clinical picture in the staphylococcal-induced and drug-induced conditions may be the same, although some have felt that the facial changes are less dramatic in the drug-induced cases.

Ulcerative lesions involving the oral cavity, trachea, esophagus, stomach and colon may occur. These complications are serious and may lead to death. Prior to the antibiotic era, skin abscesses, cellulitis, and gangrene were reported.

Ocular Findings. The skin of the eyelids and periorbital region may be involved and show skin changes similar to those observed elsewhere on the body (Fig. 4-9). Eyelashes may

be lost. A mucopurulent conjunctivitis is the most common sign. Usually this is mild, but in severe cases symblepharon formation may occur. Immobility of the lids may lead to an exposure keratitis. Corneal ulceration, scarring, and vascularization may develop (46, 80). Perforation of the globe has occurred on rare occasions.

Treatment

The treatment of TEN depends on the etiologic factors in this condition. If the disease is related to a staphylococcal infection, one of the penicillinase-resistant antistaphylococcal agents such as methicillin should be given (64). Antibiotic treatment has reduced the mortality of this form of the condition from 50% to about 10%. In the drug-induced cases of TEN, the mortality may be as high as 40%; treatment in general is supportive and is similar to the treatment of severely burned patients. Reverse isolation procedures are of value.

Ocular involvement may require nothing more than good lid hygiene and removal of crusts. Attention should be given to corneal exposure and trichiasis, since corneal ulcera-

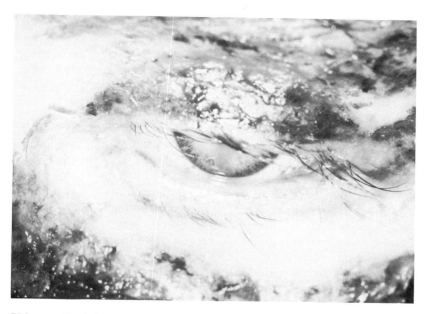

FIG. 4-9. Eyelid involvement in toxic epidermal necrolysis. (Courtesy Dr. H. B. Ostler)

tion may result. Frequently, topical lubricants and antibiotics may be helpful in preventing corneal complications.

The use of systemic corticosteroids is controversial in this condition; however, when they are given, an antibiotic should be given simultaneously in both staphylococcal and drug-related cases.

PEMPHIGUS

Pemphigus is a chronic progressive bullous disorder which has several forms based on clinical morphology. The most common and well-studied form is **pemphigus vulgaris.** A variant, **pemphigus vegetans,** is characterized by vegetative lesions in the intertriginous areas. **Pemphigus foliaceus,** which has a high incidence in Brazil, is characterized by erythematous bullous lesions and generalized exfoliation of the skin in a leaflike pattern. **Pemphigus erythematosus** has a prolonged erythematous stage and a seborrheiclike eruption.

Pemphigus affects Jewish people more frequently than others, but has been documented in all races and ethnic groups. Prior to the advent of corticosteroids, the disease was almost universally fatal as a result of fluid and electrolyte imbalance, cachexia, and sepsis.

Immunopathology

A technique which has been useful in the study of pempigus, as well as other bullous dermatoses, is immunofluorescence. Two general types of immunofluorescence procedures are used in the study of the skin. **Direct immunofluorescence** uses a skin biopsy from the patient. The tissue is incubated with fluorescein-conjugated antiserum specific for human IgG, IgM, IgA, IgE, or the complement components. **Indirect immunofluorescence** detects antibodies in the patient's serum directed against normal skin components. Epithelial tissue, usually derived from rat esophagus, is incubated with the patient's serum. After the tissues are washed, fluorescein-conjugated anti–human IgG, IgA, or IgM is applied to the sections in order to detect the already fixed anti–tissue antibodies.

To understand the pathogenesis of bullous diseases, some anatomic features of the skin should be reviewed. The epidermis is composed of layers of epidermal cells which originate in the basal layer of the epidermis. As these cells migrate into the stratum corneum they become keratinized and compacted. Epidermal cells are held together by cytoplasmic projections ending on desmosomes. An amorphous substance known as "intercellular cement" is found in the spaces between epidermal cells. If this cement substance is interfered with, epidermal cohesiveness is lost and blister formation can occur. The epidermis is attached to the dermis by the epithelial basement membrane. The basal layer of the epidermis is anchored by structures known as hemi-desmosomes. If the basement membrane or hemi-desmosomes are destroyed, the epidermis may separate from the dermis, leading to subepidermal blister formation.

Direct immunofluorescence studies in pemphigus have shown that immunoglobulins, particularly IgG, can be found in the intercellular spaces of the epidermis (15) (Table 4-2). Complement components (C1, C4, and C3), properdin factor B (C3 proactivator), and to a lesser extent properdin have also been found in the intercellular spaces (15). In addition, levels of complement in the blister fluid are markedly decreased, suggesting tissue deposition and utilization of complement. Recently, Bean and associates have demonstrated intercellular staining for IgG in the conjunctiva of a patient with pemphigus vulgaris (8).

Most patients with pemphigus also possess a circulating IgG antibody which has an affinity for the intercellular spaces of squamous epithelium. This antibody, found in approximately two-thirds of patients with pemphigus vulgaris, is believed to be directed against the intercellular cement substance (14). A strong binding of this antibody to the intercellular cement suggests that this antibody is a true autoantibody. It is possible, however, that the antibody may be secondary to damage of intercellular spaces caused by some other mechanism. The injection of circulating epithelial antibodies induced in rabbits has been shown to facilitate acantholysis (43, 123). Injection of human pemphigus serum into pri-

TABLE 4-2. PATTERNS OF DIRECT IMMUNOFLUORESCENT STAINING IN DERMATOLOGIC DISEASES

Immune reactant	Pemphigus vulgaris	Bullous pemphigoid	Dermatitis herpetiformis	Systemic lupus erythematosus
Direct intercellular staining				
IgG	++++	—	—	—
C3	+	—	—	—
Direct basement membrane staining				
IgG	—	++++ (linear)	+	++++ (granular)
IgA	—	—	++++	+
IgM	—	—	+	+
IgE	—	+	—	—
C3	—	+	+	+
C1q	ND*	+	+	+
C3PA†	—	+	+	+
Properdin	—	+	+	+
Indirect immunofluorescence (circulating antibodies)	Intercellular	Basement membrane	—	—

* Not done
† C3 proactivator (Factor B)
(Freedman SO: Clinical Immunology of the Skin. In Freedman SO, Gold P (eds): Clinical Immunology, 2nd ed. Hagerstown, Harper & Row, 1976, p 222)

mates does not produce blisters characteristic of pemphigus; however, antibody does become localized to the epidermal intercellular spaces (98). It is possible that pemphigus autoantibodies initiate a pathologic process which is followed by complement deposition, influx of white blood cells, and destructive changes leading to blister formation.

Histologically, pemphigus is characterized by loss of intercellular cement material prior to any morphologic alteration in desmosomal attachments. After losing the desmosomes, cells become acantholytic, round up, and drift into the blister cavity. Intraepidermal blister formation is the hallmark of pemphigus.

Clinical Features

General. The characteristic intraepidermal bullae of pemphigus vulgaris are thin and flaccid. They may form on any part of the body. Slight pressure over areas of normal-appearing skin may cause dislodgement of the epidermis, leaving a denuded raw area (**Nikolsky's sign;** Fig. 4-10). The mucous membranes, particularly the oral mucosa, are frequently involved. The cutaneous bullae, before rupturing, may become pustular. The ruptured blisters show little tendency to heal.

Pemphigus vulgaris may affect any age group, with the possible exception of early childhood. It seems to be more common in people between the ages of 50 and 70.

Ocular Findings. Although rare, the most common type of ocular involvement in pemphigus is inflammation of the conjunctiva presenting as a catarrhal or purulent conjunctivitis (92). Vesicles, which rapidly rupture and erode, may involve the inner canthus or palpebral conjunctiva. These are acutely painful but generally disappear in a week to 10 days, leaving no scar. Some ophthalmologists have stated that repeated bulla formation does lead to conjunctival cicatrization with progressive contraction of the conjuctival sac, especially in the lower fornix (110).

In pemphigus foliaceus, the eyelids may be involved and a mild conjunctivitis may occur (1, 76). The palpebral conjunctiva is usually affected while the bulbar conjunctiva is left intact. The cornea may be affected and vesicles, pannus, and facets may form. Infiltrative and degenerative changes of the iris as well as cataract formation have been seen in South America. In pemphigus erythematosus, the skin of the eyelids may be involved.

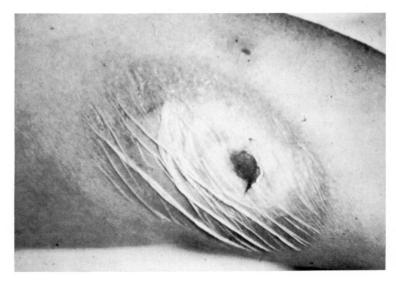

FIG. 4-10. Pemphigus vulgaris: Nikolsky's sign. (Courtesy Dr. J. U. Dy-Liacco)

Treatment

Corticosteroids are the mainstay of treatment in pemphigus and have greatly improved the prognosis of the disease. Usually prednisone is given in doses no lower than 100 mg/day, and sometimes as high as 300 mg/day (96). As the lesions heal the dose may be tapered quite rapidly. Alternate-day corticosteroid therapy has been recommended, starting with doses of 160 mg prednisone every other day (90). Cytotoxic drugs such as azathioprine, cyclophosphamide, and methotrexate have been employed in conjunction with corticosteroids. This combination allows a smaller dose of corticosteroid to be given and minimizes the corticosteroid side effects, while controlling the disease. Such combination therapy has reduced the mortality in pemphigus from 50% to about 8% (93).

Topical antibiotic–corticosteroid therapy has been used to treat the conjunctivitis accompanying pemphigus. The conjunctivitis often responds to systemic treatment at the same time the skin lesions improve. Removal of lashes when trichiasis is present may help to reduce the corneal complications. Artificial tears may be used to provide moisture in situations where tear abnormalities secondary to conjunctival changes exist (84).

CICATRICIAL PEMPHIGOID

Cicatricial pemphigoid (benign mucous membrane pemphigoid, ocular pemphigoid) is a chronic bullous dermatosis affecting primarily the mucous membranes. Wichmann (120), in 1794, reported a case of chronic bullous disease with eye involvement. In 1858, Cooper (23) described a patient having blisters of the skin and conjunctiva. Von Graefe (114) associated essential shrinkage of the conjunctiva with the end-stage of pemphigus. It was not until 1911 that Thost (109) distinguished cicatricial pemphigoid from the various forms of pemphigus. This separation from pemphigus was emphasized by Civatte (21) and Lever (70) on the basis of histopathologic studies.

Cicatricial pemphigoid can be a severe, debilitating, and blinding disease. It is characterized clinically by symblepharon formation, obliteration of the fornices, and corneal ulceration and vascularization. It is one of the most difficult ophthalmologic problems to manage successfully.

Immunopathology

Early studies failed to reveal antibodies to tissue antigens in cicatricial pemphigoid (82, 54), but recent studies (9, 12, 39, 48) have demonstrated tissue-fixed basement membrane zone antibodies, and sometimes circulating basement membrane zone antibodies in serum (Fig. 4-11). The incidence of positive direct immunofluorescence findings appears to be greater in recent years, probably owing to more sensitive techniques. Direct immunofluorescence studies show deposition of IgG or IgA in the basement membrane zone in approximately 40% of cicatricial pemphigoid patients (39). In addition, one may find deposition of IgM, components of the complement system (C1q, C4, C3), properdin, and fibrin (83).

Circulating antibodies were not found at first by indirect immunofluorescence studies (9, 12, 48). More recently, circulating basement membrane zone antibodies have been demonstrated in a small percentage of cicatricial pemphigoid patients, most of them women with extensive disease. Such antibodies may be IgG directed against the basement membrane zone of the patient's normal skin or circulating IgA directed against the patient's normal buccal mucosa (39). The antibodies are usually found in low titers and show more specificity for the patient's tissues than those of other patients. In general, patients with cicatricial pemphigoid are less likely to have circulating antibodies than patients with bullous pemphigoid, a disease in which 85%–90% of patients have positive indirect immunofluorescence findings.

Antinuclear antibodies (ANA) have been demonstrated in two-thirds of patients with ocular manifestations of cicatricial pemphigoid (116). The ANA levels do not appear to correlate with the clinical course of the disease. Circulating intercellular antibodies characteristic of pemphigus have been demonstrated in occasional patients with typical cicatricial pemphigoid (26). Bean (7) has demonstrated circulating basement membrane zone antibodies in 3 of 10 patients with cicatricial pemphigoid. Some degree of specificity exists which may allow antibody to react with one substrate tissue and not another. Thus, one serum might react only with monkey esophagus and human skin but not with other tissues. In some cases, the serum might react

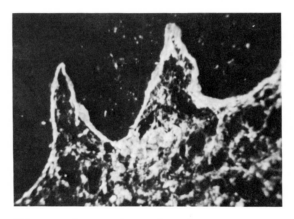

FIG. 4-11. Cicatricial pemphigoid: Basement membrane zone antibody demonstrated by immunofluorescence. (Courtesy Dr. J. U. Dy-Liacco)

only with the patient's own tissues. Such antibody specificity exists in both pemphigus and pemphigoid (7). This specificity may partially account for the small percentage of cicatricial pemphigoid patients with circulating basement membrane zone antibodies. A more likely explanation, however, seems to be that only a small amount of antibody is present and that it binds to basement membrane rather than entering the circulation (7).

The deposition of basement membrane zone antibody in both cicatricial pemphigoid and bullous pemphigoid suggests a relationship between the two diseases. These two conditions may represent a spectrum of similar disease processes with variable overlapping manifestations. Antibody directed against the patient's own tissues suggests an autoimmune pathogenesis. However, autoantibodies may be found in other types of disease associated with tissue destruction, such as viral hepatitis and myocardial infarction. Evidence for and against an autoimmune etiology in chronic bullous diseases has been presented, and currently the issue has not been resolved.

The histopathologic features of cicatricial pemphigoid are similar to those of bullous pemphigoid. Subepidermal bullae and a variably dense eosinophilic and perivascular lymphocytic infiltrate may be found. Neutrophils may also be present. The earliest histologic change found by electron microscopy is intercellular and intracellular edema of basal cells and subjacent endothelial cells. This is followed closely by eosinophil and histiocyte infiltration. The infiltrate in cicatricial pemphigoid is generally more massive, more diffuse, and less perivascular than that found in bullous pemphigoid and may have a significant plasma cell component. Neutrophils may also be plentiful while eosinophils are said to be uncommon in mucosal lesions (83).

Clinical Features

General. Cicatricial pemphigoid is a chronic blistering disease which involves mainly the mucosal epithelium. The mouth and eyes are the areas most frequently involved, but nasal, genital, and occasionally skin lesions may occur. In one series of 65 patients (83), 58 had involvement of the oral mucosa, and 34 had ocular involvement. The pharynx was affected in 30 patients, the skin in 22, and the nose in 18. Other sites of involvement included the genitalia, larynx, epiglottis, esophagus, anus, and urethra. Esophageal involvement may result in recurrent strictures, and laryngeal involvement can be life-threatening. The disease is commonest in patients aged 60 years or older and women are affected twice as often as men. There is no racial or ethnic predilection. The disease is chronic and rarely self-limited. The oral lesions are bullous and often show erosion (Fig. 4-12). The disease usually begins on the gingival or buccal mucosa and often follows dental procedures. A desquamative gingivitis is frequently the initial diagnosis. The hard and soft palate may be affected, and, less often, the uvula, tonsillar pillars, and tongue. Residual scarring may occasionally occur.

Pharyngeal involvement may lead to sore throat and difficulty in swallowing. A stenotic web between the soft palate and nasopharynx may develop and may require digital manipulation to destroy adhesions. Erosive or bullous lesions may develop within the larynx. The epiglottis and arytenoid areas are commonly affected. Life-threatening stenosis of the larynx may require tracheostomy. Esophageal strictures may prevent the patient from eating solid foods and esophageal dilation may be necessary.

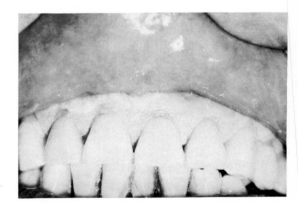

FIG. 4-12. Cicatricial pemphigoid: Bullous lesions of the oral mucosa. (Courtesy Dr. H. B. Ostler)

Genital lesions in the male are vesicular and usually involve the glans penis and foreskin. Scrotal and urethral lesions have also been observed. In the female, the labia majora and minora may be affected as well as the posterior vaginal wall. The anus and perianal tissues may show ulcerative and cicatricial lesions.

The most common sites of skin involvement are the scalp, face, and neck. Vesicular lesions may occur and may have an erythematous or urticarial base. The distal extensor surfaces, axillae, sternum, and umbilicus may be involved.

A number of diseases have been associated with cicatricial pemphigoid. Diabetes mellitus, hypertension, and tuberculosis have been reported to coexist with pemphigoid. The incidence of malignancy in patients with cicatricial pemphigoid is the same as that seen in age- and sex-matched controls with psoriasis or contact dermatitis (107). Most authors believe that no etiologic relationship exists between cicatricial pemphigoid and malignant disease (47).

Ocular Findings. Ocular involvement occurs in 50%–75% of cases in larger series (47, 83). Conjunctival involvement may occur as early as 10 years before or as late as 20 years after the onset of other mucosal or skin lesions. The conjunctiva is the main site of ocular involvement. The disease may begin as a nonspecific conjunctivitis involving one or both eyes. Early symptoms include burning, a foreign body sensation, excessive tearing, sticking to-

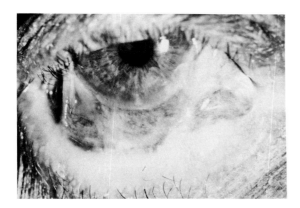

FIG. 4-13. Cicatricial pemphigoid: Symblepharon formation. (Courtesy Dr. H. B. Ostler)

gether of the eyelids, and photophobia. Occasionally, blisters may be seen on the bulbar conjunctiva or lid margins. Hyperemia and thickening of the conjunctiva may be noted and a ropy mucoid discharge may be present.

In later stages, symblepharon formation may occur (Fig. 4-13). Usually the inferior cul de sac is more involved than the superior. Symblepharon formation may progress relentlessly and lead to obliteration of the fornices, total adhesions of the bulbar and palpebral conjunctiva, and restriction of eye movements. Frequently the lacrimal puncta are obliterated. In the later stages, cicatricial entropion may be seen.

The cornea may be severely affected in the later stages of the disease. This is due to a lack of wetting by lid movement, partly from tear deficiency and entropion. The dryness results from progressive scarring of the conjunctiva, obstruction of the lacrimal ducts, and loss of goblet cells from the conjunctiva. The cornea first develops a nonspecific, diffuse, and superficial punctate epithelial keratitis. Subepithelial gray opacities subsequently appear in the periphery. Neovascularization and opacification of the entire cornea may ensue. Total dryness and epidermalization of the cornea may then develop. This can result in a relatively stable but visually disabling situation. Alternately, corneal ulcerations secondary to trichiasis or severe dry eye syndrome can lead to perforation of the cornea. Ocular involvement may be asymmetric but is usually bilateral. Approximately one-quarter of the patients with the disease become blind, most of them in both eyes (47).

Treatment

Corticosteroids are the mainstay of treatment for systemic cicatricial pemphigoid, but they are far from satisfactory in treating the ocular component. Mild cicatricial pemphigoid can frequently be controlled by topical agents. Cytotoxic drugs have been used for their immunosuppressive and steroid-sparing effects; however, their efficacy is unproven in double-blind trials (83). Azathioprine in combination with a corticosteroid is most frequently tried. Cyclophosphamide, antimalarials, sulfapyridine, and dapsone have also been used. Sulfonamides and sulfones have been recommended but not extensively used in cicatricial pemphigoid (83). These medications may be efficaceous, however, in skin lesions having significant polymorphonuclear leukocytic infiltration.

Steroid treatment seems to be of some benefit (47, 83). The risk of complications, while low, must be taken into account. The most common complication is osteoporosis; however, the other well-known complications of corticosteroid therapy may be seen.

The course of the ocular disease is variable and treatment must be adjusted accordingly. In general, the therapy of ocular pemphigoid is disappointing. Various corticosteroid preparations have been given topically, subconjunctivally, and orally but without much benefit. Both topical and systemic corticosteroid therapy may be associated with complications that worsen the course of the disease.

A major complication in ocular pemphigoid is a dry eye syndrome due to loss of goblet cells and stenosis of the lacrimal ducts. Artificial tears and mucus substitutes are often helpful for this aspect of the disease. Surgical occlusion of the puncta may be helpful in preserving the tear film. Transposition of the parotid duct has been employed in some cases to lubricate the outer eye. Soft contact lenses have been useful in maintaining a degree of corneal hydration and in preventing corneal trauma secondary to inturned lashes.

Antimicrobial agents may be necessary if cultures demonstrate colony formation of potential bacterial pathogens. Infectious corneal ulcers may develop secondary to the recurrent corneal erosion and the defective tear film. Specific antibiotic agents should be used, and long-term antimicrobial usage should be avoided if possible. Continuous wearing of soft contact lenses may, however, require long-term topical antibiotic therapy.

DRUG-INDUCED CICATRIZATION

A clinical picture similar to cicatricial pemphigoid can be induced with long-term topical drug therapy (81). Echothiophate iodide can produce symblepharon formation, foreshortening and wrinkling of the conjunctiva, punctal occlusion, epidermalization, trichiasis, and corneal opacification and vascularization when used for several years. Histologically, goblet cells are absent and basement membrane zone staining for IgG is observed. Plasma cells and lymphocytes may be present in the conjunctiva. IgG deposition may be observed between epithelial cells. Topically applied epinephrine has been also implicated in the development of cicatrization (78). Possibly other drugs will be found to induce similar changes.

BULLOUS PEMPHIGOID

This is a chronic bullous disorder which occurs in middle-aged and older patients. It is characterized by tense bullae on an erythematous base involving preferentially the flexor areas of the body. It is a milder disease than pemphigus vulgaris and is characterized by subepidermal rather than intraepidermal blisters. In addition, the mucous membranes are not prominently involved.

Immunopathology

Immunofluorescence studies of bullous pemphigoid lesions have demonstrated the presence of immunoglobulins and complement along the epidermal basement membrane (13, 59). Studies have shown deposition of IgG, IgA, IgM, IgD, and IgE (88). Components of the complement system have included Clq, C4, C3, and C5. In addition, properdin, pro-

perdin factor B, and fibrin have also been demonstrated along the skin basement membrane. The basement membrane staining demonstrated by immunofluorescence in bullous pemphigoid is linear, in contrast to the granular type of staining observed in a type III immune-complex disease such as lupus erythematosus.

The complement levels of blister fluid are markedly decreased in bullous pemphigoid. This suggests local activation of the complement system. Complement activation in this disease is thought to occur by both the classic and alternate pathways since components of both systems have been detected by immunofluorescence (88). Some patients who demonstrate the deposition of alternate pathway components also show deposition of IgE on the skin basement membrane. Since aggregated IgE can activate the complement system, this immunoglobulin may play a role in the disease (53). Serum IgE is elevated in 70% of patients with bullous pemphigoid (2). Using indirect immunofluorescence, it has been demonstrated that possibly 80% of patients have a complement-fixing IgG antibody to skin basement membrane in their serum. Unlike the case in pemphigus, the antibody titer does not seem to parallel the severity of the disease (97).

It has been postulated that antibodies develop against basement membrane; these antibodies can fix complement, causing release of chemotactic factors which bring polymorphonuclear leukocytes to the affected basement membrane (96). These cells release lysosomal enzymes which contain hydrolases and cause destruction of the basal lamina with formation of fluid-filled blisters.

Clinical Features

General. Bullous pemphigoid generally occurs after age 50. Lesions have a predilection for the intertriginous areas. Large tense bullae occur, often eroded and hemorrhagic. It is not possible to extend the blisters by firm pressure, as is the case in pemphigus. Lesions heal spontaneously with crusting. The oral mucosa is affected in about one-third of patients but lesions of other mucous membranes including the conjunctiva are uncommon. This disease should not be confused with cicatricial pemphigoid, which can cause severe ocular complications.

Ocular Findings. Ocular findings in bullous pemphigoid are rare. The lids may be incidentally affected. Conjunctival involvement is uncommon (121).

Treatment

Bullous pemphigoid is a much more benign disease than pemphigus and more amenable to treatment. A potent topical steroid may be applied to the skin lesions with tap-water wet dressings for 30–60 min three to four times a day (96). If this treatment does not control the disease, systemic prednisone 50 or 60 mg/day may be used. Cytotoxic agents have also proved useful in management of bullous pemphigoid.

DERMATITIS HERPETIFORMIS

Dermatitis herpetiformis is another chronic bullous disease which is characterized by intense itching and small groups of vesicles on the skin. The immunologic nature of this disease is supported by the findings of IgA deposition along the epidermal basement membrane in affected patients (20, 38, 111) and a predisposition in individuals with the HLA-B8 histocompatibility antigen.

Immunopathology

Direct immunofluorescence studies have demonstrated the granular deposition of IgA at the dermal–epidermal junction, and less frequently IgG and IgM deposition. C3 may also be found in areas where IgA deposition occurs, but Clq and C4 are only occasionally found. This suggests activation of the complement system mainly by the alternate pathway. In some patients, Clq has been detected in association with IgG or IgM (87). The relationship between IgA and the complement system in this disease is not well understood. IgA is incapable of activating the classic complement sequence; however, aggregated IgA myeloma

protein can activate the alternate complement pathway. Thus, IgA and the alternate complement pathway may be important in the pathogenesis of dermatitis herpetiformis.

Indirect immunofluorescence has not shown detectable anti–basement membrane antibodies in the serum of these patients, and serum complement levels are normal.

Possibly 90% of patients with dermatitis herpetiformis have the histocompatibility antigen HLA-B8, which has a frequency of less than 30% in the general population. Ninety percent of patients with adult celiac disease also have this antigen. This suggests a genetic predisposition of some individuals to develop these diseases (40).

In addition to the skin manifestations, gastrointestinal abnormalities are found in patients with dermatitis herpetiformis (55). Intestinal malabsorption and abnormalities of the jejunal mucosa are present in some patients with this disease. IgA and IgM may be increased in the gastrointestinal fluid. Gluten will induce increased synthesis of IgA in gut tissues of these patients *in vitro*. This suggests a possible relationship to gluten sensitivity. Serum IgA levels are often increased in dermatitis herpetiformis.

The pathogenesis of the disease is unknown. Possibly a hypersensitivity to gluten may develop in genetically susceptible individuals. Antigen entering the gut may stimulate the production of IgA antibody and lead to a patchy intestinal atrophy. This may allow IgA immune complexes to enter the systemic circulation and for some reason be deposited in the skin where they activate the complement system and cause basement membrane damage. Another hypothesis suggests a cross reactivity between the inciting antigen and normal skin structures. These mechanisms are only speculative, however, and the exact reason for the association between the skin disorder and gastrointestinal disease is unknown.

Histologically, the lesions of dermatitis herpetiformis show subepidermal bullous formation and eosinophilic microabscesses in the dermal papillae. Intestinal biopsies have shown a patchy duodenal or jejunal atrophy which is indistinguishable from adult celiac disease.

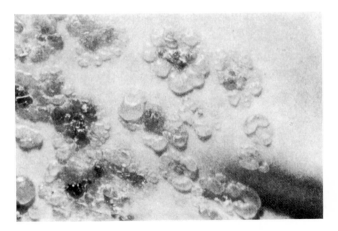

FIG. 4-14. Dermatitis herpetiformis: Typical grouped arrangement of blisters. (Korting GW: The Skin and Eye. Engl. ed. 1973, Georg Thieme Verlag, Stuttgart, Germany)

Clinical Features

Dermatitis herpetiformis may occur at any age. Groups of polymorphous papulovesicular lesions occur on the buttocks, elbows, knees, back, and head (Fig. 4-14). An intense burning pruritus is characteristic of this disease. If untreated, the disease may persist for several years with chronic low-grade activity and acute exacerbations. Although the jejunum and duodenal mucosa may show findings similar to those seen in adult celiac disease, frank malabsorption syndrome is only occasionally observed.

The lids may be involved incidentally, while the conjunctiva is only rarely affected (31).

Treatment

The skin disease may be controlled with dapsone or sulfapyridine. Sytemic corticosteroids are of little value; however, topical steroid creams may reduce the skin irritation. Sulfonamide compounds do not affect the gastrointestinal disease. A gluten-free diet has been associated with improvement of the gastrointestinal lesions, and in one case a prolonged gluten-free diet resulted in clearance of skin lesions (86).

When treated with dapsone, patients may be free of disease for many years but can experience a recurrence within 3–4 days if the medication is discontinued. Prognosis is excellent and no deaths have been reported in this disease.

ERYTHEMA MULTIFORME

Erythema multiforme is an acute bullous eruption which involves the skin and mucous membranes. The cause is unknown, but it is frequently felt to be related to a drug reaction or an infection. It has a minor and a major form. The minor form is milder and associated mainly with cutaneous lesions. The more severe major form frequently shows conjunctival involvement and is therefore of greater concern to the ophthalmologist. It is this latter form of the disease which is often referred to as the **Stevens–Johnson syndrome** (105).

Immunopathology

Erythema multiforme has long been suspected of being a hypersensitivity disease. The precipitating causes may include infectious agents, reactions to drugs, physical factors such as sunlight, cold, or x-ray, and malignancy.

Of the infectious agents associated with

erythema multiforme, one that is commonly mentioned is herpes simplex. Herpes simplex virus has been isolated from throat swabbings in patients with erythema multiforme and there may be a rise in antibody titer to herpes virus in afflicted patients. Additionally, the vesiculobullous lesions of erythema multiforme can be reproduced by intradermal injection of antigen prepared from killed herpes simplex organisms (101). Other organisms have been implicated as well. *Mycoplasma pneumoniae* has been recovered from blister fluid in cases of erythema multiforme. Complement-fixing antibodies to *M. pneumoniae* may also be present. An association also exists between acute histoplasmosis and erythema multiforme. Other viruses (mumps, variola, vaccinia, poliomyelitis), various bacteria (tubercle baccillus, gonococcus), fungi, and protozoa have also been considered etiologic agents (119).

The drugs most often associated with erythema multiforme are the sulfonamides. Long-acting sulfonamides have been suspected for many years as triggering factors, in the Stevens–Johnson syndrome. Other commonly implicated drugs include tetracyclines, penicillin, bromides, iodides, salicylates, barbiturates, phenylbutazone, corticosteroids, and vaccines against poliomyelitis, smallpox, influenza, diphtheria, and tetanus. While many possible etiologies have been proposed in erythema multiforme, none is clearly established as a cause. The disease may represent pathophysiologic events which are precipitated by multiple causes.

The definitive histopathologic lesion of erythema multiforme is not clearly defined. Some feel that diffuse vasculitis and release of necrotizing toxins within the epidermis may occur. The early bullae are formed subdermally and are similar to those seen in cicatricial pemphigoid. The basement membrane of the epidermis may be found in the roofs of the bullae. Severe dermal inflammation may be seen and often the overlying epidermis shows necrosis.

Conjunctival scrapings in these patients show numerous inflammatory cells, including neutrophils and eosinophils. No bacteria are generally seen on scrapings, and cultures usually reveal the normal flora.

Clinical Features

General. Although erythema multiforme may occur at any age, it is most frequently seen in children and young adults. The disease begins with prodromal symptoms that last for several days before the skin lesions appear. During this period, fever, malaise, headache, transient joint pain and swelling, and symptoms of an upper respiratory infection may occur. In the minor form, cutaneous lesions predominate, but in the major form, mucous membranes show extensive involvement. The cutaneous lesions are red in color and have a symmetric distribution, particularly on the extensor surfaces and distal parts of the extremities. The palms and soles are usually involved (Fig. 4–15). The trunk is spared except in severe cases. Typical "iris" or "target" lesions consist of concentric zones of red and white. The central zone is bright red and is surrounded by a pale zone. Peripheral to this pale zone is another red ring. In the major form, tense bullae form beneath these target lesions.

The lips and oral mucosa may show extensive involvement. Raw, painful areas appear where bullae have broken and there may be crusting and a bloody serous exudate. The process may extend to the pharynx, larynx, trachea, and bronchi.

Ocular Findings. Ocular involvement is common in the severe bullous form with mucous membrane involvement (3, 29, 49). The eyelids may be involved in the general eruption and the lid margins may show a hemorrhagic crusting. The conjunctiva is frequently involved in the severe form of the disease (Fig. 4-16). There may be a mild conjunctivitis which resolves without complications, or there may be severe involvement with formation of blisters, pseudomembranes, and symblepharon. A purulent conjunctivitis may develop as a result of secondary infection; the raw conjunctival surfaces may heal with formation of symblepharon or ankyloblepharon. Lid deformities and trichiasis result from cicatricial changes. Loss of the conjunctival goblet cells leads to a tear deficiency and a dry eye syndrome. Corneal complications follow and represent the most serious ocular complication of

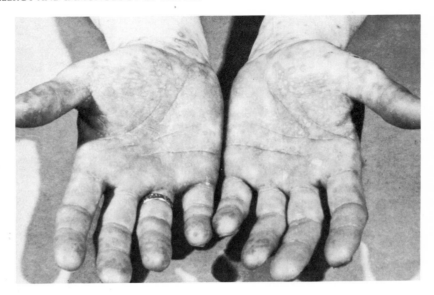

FIG. 4-15. Erythema multiforme: Erythematous rash involving the hands. (Courtesy Dr. G. Mintsioulis)

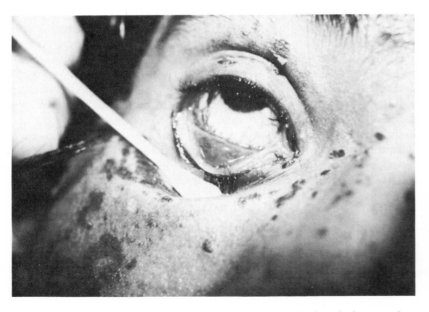

FIG. 4-16. Stevens–Johnson syndrome. Note conjunctival and skin involvement. (Courtesy Dr. R. F. Dennis.)

the disease. Corneal ulceration and even perforation can result. Corneal scarring and vascularization may also develop. Ocular complications are said to occur in as many as 50% of patients with the Stevens–Johnson syndrome (3).

Treatment

During the acute systemic disease, supportive measures and often systemic corticosteroids are used by the internist or dermatologist. Topical corticosteroids have been used to quiet the acute inflammatory ocular disease, but their efficacy has not been proven. Topical antibiotics should be used to treat secondary infections and some have advocated their use to prevent infection. Various measures have been used to prevent the formation of symblepharon, including sweeping the fornices with a glass rod and early tarsorrhaphy (3). There is no concrete evidence that any of these measures will prevent symblepharon formation. It would seem reasonable to maintain good hygiene in these cases and to prevent corneal exposure and epithelial breakdown. Reverse sterile precautions are sometimes used during the acute phase of the disease.

In chronic cases, tear supplements should be used frequently to prevent corneal epithelial breakdown. Soft contact lenses are often useful to help maintain corneal hydration and to prevent erosion by inturned lashes. Lid deformities may be corrected by surgical procedures.

ERYTHEMA NODOSUM

Erythema nodosum is a cutaneous complication of a wide variety of systemic disorders (16, 27). Many of these systemic conditions have ocular manifestations, including sarcoid, Behçet's disease, coccidioidomycosis and cat-scratch fever. Erythema nodosum is characterized by acute, red, painful nodules on the extensor surfaces of the legs and forearms. Immunologic mechanisms are probably important in its pathogenesis.

During the 1930s erythema nodosum was common among patients with active tuberculosis. This association was particularly prevalent in children. Today, erythema nodosum is frequently associated with sarcoid, especially in the Scandinavian countries. In North America, erythema nodosum is more frequently associated with β-hemolytic streptococcal infections and other upper respiratory infections. A list of associated conditions is presented in Table 4-3.

Immunopathology

Erythema nodosum is characterized histologically by a vasculitis. An Arthus-type reaction

TABLE 4-3. CONDITIONS ASSOCIATED WITH ERYTHEMA NODOSUM

Infectious diseases
  Streptococcal infection
  Tuberculosis
  Systemic fungal infections (*e.g.*, coccidioidomycosis, North American blastomycosis, histoplasmosis)
  Psittacosis
  Lymphogranuloma venereum
  Yersinia infections
  Cat-scratch disease
Systemic diseases
  Sarcoidosis
  Inflammatory bowel disease (*e.g.*, ulcerative colitis, regional enteritis)
  Behçet's syndrome
Drugs
  Oral contraceptive agents
  Sulfonamides
  Bromides
  Iodides

(Blomgren SE: Semin Rheumatol 4:1, 1974)

with deposition of circulating immune complexes has been suggested as a possible mechanism. Attempts to demonstrate IgG and IgM antibodies as well as complement components by immunofluorescence techniques have not, however, been successful. Patients with erythema nodosum have a factor in their serum which causes guinea pig macrophages to aggregate (66). This finding suggests the possibility that mediators of cellular immunity may be produced in excess.

Lesions of erythema nodosum are also characterized histologically by the accumulation of leukocytes and by edema and swelling of collagen bundles. The walls of veins are frequently edematous and infiltrated by inflammatory cells. Endothelial cell proliferation and narrowing of vessel lumens may be seen as well.

Clinical Features

The lesions of erythema nodosum are subcutaneous nodules which are red and painful. The extensor surfaces of the legs and arms are most frequently involved. Occasionally, the face, buttocks, and trunk are involved as well. Often, a low-grade fever and migratory polyarthritis may accompany the skin lesions. Women are affected three times more frequently than men. The course is self-limited and lasts approximately 3–5 weeks. Since erythema nodosum generally accompanies a systemic disorder or infectious process, a search should be made for an underlying primary condition.

Treatment

The disease is generally self-limited and does not require drug therapy. Antiinflammatory agents such as aspirin can be given for arthralgias and other discomfort. Corticosteroids are generally not given because of the frequent association of erythema nodosum with an underlying infection. There is also no evidence that they shorten the course of the disease.

VITILIGO

Patients with vitiligo (Fig. 4-17) have a tendency to form autoantibodies directed against thyroid cytoplasm, thyroglobulin, gastric pari-

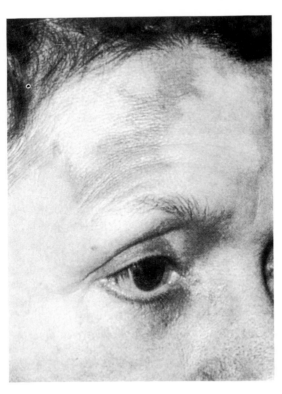

FIG. 4-17. Vitiligo. (Korting GW: The Skin and Eye. Engl. ed. 1973, Georg Thieme Verlag, Stuttgart, Germany)

etal cells, and adrenal cytoplasm (17). Vitiligo is associated clinically with the Vogt–Koyanagi–Harada syndrome, thyroiditis, pernicious anemia, and diabetes mellitus.

REFERENCES

1. Amendola F: Ocular manifestations of pemphigus foliaceus. Am J Ophthalmol 32:35, 1949
2. Arbesman CE, Wypych JI, Reisman RE: Serum IgE in human diseases. In Goodfriend L, Sehon AH, Orange R (eds): Mechanisms in Allergy (Reagin Mediated Hypersensitivity) Immunology (series), Vol 1. New York, Marcel Dekker, 1973, p 163
3. Arstikaitis M: Ocular aftermath of Stevens-Johnson syndrome. Arch Ophthalmol 90:376, 1973
4. Austen KF, Sheffer AL: Detection of hereditary angioneurotic edema by demonstration of a reduction in the second component of human complement. N Engl J Med 272–649, 1965
5. Baker H: Psoriasis: A review, Part II. Dermatologica 150:136, 1975
6. Beall GN: Urticaria: a review of laboratory and clinical observations. Medicine 43:131, 1964
7. Bean SF: Cicatricial pemphigoid. Int J Dermatol 14:23, 1975
8. Bean SF, Holubar K, Gillett RB: Pemphigus involving the eyes. Arch Dermatol 111:1484, 1975
9. Bean SF, Waisman M, Michel B et al: Cicatricial pemphigoid. Arch Dermatol 106:195, 1972
10. Beetham WP: Atopic cataract. Arch Ophthalmol 24:21, 1940
11. Bernstein MJ: A dermatitis caused by dinitrochlor benzole. Lancet 1:1534, 1912
12. Bettelheim H, Zehetbauer G, Kokoschka E et al: Direkte immunofluorescenzoptische Untersuchungenbeim Pemphigus ocularis (narbenbildendes Pemphigoid). Klin Monatsbl Augenheilkd 163:361, 1973
13. Beutner EH, Chorzelski TB, Jordan RE: Autosensitization in pemphigus and bullous pemphigoid. Springfield IL, CC Thomas, 1971, p 143
14. Beutner EH, Jordan RE: Demonstration of skin antibodies in serum of pemphigus vulgaris patients by indirect immunofluorescent staining. Proc Soc Exp Biol Med 117:505, 1964
15. Beutner EH, Lever WF, Witebsky E, Jordan RE, Chertok B: Autoantibodies in pemphigus vulgaris. JAMA 192:682, 1965
16. Blomgren SE: Erythema nodosum. Semin Arthritis Rheum 4:1, 1974
17. Brostoff J: Autoantibodies in patients with vitiligo. Lancet 2:177, 1969

18. Buckley RH, Dees SC: Serum immunoglobulins. III. Abnormalities associated with chronic urticaria in children. J Allergy 40:294, 1967
19. Chase MW: The cellular transfer of cutaneous hypersensitivity to tuberculin. Proc Soc Exp Biol Med 59:134, 1945
20. Chlorzelski TP, Beutner EH, Jablonska S et al: Immunofluorescence studies in the diagnosis of dermatitis herpetiformis and its differentiation from bullous pemphigoid. J Invest Dermatol 56:373, 1971
21. Civatte A: Le diagnostic des dermatoses bulleuses au laboratoire. Arch Belg Derm Syph 5:273, 1949
22. Coles RS, Laval J: Retinal detachments occurring in cataract associated with neurodermatitis. Arch Ophthalmol 48:30, 1952
23. Cooper W: Pemphigus of the conjunctiva. Ophthalmol Hosp Rep 1:155, 1858
24. Copeman PWM: Eczema and keratoconus. Br Med J 2:977, 1965
25. Copeman PW, Winkelman RK: Vascular changes accompanying white dermographism and delayed blanch in atopic dermatitis. Br J Dermatol 81:944, 1969
26. Cram DL, Griffith MR, Fukuyama K: Pemphigus-like antibodies in cicatricial pemphigoid. Arch Dermatol 109:235, 1974
27. Darlington LG: Erythema nodosum and oral contraceptives. Br J Dermatol 90:209, 1974
28. Donaldson V, Evans RR: A biochemical abnormality in hereditary angioneurotic edema. Am J Med 35:37, 1963
29. Duke-Elder S: System of Ophthalmology, Vol 8, Part 1. London, Henry Kimpton, 1965, pp 517–523
30. Duke-Elder S: The Ocular Adnexa. In System of Ophthalmology, Vol 13, Part 1. London, Henry Kimpton, 1974, pp 58–70
31. Duke-Elder S: The Ocular Adnexa. In System of Ophthalmology, Vol 13. London, Henry Kimpton, 1974, p 281
32. Dvorak HF, Dvorak AM: Basophilic leukocytes: structure, function and role in disease. Clin Hematol 4:651, 1975
33. Dvorak HF, Dvorak AM, Simpson BA et al: Cutaneous basophil hypersensitivity. II. A light and electron microscopic study. J Exp Med 132:558, 1970
34. Epstein WL, Maibach HI: Immunologic competence of patients with psoriasis receiving cytotoxic therapy. Arch Dermatol 91:599, 1965
35. Freedman SO, Gold P: Clinical Immunology, 2nd ed. Hagerstown, Harper & Row, 1976, p 204
36. Frank MM, Gelfand JA, Atkinson JP: Hereditary angioedema: the clinical syndrome and its management. Ann Intern Med 84:580, 1976
37. Frank MM, Sergent JS, Kane MA, Alling DW: Epsilon aminocaproic acid therapy of hereditary angioneurotic edema. N Engl J Med 286:808, 1972
38. Fraser NG, Dick HM, Crichton WB: Immunoglobulins in dermatitis herpetiformis and various other skin diseases. Br J Dermatol 81:89, 1969
39. Furey N, West C, Andrews T et al.: Immunofluorescent studies of ocular cicatricial pemphigoid. Am J Ophthalmol 80:825, 1975
40. Gebhard RL, Falchuk ZM, Katz SI et al: Dermatitis herpetiformis: immunologic concomitants of small intestinal disease and relationship to histocompatibility antigen HL–A8. J Clin Invest 54:98, 1974
41. Greaves MW, Plummer VM, McLaughlin P, Stanworth DR: Serum and cell bound IgE in chronic urticaria. Clin Allergy 4:265, 1974
42. Green GR, Koelsche GA, Kerland RR: Etiology and pathogenesis of chronic urticaria. Ann Allergy 23:30, 1965
43. Grob PJ, Inderbitzin TM: Experimental production in rabbits of antiepithelial antibodies. J Invest Dermatol 49:637, 1967
44. Guilhou JJ, Clot J, Meynadier J, Lapinski H: Immunological aspects of psoriasis. I. Immunoglobulins and anti-IgG factors. Br J Dermatol 94:501. 1976
45. Gutterman JU, Maglivit G, Reed R et al: Immunology and immunotherapy of human malignant melanomas: historic review and perspectives for the future. Semin Oncol 2:155, 1975
46. Halprin K: Toxic epidermal necrolysis. In Demis D (ed): Clinical Dermatology, Vol 1. Hagerstown, Harper & Row, 1972
47. Hardy KM, Perry HO, Pingree GC, Kirby TJ Jr: Benign mucous membrane pemphigoid. Arch Dermatol 104:467, 1971
48. Herron BE: Immunologic aspects of cicatricial pemphigoid. Am J Ophthalmol 79:271, 1975
49. Howard G: The Stevens-Johnson syndrome: ocular prognosis and treatment. Am J Opthalmol 55:893, 1963
50. Husz S, Berko G, Schneider I, Simon N: Immunoelectrophoretic changes in Lyell syndrome. Int J Dermatol 13:205, 1974
51. Ingram RM: Retinal detachment associated with atopic dermatitis and cataract. Br J Ophthalmol 49:96, 1965
52. Ishizaka K, Ishizaka T: Identification of IgE antibodies as a carrier of reaginic activity. J Immunol 99:1187, 1967
53. Ishizaka T, Sian CM, Ishizaka K: Complement fixation by aggregated IgE through alternate pathway. J Immunol 108:848, 1972
54. Jablonska S: Immunopathology of bullous diseases. Ann Clin Res 2:7, 1970
55. Jablonska S, Chorzelski TP, Beutner EH et al: Dermatitis herpetiformis and bullous pemphigoid. Arch Dermatol 112:45, 1976
56. Jenner E: An Inquiry into the Causes and Ef-

fects of the Variolae Vaccine, a Disease Discovered in Some Western Counties of England, Particularly Gloucestershire, and Known by the Name of Cow Pox. London, Sampson Low, 1798

57. Johansson SGO, Bennich H, Wide L: A new class of immunoglobulin in human serum. Immunology 14:265, 1968

58. Johannson SGO, Juhlin L: Immunoglobulin E in healed atopic dermatitis and after treatment with corticosteroids and azathioprine. Br J Dermatol 82:10, 1970

59. Jordan RE, Beutner EH, Witebsky E: Basement zone antibodies in bullous pemphigoid. JAMA 200:751, 1971

60. Jordan RE, Schoeter AK, Rogers RS III, Perry HO: Classical and alternate pathway activation of complement in pemphigus vulgaris lesions. J Invest Dermatol 63:256, 1974

61. Kahn G: Eczematoid eruptions in children. Pediatr Clin North Am 22:203, 1975

62. Kaldeck R: Ocular psoriasis. Arch Dermatol 68:44, 1953

63. Karseras AG, Ruben M: Aetiology of keratoconus. Br J Ophthalmol 60:522, 1976

64. Koblenzer PJ: Toxic epidermal necrolysis (TEN, Ritter's Disease) and staphylococcal scalded skin syndrome (SSSS). A description and review. Clin Pediatr 15:724, 1976

65. Koranda FC, Dehmel EM, Kahn CM et al: Cutaneous complications in immunosuppressed renal homograft recipients. JAMA 229:419, 1974

66. Kruger GG, Weston WL, Thorne EG et al: A phenomenon of macrophage aggregation activity in sera of patients with exfoliative erythroderma, erythema multiforme, and erythema nodosum. J Invest Dermatol 60:282, 1973

67. Landsteiner K, Chase MW: Experiments on transfer of cutaneous sensitivity to simple compounds. Proc Soc Exp Biol Med 71:516, 1942

68. Lawrence HS: Transfer in humans of skin sensitivity of tuberculin type with components of disrupted leukocytes. Bull NY Acad Med 32:236, 1956

69. Levantine A, Brostoff J: Immunological responses of patients with psoriasis and the effect of treatment with methotrexate. 93:659, 1975

70. Lever WF: Pemphigus: a histopathologic study. Arch Dermatol 64:727, 1951

71. Levine MI: Chronic urticaria. J Allergy Clin Immunol 55:276, 1975

72. Lobitz WC Jr, Campbell DJ: Physiologic studies in atopic dermatitis (disseminated neurodermatitis). I. The local cutaneous response to intradermally injected acetylcholine and epinephrine. Arch Dermatol 67:575, 1953

73. Lobitz WC, Honeyman JF, Winkler NW: Suppressed cell-mediated immunity in two adults with atopic dermatitis. Br J Dermatol 86:317, 1972

74. Manganotti G, Silvestri U: Contributo allo studio della sindrome di Lyell. Arch Ital Dermatol 32:192, 1964

74a. Mathias CGT, Maibach HI, Irvine A, Adler W: Allergic contact dermatitis to echothiophate iodide and phenylephrine. Arch Ophthalmol 97:286, 1979

75. McGready SJ, Buckley RH: Depression of cell mediated immunity in atopic eczema. J Allergy Clin Immunol 56:393, 1975

76. Michel B, Thomas C, Levine M et al: Cicatricial pemphigoid and its relationship to ocular pemphigus and essential shrinkage of the conjunctiva. Ann Ophthalmol 7:11, 1975

77. Michel RG, Hudson WR, Pope TH: Angioneurotic edema. Arch Otolaryngol 101:544, 1975

78. Norn MS: Pemphigoid related to epinephrine treatment. Am J Ophthalmol 83:138, 1977

79. Osler W: Hereditary angioneurotic edema. Am J Med Sci 95:362, 1888

80. Ostler HB, Conant M, Groundwater J: Lyell's disease, the Stevens-Johnson syndrome and exfoliative dermatitis. Trans Am Acad Ophthalmol Otolaryngol 74:1254, 1970

81. Patten JT, Cavanagh HD, Allansmith MR: Induced ocular pseudopemphigoid. Am J Ophthalmol 82:272, 1976

82. Peck SM, Osserman KE, Weiner LB et al: Studies in bullous diseases. Immunofluorescent serologic tests. N Engl J Med 279:951, 1968

83. Person J, Rogers RS: Bullous and cicatricial pemphigoid. Clinical, histopathologic and immunopathologic correlations. Mayo Clin Proc 52:54, 1977

84. Podos S: Oculocutaneous disease. In Demis D (ed): Clinical Dermatology, Vol 4. Hagerstown, Harper & Row, 1972

85. Prausnitz C, Kustner H: Studien Uber die Uberempfindlichkeit. Zentralbe Bakteriol. Parasitol, Infekt Hyg 86:160–169, 1921

86. Provost TT: Dermatologic Diseases. In Fudenberg HH, Stites DP, Caldwell JC, Wells JV (eds): Basic and Clinical Immunology. Los Altos, Lange, 1976, p 506

87. Provost TT, Tomasi TB: Evidence for the activation of complement via the alternate pathway in skin disease. II. Dermatitis herpetiformis. Clin Immunol Immunopathol 3:178, 1974

88. Provost TT, Tomasi TB: Immunopathology of bullous pemphigoid. Clin Exp Immunol 18:193, 1974

89. Psoriatic arthritis (editorial). Lancet 2:554, 1976

90. Rabhan NB, Kopf AW: Alternate-day prednisone therapy for pemphigus vulgaris. Arch Dermatol 103:615, 1971

91. Rachelefsky GS, Opelz G, Mickey MR et al:

Defective T cell function in atopic dermatitis. J Allergy Clin Immunol 57:569, 1976

92. Rook A, Wilkinson D, Ebling F (eds): Textbook of Dermatology, 2nd ed. Oxford, Blackwell, 1972

93. Rosenberg FR, Sanders S, Nelson CT: Pemphigus: a 20-year review of 107 patients treated with corticosteroids. Arch Dermatol 112:962, 1976

94. Ruddy S, Gigli I, Austen KF: The complement system of man. N Engl J Med 287:489, 545, 592, 632, 1972

95. Russell TF, Schultes LM, Kuban DJ: Histocompatibility (HL-A) antigens associated with psoriasis. N Engl J Med 287:738, 1972

96. Sams WM: Pemphigus and pemphigoid: dermatologic example of Type II immune reactivity. Ann Allergy 37:255, 1976

97. Sams WM, Jordan RE: Correlation of pemphigoid and pemphigus antibody titers with activity of the disease. Br J Dermatol 84:7, 1971

98. Sams WM, Jordan RE: Pemphigus antibodies: their role in disease. J Invest Dermatol 56:474, 1971

99. Schorr WF, Mohajerin AH: Paraben sensitivity. Arch Dermatol 93:721, 1966

100. Sheffer AC: Urticaria and angioedema. Pediatr Clin North Am 22:193, 1975

101. Shelley WB: Herpes simplex virus as a cause of erythema multiforme. JAMA 201:153, 1967

102. Solomon LM, Nadler NJ: Radioautography of nor-adrenaline-14$_c$ in atopic dermatitis. Can Med Assoc J 96:1147, 1967

103. Spencer WH, Fisher JJ: The association of keratoconus with atopic dermatitis. Am J Ophthalmol 47:332, 1959

104. Stein J, Turk E: Beitrag zum Epidermolyse-Syndrome (Lyell) im Kindesalter. Dtsch Ges Wes 22:2125, 1963

105. Stevens AM, Johnson FC: A new eruptive fever associated with stomatitis and ophthalmia: report of two cases in children. Am J Dis Child 24:526, 1922

106. Stone SP, Muller SA, Gleich GJ: IgE levels in atopic dermatitis. Arch Dermatol 108:806, 1973

107. Stone SP, Shroeter AL: Bullous pemphigoid and associated malignant neoplasms. Arch Dermatol 111:991, 1975

108. Stuart JA: Ocular psoriasis. Am J Ophthalmol 55:615, 1963

109. Thost A: Der chronische Schleimhautpemphigus der oberen Luftwege. Arch Otorhinolaryngol (NY) 25:459, 1911

110. Thygeson P: Dermatosis with ocular manifestations. In Sorsby A (ed): Modern Ophthalmology, Vol 2. Philadelphia, Lippincott, pp 559–586

111. Van Der Meer JB: Granular deposits of immunoglobulins in the skin of patients with dermatitis herpetiformis: an immunofluorescent study. Br J Dermatol 81:493, 1969

112. Van Scott EJ: Therapy of psoriasis 1975. JAMA 235:197, 1976

113. Van Scott EJ, Farber EM: Disorders with epidermal proliferation. In Fitzpatrick T, et al (eds): Dermatology in General Medicine. New York, McGraw-Hill, 1971, pp 228–230

114. Von Graefe A (Cited by Taylor RF): Modern treatment of severe shrinkage of the conjunctiva. Br J Ophthalmol 51:31, 1967

115. Walinder PE, Gip L, Stempa M: Corneal changes in patients treated with clofazimine. Br J Ophthalmol 60:526, 1976

116. Waltman S, Yarian D: Circulating autoantibodies in ocular pemphigoid. Am J Ophthalmol 77:891, 1974

117. Wenner HA: Complications of infantile eczema caused by the virus of herpes simplex. Am J Dis Child 67:247, 1944

118. White SH, Newcomer V, Mickey M, Terasaki P: Disturbance of HL-A antigen frequency in psoriasis. N Engl J Med 287:740, 1972

119. Whitmore PV: Skin and mucous membrane disorders. In Duane T (ed): Clinical Ophthalmology. Hagerstown, Harper & Row, 1976

120. Wichmann JE: Ibdeen zur Diagnostik: Beobachtenden Aertzen Mitgetheilet, Vol 1. Hanover, Germany, Helwing 1794, p 89

121. Wilson LA, Grayson M: Oculodermatologic disorders. In Duane T (ed): Clinical Ophthalmology. Hagerstown, Harper & Row, 1976

122. Winkelman RK: Nonallergic factors in atopic dermatitis. J Allergy 37:29, 1966

123. Wood GW, Beutner EH, Chorzelski TP: Studies in immunodermatology. II. Production of pemphigus-like lesions by intradermal injection of monkeys with Brazilian pemphigus foliaceous sera. Int Arch Allergy 42:456, 1972

FIVE
FIVE
FIVE

immunology of ocular infections

We live in close contact with a large variety of microorganisms. They are present everywhere in our environment and they populate the body surfaces exposed to that environment. An individual with a normally functioning immune system can live in harmony with these bacteria, viruses, and fungi, but when the immune system is compromised, the body's microflora can invade its host and produce disease. A normally functioning immune system is also required to ward off certain pathogenic microorganisms which are not part of the normal flora of the skin and mucous membranes. Defense against these organisms requires augmentation of the normal immune response. In this chapter, we will examine the defenses which prevent the invasion of the host by microorganisms. We will also consider the specific agents which infect the eye and the mechanisms by which the immune system responds to these assaults.

RESISTANCE TO INFECTION

HOST DEFENSES AT BODY SURFACES

The first-line defenses against microorganisms are an impressive group of relatively nonspecific factors which operate wherever there is contact between the host and the outside environment. Microorganisms are discharged from the conjunctiva by tearing, from the oral cavity by salivation, and from the respiratory tract by coughing and sneezing. In a similar manner, desquamation of the skin sheds large numbers of adherent microorganisms.

Any disturbance in the barrier function of the skin or mucous membranes can influence the local invasion by microorganisms (48). Trauma, moisture, a change in temperature, or chemical irritation can all affect local resistance to bacterial invasion. In Sjögren's syndrome, a decrease in the natural flow of tears diminishes the resistance of the surface of the eye to microbial invasion. In addition, lysozyme, a cationic low-molecular-weight enzyme normally present in tears, saliva, and nasal secretions, is markedly reduced in Sjögren's syndrome (see Ch. 3).

The body may prevent invasion of certain microorganisms by other local factors such as pH and the composition of the normal flora. Secretory IgA appears to play a key role in preventing mucosal invasion of several microorganisms, but the exact mechanism for this activity is unknown. Secretory IgA seems to prevent bacterial attachment to mucosal cells. It may also produce lysis of bacteria in the presence of complement and lysozyme, and augment phagocytosis and opsonization of microorganisms (see Polymorphonuclear Neutrophils). The mucous membranes are often a portal of entry for microbial pathogens and are in general more easily penetrated by microorganisms than the skin is. In order for a pathogen to infect a mucosal surface, it must first attach to an epithelial cell surface. Attachment is influenced by the structure of the microorganism. For example, the gonococcus has specialized pili (hairlike proteinaceous appendages) which facilitate adherence to the mucosal surface. Some organisms are capable of synthesizing polymers or antiphagocytic substances which prevent their destruction. For example, *Neisseria meningitidis* produces an IgA protease which inactivates secretory IgA.

SYSTEMIC IMMUNITY TO INFECTION

Cellular Responses

Once the microorganism has succeeded in penetrating the surface defenses of the host, it must face the second line of defense, the phagocytic cells (12). These wandering cells are capable of ingesting the invading microorganisms. Those which escape ingestion evoke an inflammatory response characterized by dilatation of blood vessels, increased vascular permeability, and migration of inflammatory cells. The two main types of phagocytic cells are the neutrophil and the mononuclear phagocyte, although endothelial cells, epithelial cells, and fibroblasts also have phagocytic properties under specialized conditions. The neutrophil and monocyte have specialized receptors which enhance their phagocytic abilities. The neutrophil is particularly concerned with ingestion of extracellular pathogens such as the pneumococcus. The mononuclear phagocyte is capable of eliminating microorganisms which reside intracellularly. Thus, mononuclear cells are most important in chronic infections, and their activity can be further augmented by sensitized lymphocytes.

Polymorphonuclear Neutrophils

Neutrophils are produced in the bone marrow and circulate with a half-life of 6–7 h. These actively phagocytic cells are brought to a site of inflammation by chemotactic factors which are mostly of host origin. Components of the complement system (C3a, C5a, and C567) are the most important chemotactic factors for neutrophils (137). Activated lymphocytes also generate a chemotactic factor for neutrophils. Neutrophils are highly mobile cells and are the first cells to accumulate at the site of inflammation.

Phagocytosis of microorganisms by neutrophils is enhanced by the process known as **opsonization. Opsonins** are substances which coat bacteria and make them more susceptible to phagocytosis. The two main opsonins are

antibody and complement. Opsonization may take place by a coating of the microorganism 1) with specific antibody alone, 2) with specific antibody in the presence of components of the classic complement pathway, or 3) by nonspecific, heat-labile antibody acting in conjunction with components of the alternate complement pathway. The third mechanism is important in the early preimmune stages of infection. Natural antibodies, normally present in serum, may also act as opsonins. Ingestion may also be accomplished by surface phagocytosis, in which encapsulated bacteria are trapped between leukocytes, between leukocytes and tissue surfaces, or with fibrin clots.

Neutrophils process microorganisms through a series of four steps: 1) Ingestion is accomplished when a microbe comes in contact with the neutrophil cell membrane. The particle becomes encased in a phagocytic vesicle, or phagosome, which buds off from the cell periphery and moves into the cell. 2) Cytoplasmic granules containing hydrolytic lysosomal enzymes fuse with the phagosome and degranulate, releasing the granule contents into the phagosome. 3) The microorganism is destroyed by oxidative and nonoxidative killing mechanisms. 4) Digestion takes place and the phagocytic process is terminated (19).

Mononuclear Phagocytes

Mononuclear phagocytes are produced in the bone marrow, circulate with a half-life of 8½h, and leave the circulation to become mature tissue macrophages. Components of the complement system, especially C5a, are chemotactic for monocytes, as are lymphokines from sensitized lymphocytes. Monocytes and macrophages ingest microorganisms and are capable of destroying them with lysosomal enzymes. Some microorganisms may escape this type of killing and survive intracellularly by preventing fusion between the phagosome and lysosome.

Humoral Immunity

Antibodies may participate in bacterial cell lysis, particularly in gram-negative infections where antibodies may be directed against cell wall antigens. This type of lysis occurs in the presence of complement. Antibodies to gram-positive bacteria more often act as opsonins, coating the microorganisms and making them more susceptible to phagocytosis (10). Antibodies are also important in controlling certain viral infections, especially those in which virus spreads extracellularly. In other types of viral infection, cellular immunity and interferon seem to be of greater importance than antibody.

Cell-Mediated Immunity

Sensitized T lymphocytes and cell-mediated immunity are important in acquired resistance to a wide variety of intracellular microorganisms. Macrophages process antigen and facilitate the engagement of antigen-sensitive T lymphocytes. As noted previously, activated T lymphocytes can produce the soluble mediators, lymphokines, which control the accumulation of mononuclear phagocytes at the focus of infection. Sensitized lymphocytes may also activate the hydrolytic granules within macrophages and stimulate these cells to destroy microorganisms. Such activated macrophages can act nonspecifically to limit infection by organisms other than those responsible for their activation. However, they are usually more efficient at eliminating the sensitizing microorganisms than an organism not previously encountered. Immunity to intracellular organisms can often be transferred to unsensitized animals with activated lymphocytes. This process, known as **adoptive immunity,** confers specific immunity on the recipient animal.

MAJOR TRANSPLANTATION ANTIGENS IN HOST RESPONSES TO INFECTION

All known T cell functions depend on recognizing a foreign (*e.g.,* viral) antigen as well as host, antigen. Virus-specific cytotoxic T cells are thus "genetically restricted" cells and will act only upon the host's target cells since they are genetically identical to the host's T cells (174). Cell surface transplantation antigens appear to be important in the T cell's recognition of the host; these cell surface antigens are de-termined by the major histocompatibility complex.

The concept of dual specificity seems to apply also to destruction of intracellular bacteria such as *Listeria monocytogenes.* Unlike cell-mediated responses, antibody-mediated immune phenomena (opsonization, antibody-plus-complement–mediated lysis, and antibody-dependent cytolytic cell activity) are not restricted genetically and are responsive only to foreign antigenic determinants characteristic of the pathogen.

BACTERIAL INFECTIONS

STAPHYLOCOCCAL INFECTIONS

The staphylococcus is one of the most commonly encountered ocular pathogens. It can cause disease of the lids, conjunctiva or cornea. The organism contains several virulent factors, such as coagulase, α-toxin, lipase, leukocidin, enterotoxin, exfoliatin, and protein A. Coagulase production is the major feature which distinguishes *S. aureus* from the less virulent *S. epidermidis* (96). α-Toxin is thought to be important as the cause of dermal necrosis. Exfoliatin causes separation of the epidermis at the granular cell layer and is important in producing the skin lesions of toxic epidermal necrolysis.

Immunopathology

Neutrophils are considered to be the major defense against infection due to *S. aureus* (96). They appear rapidly, ingest the organism, and kill it. Protein A and other components of the bacterium seem to be chemotactic for neutrophils. Protein A has the unique ability to bind the Fc portion of opsonic IgG and to act essentially as an antiphagocytic surface factor.

IgG antibodies to various components of *S. aureus* appear during the acute and chronic phases of staphylococcal infection. Specific antibodies do not lead to bacterial lysis, but phagocytosis is enhanced by the presence of specific opsonizing antibody and complement. Cellular immune responses may help to localize staphylococcal infections and limit their spread but such inflammatory responses may also contribute to tissue damage. It is not precisely known to what extent humoral and cellular immune mechanisms participate in limiting staphylococcal infections.

Clinical Features

S. aureus may be cultured from the lid margins of at least one-third of subjects without apparent lid disease (9). The staphylococcus is probably the most common cause of blepharitis and is often refractory to treatment. Staphylococcal blepharitis is characterized by ulceration of the lid margins, formation of collarettes and fibrinous scales around the eyelashes, localized poliosis, broken, misdirected, and sparse eyelashes, multiple recurrent chalazions, and fine epithelial keratitis or catarrhal corneal ulcers (129). Staphylococcal blepharitis may be associated with other conditions which impair the local immunity of the lid margins (Fig. 5-1). Patients with atopic dermatitis have a higher than normal incidence of staphylococcal infection, as do patients with keratoconjunctivitis sicca, rosacea, and seborrheic dermatitis. A chronic papillary conjunctivitis is often seen and is probably due to the necrotizing toxin produced by the organism (rather than to colonization of the conjunctiva by staphylococci).

Internal and external hordeolums and possibly meibomianitis may result from staphylococcal infection of the lids. These infections are chronic and often difficult to eradicate. An **external hordeolum** (or **stye**) is essentially a staphylococcal abscess inside the lumen of a gland of Zeis which points to the skin side of the eyelid. An **internal hordeolum** (or **acute chalazion**) is usually caused by an acute staphylococcal infection of a meibomian gland. It may point to either the skin side or the conjunctival side.

Catarrhal infiltrates occur just inside the limbus at the 2, 4, 8, and 10 o'clock positions—sites of contact between the lid margins and cornea (Fig. 5-2). These infiltrates probably represent reactions between antibody and staphylococcal antigens or exotoxin. A lucid interval is seen between the infiltrate and the limbus, possibly because of the removal of antigen by the limbal blood vessels. Occasionally, multiple staphylococcal infiltrates coalesce to form a ring just inside the limbus. There have been some reports of catarrhal marginal ulcers associated with *Haemophilus aegyptius*, *Moraxella lacunata*, and hemolytic streptococci (145).

Toxic keratoconjunctivitis has been produced in rabbits and in human volunteers by the topical application of a filtrate prepared from a culture of *S. aureus* (3, 144). A necrotizing toxin is thought to be responsible for the keratoconjunctivitis, which affects the conjunctiva and predominantly the lower half of the cornea. A less severe clinical picture is

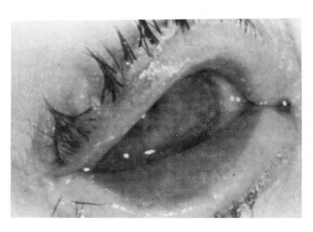

FIG. 5-1. Staphylococcal blepharitis in 10-year-old child with panhypogammaglobulinemia.

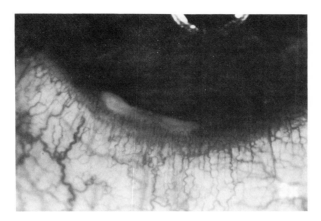

FIG. 5-2. Catarrhal infiltrate accompanying staphylococcal blepharitis. (Courtesy Dr. G. Mintsioulis)

produced by topical application of filtrates from *S. epidermidis* (157).

Phlyctenulosis is most commonly seen as a sequela of staphylococcal infection, although at one time tuberculosis was most commonly associated with this condition. Phlyctenulosis is thought to represent a delayed hypersensitivity reaction to bacterial antigen. The first phlyctenule appears at the limbus but subsequent ones may affect the conjunctiva, cornea, or both. The lesion ulcerates late in its 10- to 14-day course, leaving a limbus-based triangular scar which is pathognomonic. Corneal perforations occasionally occur (107) but are rare. Other causes of phlyctenulosis include *Candida albicans, Coccidioides immitis,* the organism of lymphogranuloma venereum, and certain nematodes (58, 147).

Central corneal ulcers and postoperative endophthalmitis are frequently caused by the staphylococcus (9), and in some areas it is the most common pathogen associated with these two entities. Skin diseases caused by staphylococci may affect the eyelids. These include impetigo contagiosa (see Streptococcal Infections), infectious eczematoid dermatitis, and toxic epidermal necrolysis (see in Ch. 4).

Treatment

Treatment of chronic staphylococcal blepharitis consists of lid hygiene and application of topical antibiotic ointments. Erythromycin and bacitracin are particularly effective, but the choice of an antibiotic should be based on cultures and antibiotic sensitivity patterns. In recalcitrant cases, systemic antibiotic therapy may be of value. Catarrhal infiltrates may respond dramatically to low-dose topical corticosteroids but those associated with staphylococci do not respond as dramatically as other types (107). Staphage lysate has been useful in those patients with persistent staphylococcal infections who have a marked reaction to the first subcutaneous injection of the lysate. This material is prepared from a broth culture of virulent staphylococci that have been completely lysed by a bacteriophage, causing the organism's entire cytoplasm to be released (127). Increasing doses of staphage lysate are injected until clinical improvement is seen. The mechanism of action of this material is unknown, but presumably stimulation of the immune system is involved.

Nonpathogenic staphylococci can be used to colonize the lids and to overgrow and crowd out the pathogenic organisms. This method has been used successfully in chronic staphylococcal skin infections but has not been widely used in the treatment of ocular disease.

STREPTOCOCCAL INFECTIONS

The genus *Streptococcus* can be divided into a number of immunologically specific groups (designated A through O) on the basis of the

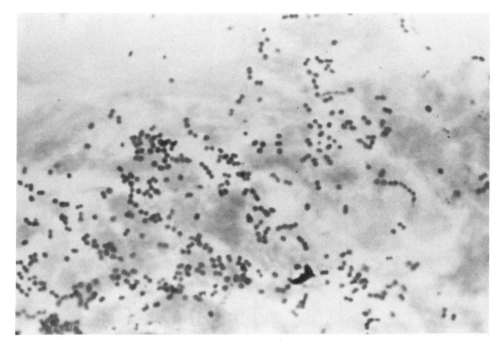

FIG. 5-3. Streptococci in scraping from corneal ulcer. Note tendency of organisms to form chains. (Courtesy Mr. M. Okumoto)

presence of group-specific carbohydrate antigens in their cell walls. The important etiologic agents in human infections are groups A, B, and D. The streptococcus is a gram-positive coccus found in chains of varying length (Fig. 5-3). They may be very fastidious organisms and require blood or an enriched medium for growth. In the eye, they can produce conjunctivitis, keratitis, or an endophthalmitis.

Immunopathology

The streptococcus possesses two antiphagocytic surface components: hyaluronic acid, which is not immunogenic, and M protein. M proteins are cell wall components associated with virulence. The M protein and the hyaluronate capsule are the chief factors that protect the organism locally from ingestion and phagocytosis (14). Organisms lacking M protein are readily phagocytized and killed in the absence of type-specific antibody.

Streptolysins are responsible for β-hemolysis. Except for streptolysin S, all known extracellular products of group A streptococci are antigenic. Antibody titers to one or more of

these antigens can be determined if a recent streptococcal infection has occurred. The antibody most commonly measured is streptolysin O, which usually increases 3 weeks after most streptococcal pharyngitis. One exception is in patients with impetigo. Here, a feeble antistreptolysin O response occurs, owing to binding of streptolysin O by skin cholesterol, which thus prevents the enzyme from serving as an effective antigen.

Several other streptococcal enzymes are antigenic and elicit good antibody responses (14). These include hyaluronidase, desoxyribonuclease B, and diphosphopyridine nucleotidase. Measurements of these antibodies are useful clinically in determining past streptococcal infection. Erythrogenic toxin is another extracellular product produced by the streptococcus. It is responsible for the rash of scarlet fever and probably some of the toxic symptoms of that disease.

Clinical Features

The eyelids may be affected by impetigo contagiosa and facial erysipelas. **Impetigo conta-**

giosa is a superficial pyoderma occurring primarily in children. The lesions begin as small vesicles which rapidly evolve into discrete pustules with little or no erythema. They acquire an amber crust and then develop a thick purulent crust tacked onto an erythematous base. Streptococci, staphylococci, or in some cases both organisms can be isolated. Acute glomerulonephritis may sometimes be associated with streptococcal impetigo (30). **Erysipelas** is a superficial cellulitis caused mainly by group A streptococci and affecting children and the elderly. The lesions begin with small breaks in the skin, often on the head and face. They become hot and red, and develop sharply raised, indurated borders. There may be vesicles or bullae containing seropurulent material and often systemic signs of chills, fever, headaches, and joint pains. In erysipelas, eyelid involvement occurs frequently since the disease most commonly affects the face and spreads easily to the lids. Erysipelas often arises through small excoriations of the skin such as those caused by a shield after cataract surgery or by poorly fitting eyeglasses. The cornea and conjunctiva may also be affected, and a pseudomembranous or membranous keratoconjunctivitis may develop. Orbital and cavernous sinus involvement have on occasion supervened.

Infectious eczematoid dermatitis may in rare instances be caused by streptococcal infection but this can only be differentiated from staphylococcal disease by culture. Acute cellulitis may be caused by streptococci; it usually begins in traumatized areas. As the affected area enlarges it may be accompanied by systemic symptoms. Streptococcal gangrene can occasionally affect the eyelids following cellulitis. The central area becomes blue-black or necrotic 3–4 days after the cellulitis begins.

Treatment

Streptococcal impetigo and infectious eczematoid dermatitis are easily treated with topical erythromycin or bacitracin ointment. Erysipelas, a comparatively deep infection, requires the use of systemic antibiotics or sulfonamides. Cellulitis and gangrene also require systemic treatment, with penicillin.

PNEUMOCOCCAL INFECTIONS

Streptococcus pneumoniae (pneumococcus) is a true corneal pathogen and one of the most frequent causes of central bacterial corneal ulcers. Unlike the case with opportunistic pathogens, pneumococcal corneal infection may occur in the absence of immunosuppression or when an overwhelming inoculum of the infectious agent is encountered.

Immunopathology

S. pneumoniae is a gram-positive, lancet-shaped diplococcus. The organism possesses a capsule, and 82 antigenically specific capsular polysaccharides have been recognized. These capsular polysaccharides serve an antiphagocytic function but the precise method by which they inhibit phagocytosis is unknown. The amount of capsular material appears to be directly proportionate to the organism's virulence. The pneumococcal polysaccharide may be dissociated from the surface of the microorganism, and a high level of capsular antigen in the bloodstream is associated with a less favorable prognosis in pneumococcal pneumonia. Other immunogenic constituents of the microorganism (C substance, M protein) have been identified but do not appear to play an important role in virulence or host responses.

Immunologic diagnosis is often helpful in pneumococcal infection. The **Quellung phenomenon** is a swelling of the polysaccharide capsule in the presence of specific antiserum. Pneumococcal capsular polysaccharide antigen can be detected in the blood and other body fluids by a variety of immunologic techniques. A polyvalent antiserum also assists in the rapid identification of the organism.

Clinical Features

S. pneumoniae has historically been a common cause of central corneal ulcers even in the absence of a compromised cornea (146). Type 4 pneumococcus has been the agent most often associated with such infections (101). The ulcer begins rapidly, after an abrasion, often within 24–48 h. It spreads in a serpiginous fashion from the original site of infection to the center of the cornea. The advancing border has a gray or yellow cloudy infiltrative appearance. Active ulceration occurs at the advancing edge, while the trailing edge shows signs of healing. The lesion begins superficially but deep involvement may follow quite rapidly. The surrounding cornea will often remain relatively clear. A moderately large hypopyon is frequently present. Marked thinning and ectasia of the cornea may be recognized early by hypotony and by the appearance of tiny points of blood at the base of the ulcer (143).

S. pneumoniae may be found on the lid margins or in the conjunctival sac. It often is harbored in the lacrimal sac of patients who have intermittent or continuous occlusion of the nasolacrimal duct. The organism may be associated with a conjunctivitis but there have been no reports of a corneal ulcer arising from a preexisting pneumococcal conjunctivitis. This may be due to the lack of capsule formation in organisms causing conjunctivitis.

Treatment

Penicillin is the drug of choice in pneumococcal infections, although erythromycin and bacitracin are also effective. Tetracycline-resistant and erythromycin-resistant strains have occasionally been encountered.

PSEUDOMONAS INFECTIONS

Pseudomonas aeruginosa is a slender, gram-negative rod (Fig. 5-4). It is a frequent cause of ocular infections such as corneal ulcers, endophthalmitis, meibomianitis, and blepharoconjunctivitis.

Immunopathology

Pseudomonas infection is common in the compromised host. Conditions predisposing to *Pseudomonas* infection include congenital immunologic deficiency (*e.g.*, agammaglobulinemia), immunologic immaturity (*e.g.*, prematurity in infants), and immunologic suppression (*e.g.*, from many cancers; in transplant patients, particularly those with granulocytopenia) (171). A special predisposing condition is cystic fibrosis. The organism has the ability to invade vascular walls, which often leads to gangrenous skin lesions, and it may produce a local vasculitis with necrotic, hemolytic lesions

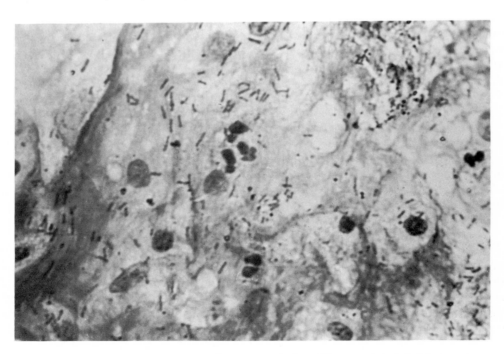

FIG. 5-4. *Pseudomonas* in scraping from corneal ulcer (Courtesy Mr. M. Okumoto)

of the skin and underlying tissues. The organism can produce rapid and extensive liquefaction necrosis. This is thought to be due to the production of pseudomonal proteases. These enzymes can attack corneal proteoglycans, which ordinarily insulate the corneal collagen and maintain interfibrillar attachments (73). The enzymatic attack leads to dispersal of collagen fibers, weakening of the corneal stroma, and, ultimately, corneal perforation. A serious problem with hospital-acquired *Pseudomonas* infections is that the causative organism has frequently been subjected to intense unnatural selection so that the predominate strains tend to be those most resistant to drug therapy (171). The development of drug resistance appears to be associated with the so-called R factors, which can be passed from strain to strain or from species to species.

Clinical Features

Pseudomonas is the most frequent cause of central bacterial corneal ulcers today. The lesion begins with a gray infiltrate around an abrasion or laceration and is associated with severe pain. Owing to the production of proteases, the ulcer spreads rapidly in all directions, accompanied by a loss of corneal stromal substance. The ulcer usually is round and has a gray center. A large hypopyon is typically seen. A mucopurulent discharge with a greenish color is sometimes present. Corneal rings have been described in association with gram-negative organisms, particularly *Pseudomonas*, and recent studies suggest that endotoxin and components of the alternate complement pathway are involved in their production (92).

    Pseudomonas is a ubiquitous organism and may be cultured from many sites. It is a frequent contaminant of eye solutions, especially those containing fluorescein and physostigmine (eserine) (159). It may also be cultured from mascara and has been associated with corneal ulcers following corneal abrasions with mascara brushes (167).

    Pseudomonas is a common inhabitant of the meibomian glands in patients who have recovered from erythema multiforme with mucous membrane involvement. Occasionally it is associated with chronic dacryocystitis or chronic meibomian infection (143).

Treatment

Pseudomonas usually responds well to treatment with gentamicin or carbenicillin. The latter drug is more effective if there is a deficiency of granulocytes (171). Tobramycin is also an effective drug in the treatment of *Pseudomonas* infections and has been used to treat experimental *Pseudomonas* keratitis (24). Effective therapy calls for rapid identification of the organism and intensive treatment with topical and periocular antibiotics.

NEISSERIA INFECTIONS

Acute purulent conjunctivitis results from infection with *Neisseria gonorrhoeae*. A much rarer and usually milder conjunctivitis may be caused by *Neisseria meningitidis*. Gonococcal conjunctivitis is becoming more important because of its increasing incidence and the development of penicillin-resistant strains.

Immunopathology

Neisseria is a gram-negative diplococcus which resides both intra- and extracellularly. It is most easily cultured on chocolate or Thayer–Martin medium. The gonococcus attaches to mucosal surfaces by means of pili, hairlike proteinaceous appendages which are present on virulent gonococci. These pili are believed to have an antiphagocytic function. A local immune response to the gonococcus is indicated by the appearance of IgG and secretory IgA antibody in external secretions. Both types of antibody appear to be capable of inhibiting gonococcal attachment to mucosal surfaces in a strain-specific manner *in vitro*. Serum antibody to *N. gonorrhoeae* may have both an opsonic and bactericidal effect. Locally produced IgA antibody, however, does not seem to be bactericidal. Complement components do participate in the destruction of the gonococcus.

    The meningococcus possesses group-specific capsular polysaccharides with antiphagocytic capacity and a lipopolysaccharide–endotoxin complex which may play a role in disseminated infections. The organism is classified into nine groups on the basis of agglutination reactions. Direct meningococcal bacteriolysis occurs *in vitro* through interaction of the organism with circulating meningococcal antibody and complement. Whether actual bacteriolysis occurs *in vivo* or whether opsonic antibody alone is important is unclear.

No serologic test exists for detection of *Neisseria* infection, mainly because of the difficulties in making a purified antigen. No specific immunity results from a gonococcal infection, and the development of a gonococcal vaccine seems impractical at the present time.

Clinical Features

An acute purulent conjunctivitis is the hallmark of ocular gonococcal infection (Fig. 5-5). Meningococcal conjunctivitis is usually milder and has fewer sequelae. Any severe, profusely exudative conjunctivitis demands immediate laboratory investigation and treatment, since any delay may lead to corneal damage and hematogenous dissemination. Marginal corneal ulceration may follow acute infection and if toxic products of *N. gonorrhoeae* diffuse through the cornea into the anterior chamber they may cause a toxic iritis.

Diagnosis and Treatment

A Gram stain should be done on all suspected cases. The finding of a gram-negative intracellular or extracellular diplococcus is sufficient evidence of infection and treatment should be instituted at once. A culture should be done on Thayer–Martin medium or chocolate agar.

Both systemic and topical antibiotic therapy are indicated for *Neisseria* infection. The current recommendations for therapy are as follows (142): 1) For adults, 4.8 million units of procaine penicillin G should be given intramuscularly daily for 3–5 days. 2) To increase the serum level of penicillin, probenecid 0.5 g should be given orally 1 h before the initial dose of penicillin and every 6 h thereafter. 3) For newborns, aqueous penicillin 50,000 units/kg of body weight should be given for 3–5 days without probenecid. 4) Chloramphenicol drops, tetracycline ointment, or tetracycline-in-oil drops should administered every 5–15 min and this therapy should be decreased when a response is seen. Atropine may be given for mydriasis.

HAEMOPHILUS INFECTIONS

Haemophilus is a cause of acute bacterial conjunctivitis and occasionally of orbital cellulitis. Two species are important in ophthalmology:

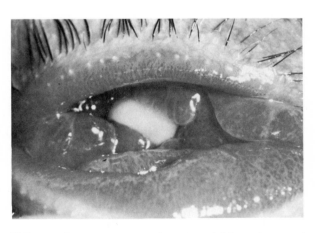

FIG. 5-5. Severe gonococcal conjunctivitis and corneal infiltrate in an adult. (Courtesy Dr. H. B. Ostler)

H. influenzae and *H. aegyptius*. The latter is also known as the Koch–Weeks bacillus.

Immunopathology

Haemophilus is classified as a gram-negative, facultative, anaerobic rod. *H. influenzae* is a coccobacillus which may be capsulated, and *H. aegyptius* is a slender rod. There are six serologic types of *H. influenzae*, with type B being the most pathogenic. The organism is far more pathogenic in children than in adults, and protective antibody as a result of previous contact with *Haemophilus* may account for the relative age-specificity of infection.

Capsular polysaccharides of *H. influenzae* are considered to serve an antiphagocytic function, and detection of capsular antigen in the serum by a variety of techniques is a useful diagnostic procedure.

Host responses to *H. influenzae* are primarily mediated by antibody. Opsonization and phagocytosis are the principal protective mechanisms. Antibody- and complement-mediated bacteriolysis can be demonstrated *in vitro* in the presence of complement but the role of this mechanism *in vivo* is uncertain.

Clinical Features

H. influenzae is the most common cause of bacterial meningitis in the first years of life. It may also be responsible for arthritis, cellulitis, episcleritis, and otitis media in children. *H. influenzae* causes a mild mucopurulent or catarrhal conjunctivitis in cool climates. *H. aegyptius* causes a more severe, purulent conjunctivitis in warm climates which may be accompanied by subconjunctival hemorrhages and may be followed by marginal corneal ulceration (25). *H. influenzae* is also a common cause of dacryocystitis, and may also cause orbital cellulitis (81).

Treatment

Broad-spectrum antibiotics, particularly ampicillin, are the drugs of choice in the treatment of *Haemophilus* infection (41). Ampicillin resistance, mediated by a plasmid which codes for penicillinase production, has recently been reported. Chloramphenicol or sulfonamides may also be used in the treatment of *Haemophilus* infection. A vaccine for *H. influenzae* has recently been developed, but adults respond to the vaccine much better than children do.

MORAXELLA INFECTIONS

Moraxella lacunata is a frequent cause of chronic catarrhal conjunctivitis in warm climates. The organism may also produce an angular conjunctivitis associated with dermatitis of the external or internal canthus. *Moraxella* is typically found as a diplobacillus (Fig. 5-6). It is gram-negative but has a tendency to retain crystal violet and may sometimes appear gram-positive. It may be capsulated and is an obligate aerobe.

Clinical Features

M. lacunata usually produces an angular blepharitis but it can also cause a follicular conjunctivitis involving especially the upper tarsal plate. A moderate mucopurulent discharge and a keratitis may be present.

Moraxella liquefaciens produces an indolent corneal ulcer which is most often found in alcoholics, diabetics, or debilitated patients (36). The frequency of *Moraxella* corneal ulcers varies greatly in different parts of the country, but at one time *M. liquefaciens* was responsible for half the corneal ulcers in the New York area. The ulcer causes little pain and tends to be oval in shape. It may follow mild trauma and progress toward the deep stroma over a period of days or weeks. There may be a mild hypopyon or no hypopyon at all. The lesion progresses slowly and the unaffected part of the cornea remains relatively clear. Occasionally, *Moraxella* may be the cause of endophthalmitis (23).

Treatment

Moraxella conjunctivitis will respond to treatment with topically applied zinc sulfate solution but sulfonamides, tetracyclines, or erythromycin may be even more effective. *Moraxella* corneal ulcers will also respond to treatment with sulfonamides, tetracycline,

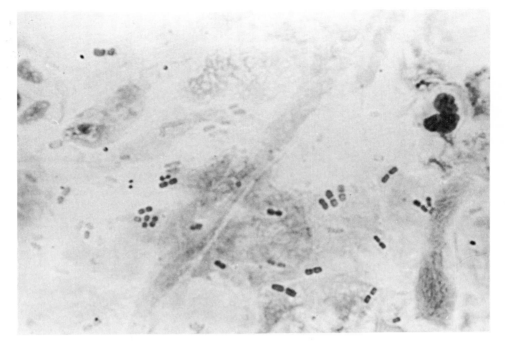

FIG. 5-6. *Moraxella* in scraping from corneal ulcer. Note typical diplobacillus appearance. (Courtesy Mr. M. Okumoto)

chloramphenicol, or gentamicin. Initially, topical medication should be applied every 30 min while awake and every hour during the night.

CHLAMYDIAL INFECTIONS

The chlamydia are a major cause of follicular conjunctivitis (151). These organisms are more closely related to bacteria than to viruses since they possess DNA and RNA, are sensitive to antibiotics, and possess muramic acid, a unique component of bacterial cell walls (112). *Chlamydia* organisms are responsible for inclusion conjunctivitis in adults and newborns, and for trachoma and lymphogranuloma venereum. A number of zoonotic infections are also caused by chlamydia.

Immunopathology

Two species of *Chlamydia* are officially recognized: *C. trachomatis* and *C. psittaci.* All members of the genus share a common "group" antigen. *C. trachomatis* has 15 antigenic serotypes, with types A, B, Ba, and C being mainly responsible for trachoma. Types D, E, F, G, H, I, J, and K are responsible for inclusion conjunctivitis and genital infections. Types L-1, L-2, and L-3 are associated with lymphogranuloma venereum. It has often been stated that the species designation for *C. trachomatis* is too broad (121). An unofficial classification (114) which would distinguish the agent responsible for oculogenital disease (*C. oculogenitalis*) from the agents which produce trachoma (*C. trachomatis*) and lymphogranuloma venereum (*C. lymphogranulomatosis*) has yet to be officially adopted. Such a classification would be useful since it would distinguish the chlamydia on the basis of serotypes and pathogenicity patterns (149). Chlamydia are obligate intracellular parasites which are incapable of synthesizing ATP. When they infect the host cell, they divert its synthetic capabilities to meet their own metabolic requirements and they direct the cell toward the production of more chlamydia (2). The organism is often identified by the presence of elementary or initial bodies within cells. Chlamydia are capable of specifically inducing their own phagocytosis by "nonprofessional" phagocytic host cells (16). They also have the ability to resist the normal defense mechanisms of the cell. Although they are found within phagosomes, they can prevent fusion of the phagosome with a lysosome (71).

Antibodies to chlamydia of the IgG or IgA class may be found in the tears of patients with trachoma or inclusion conjunctivitis (42, 84). Antibodies may be detected in serum by the group complement fixation test, which is useful in the diagnosis of trachoma, inclusion conjunctivitis, or the genital tract infection caused by these agents. A microimmunofluorescent test, which uses a number of specific antigens, was first used for serotyping and has some value in diagnosing chlamydial infections. A problem in diagnosing chlamydial infections by serologic methods is the difficulty in obtaining appropriately timed samples to demonstrate rising titers of antibody (121). IgM antibodies, which are short-lived, are useful in diagnosing first attacks of urethritis or chlamydial disease in infants (121).

It has been adequately demonstrated that antibody to an infecting chlamydia strain is present in the patient's serum and less frequently in tears (26). In humans and guinea pigs immunized with the trachoma agent, a cellular immune response is also elicited (74, 133). Although IgG and IgM have been detected in the serum of animals infected experimentally with chlamydia (53, 161), it appears that any resistance to infection offered by antibody is attributable to locally formed secretory IgA (95). There is no convincing evidence, however, that antichlamydial antibody exerts any significant effect on the disease process (21).

Guinea pig inclusion conjunctivitis (GPIC) is an animal model for chlamydial disease and extensive immunologic studies have been performed on this model to determine the relative roles of humoral and cellular immune mechanisms in chlamydial disease. High levels of serum antibody produced by intraperitoneal injections of killed GPIC organisms do not offer any protection against conjunctival challenge with the live agent (95). Passive immunization with serum antibody from prev-

iously infected animals does not render the recipients resistant to challenge with the agent of GPIC, indicating that serum antibody may not be important in conferring immunity against the local infection (162). In contrast, cyclophosphamide-treated, B-lymphocyte–depleted guinea pigs have a delayed appearance of secretory IgA antibody to GPIC in tears and a prolonged infection (91). This indicates that B cells may play a role in the control of chlamydial infection.

Clinical Features

Trachoma. Trachoma is one of the most common of all human diseases and the leading cause of preventable blindness in the world today. The disease is a major public health problem in North Africa, sub-Saharan Africa, the Middle East, and Southeast Asia. Sporadic cases are seen in the white population in the United States although trachoma is now rare in the United States except in the rural Mexican-American population and to a lesser extent in the Southwest American Indians.

Trachoma has a special affinity for the eye and is usually bilateral. It spreads by direct contact, especially among families. Insects, especially flies, may also play a role in transmission. The most active disease is seen in relatively young children.

The natural course of uncomplicated trachoma appears to be relatively self-limiting in terms of active disease or inflammation due to infection (121). Reinfection unfortunately is common and secondary bacterial infection may prolong the inflammatory disease for many years. The end result may be conjunctival scarring and distortion of the lids, producing corneal trauma and blinding sequelae.

Clinically, trachoma produces a chronic follicular conjunctivitis that leads to conjunctival scarring and superficial vascularization of the cornea. The disease resembles a bacterial conjunctivitis at the onset, with tearing, photophobia, and discharge. Examination reveals papillary hypertrophy, tarsal and limbal follicles, and injection and chemosis of the conjunctiva. Corneal involvement produces a superior keratitis and pannus formation. A tender preauricular node may be palpable.

Trachoma is usually described by the Mac-Callan classification in the following stages: stage 0: no sign of trachoma; stage I (early lymphoid hyperplasia): papillary hypertrophy and immature (small) follicles on the upper tarsus; stage IIa (established trachoma): papillary hypertrophy and mature (large) follicles on the tarsus; stage IIb (established trachoma): papillary hypertrophy predominating and masking the follicles on the upper tarsus; stage III (cicatricial trachoma): early conjunctival scarring shown by fine white lines in the subepithelial conjunctiva; and stage IV (healed trachoma): conjunctival stellate and linear scarring without inflammation of the upper tarsus.

In established trachoma, there may be superior epithelial keratitis, subepithelial keratitis, pannus, superior limbal follicles, and ultimately the cicatricial remains of these follicles known as Herbert's pits (Fig. 5-7). Both limbal follicles and Herbert's pits are pathognomonic for trachoma. Late complications of trachoma include dacryostenosis and a dry eye syndrome.

Inclusion Conjunctivitis. Inclusion conjunctivitis in infants begins 4–12 days after birth but may have an earlier onset if the placental membranes have been ruptured prematurely. The disease is characterized by swelling of the lids, papillary conjunctivitis, and a purulent discharge. Pseudomembranes may occasion-

ally form and lead to scarring. Follicle formation is not seen in the newborn, but if the conjunctivitis persists for 2–3 months, follicles will typically form.

In the adult, a follicular conjunctivitis of acute onset with a preauricular node usually develops (Fig. 5-8). The lower tarsus usually contains many papillae and follicles. Pseudomembranes do not form in the adult, so that scarring is not seen. A superficial keratitis may be present superiorly, and, less often, a superior micropannus (less than 1–2 mm) may form. Occasionally, subepithelial opacities develop, especially in the peripheral cornea. The disease can be differentiated from adenovirus infection because it persists for 3–12 months if untreated (155). Chlamydia can usually be cultured from the cervix of infectd women and from the urethra of infected men (121). Ocular infection can be diagnosed by demonstration of the agent in Giemsa-stained smears from the conjunctiva (Fig. 5-9).

Lymphogranuloma Venereum (LGV). Lymphogranuloma venereum (LGV) infections of the conjunctiva can result from laboratory accidents, although venereal transmission is occasionally seen. A granulomatous, conjunctival reaction with a large preauricular node is characteristic. The eyelids become greatly edematous as a result of lymphatic blockage, and the conjunctiva may become diffusely scarred. Optic neuritis, uveitis, epi-

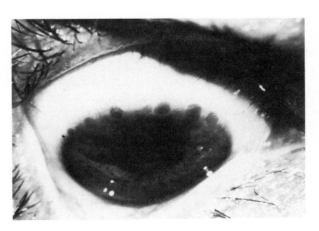

FIG. 5-7. Herbert's pits in patient with stage IV trachoma.

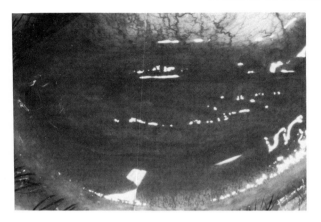

FIG. 5-8. Follicular conjunctivitis in patient with inclusion conjunctivitis.

scleritis, and phlyctenulosis have also been reported.

Treatment

An ideal antimicrobial treatment for trachoma has not yet been developed (55). Useful drugs include tetracycline, erythromycin, rifampin, and the sulfonamides. All are effective when administered systemically (121). Tetracycline cannot be given to young children, and in these cases erythromycin and rifampin can be used. Topical application of tetracycline once or twice daily for 6–10 weeks has been recommended, or, alternatively, the drug can be administered daily for 5 consecutive days each month for 6 months (75). Naturally occurring trachoma confers no immunity to recurrent

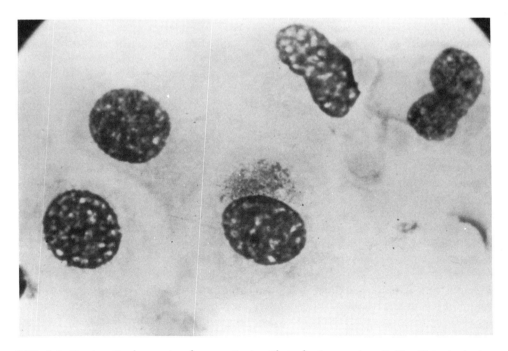

FIG. 5-9. Conjunctival scraping from patient with inclusion conjunctivitis. Note inclusion in central epithelial cell. (Courtesy of Mr. M. Okumoto)

disease, but interest in a vaccine for trachoma has still persisted for many years (20, 43). Immunity with such vaccines is short-lived and can be broken with higher inoculating doses. It has even been suggested that hypersensitization may be produced by immunization and actually make the disease worse (160).

Inclusion conjunctivitis in infants may be treated with 1% tetracycline drops in oil, erythromycin ophthalmic ointment, or sulfonamide drops instilled five to six times a day for 14 days. In adults a 3-week course of oral tetracycline 1–1½ g/day, or erythromycin 1 g/day, is curative. Systemic tetracycline should not be given to gravid women or to children under the age of 7. The consorts of patients should be examined and treated if infected.

Lymphogranuloma venereum responds to treatment with a sulfonamide or a broad-spectrum antibiotic given systemically for 3–4 weeks.

VIRAL INFECTIONS

SPECIAL ASPECTS OF VIRAL IMMUNITY

Viruses which spread extracellularly and do not alter the plasma membrane of the host cell are controlled mainly by secretory IgA. Viruses of this type include the enteroviruses and the rhinoviruses. Viruses which spread by fusion of infected cells with their neighbors are controlled mainly by cell-mediated immunity. Herpes simplex and vaccinia are two such viruses which incorporate their antigens directly into the host cell's surface. Myxo- and paramyxoviruses mature by budding off from the host cell membrane and elicit both a cell-mediated and a humoral immune response.

Antibody, cell-mediated immunity, and interferon all play a role in viral immunity. Antibody prevents adsorption of virus onto host cells and neutralizes the virus in some unknown way. Antibody is not thought to have the same important opsonic function in viral immunity that it has in antibacterial immunity. T lymphocytes can destroy virus-infected cells by direct cytotoxicity or they can induce macrophages to destroy the virus. Interferon, a protein of low molecular weight, prevents translation of viral but not host messenger RNA (169). It can prevent viral multiplication and thereby inhibit the spread of a virus. Interferon is not virus-specific, having activity against a wide range of viruses. Synthetic interferon inducers such as polyinosinic: polycytidilic acid (poly I:C) are currently being investigated.

Some viruses can infect host cells and replicate but do not actually cause damage to host tissues. Instead, the humoral or cellular immune response to the infection causes disease by attacking the infected cells. Lymphocytic choriomeningitis (LCM) virus produces a disease in mice in which cytotoxic T lymphocytes rather than the virus itself cause the disease. Certain autoimmune diseases are thought to develop by this same mechanism. In contrast, the immune response to poxvirus (vaccinia) or influenza virus in humans is mainly protective and directed at preventing cell destruction by the virus.

The interaction of antiviral antibodies with virus-infected cells can have several possible consequences (88): 1) Antiviral antibody can lead to the destruction of virus-infected cells in the presence of serum complement (89, 102). 2) Antiviral IgG can direct cell-mediated cytotoxicity in a non–complement-mediated manner (113, 126). 3) Antiviral antibody or antigen–antibody complexes could block cell-mediated immune responses by preventing sensitized lymphocytes from recognizing and reacting with viral antigens (4). 4) Antibody attached to virus-infected host cells could recruit activated macrophages to the site of infection and lead to enhancement of phagocytosis (4). 5) An antibody-mediated reaction in which infected cells are killed by a population of non–immune adherent killer (K) cells has recently been suggested both in an animal model (113) and in a model using human monocytes in the presence of antibody (126). Thus, antiviral antibodies may alter the immune response to herpes simplex virus in several possible ways. Antibody may play a role in the elimination of HSV or it may assist and augment cellular immune responses in some fashion.

HERPES SIMPLEX

Herpes simplex virus (HSV) belongs to a large group of DNA viruses which include cytomegalovirus, varicella-zoster, and the Epstein–Barr virus. It can infect a variety of species and has the ability to persist throughout the life of the infected host. HSV can be differentiated into two major antigenic types: HSV-1, which infects primarily nongenital body sites, and HSV-2, which usually affects genital sites. Herpes simplex is one of the most important infectious agents producing ocular disease, and corneal scarring secondary to herpes simplex keratitis is one of the leading indications for keratoplasty.

Immunopathology

Clinically, it is well known that immunosuppressed patients are susceptible to a great many opportunistic infections, including many viral infections. Early workers recognized that the frequency of herpes simplex keratitis was high in patients with atopic dermatitis and in patients with malaria (35). An increased incidence of HSV infection is also found among patients with primary or secondary immunodeficiencies of thymus-dependent lymphoid function or of the reticuloendothelial system. Patients with lymphoreticular malignancies, those receiving immunosuppressive drugs for transplantation (72, 93) or malignancy (6, 94), and patients with primary immunodeficiencies such as Wiskott–Aldrich syndrome (136) have an increased susceptibility to herpetic infection.

Unlike the case in patients with compromised cellular immunity, HSV infection runs a relatively benign course in the uncompromised host (150). Much of the morbidity associated with herpetic infection in man appears to be related to complications, many of which are secondary to the use of immunosuppressive therapy capable of impairing the host's natural defenses against viral disease. A striking example of this is seen in herpes simplex keratitis, a disease associated with particularly severe complications since the introduction of corticosteroids in 1952 (150).

Humoral Immunity. Neutralization of herpes simplex virus by antibody is known to occur. Antibody responses to HSV are generally measured by serologic testing procedures which detect complement-fixing or neutralizing antibodies. A number of problems exist with respect to the sensitivity and specificity of these tests and it is not always possible to differentiate primary from secondary antibody responses or to differentiate between antibodies to type 1 and type 2 HSV.

Infection in newborns leads to production of herpes-specific IgM antibodies within 1–3 weeks (97). These antibodies increase during the first 2–3 months of life and are detectable for at least a year. IgM antibodies neutralize herpesvirus poorly, but IgG and IgA antibodies, detectable at a later time period, correlate better with neutralizing activity. A depression of IgA antibodies in patients with recurrent herpes infection has been suggested (156) but not confirmed. Secretory IgA in tears has been cited as a possible factor in preventing local recurrences of herpes, but antiviral IgA antibodies in rabbit tears do not appear to reduce the severity or frequency of herpetic disease (17). The role of IgG in herpes infection is currently unclear. IgG antibodies may possibly interact with HSV and prevent its complete neutralization by antiviral IgA (17). It has also been proposed that antiviral IgG antibodies may in fact prevent reactivation of viral infection and contribute to the maintenance of a latent herpetic infection (135). While the exact role of antibody in HSV infection is unclear, it is apparent that humoral immune responses, including production of neutralizing antibody, are neither effective in preventing clinical recurrences nor capable of inhibiting direct cell-to-cell virus propagation (51, 79). As discussed later, cell-mediated immunity appears to be crucial but may not alone be sufficient to prevent recurrent attacks.

Cell-Mediated Immunity. Delayed-type hypersensitivity reactions to herpetic antigens can readily be elicited in herpes-immunized experimental animals (90) and in man (56). Cutaneous hypersensitivity, like circulating antibody, is predictably present in recurrent disease. The precise way in which cell-mediated immunity operates to protect the host from damage by HSV is far from clear. Various methods of studying cellular immune responses in animals and man have been carried out which in general support the concept that cellular immunity is a key mechanism to the recovery from HSV infection. These studies have measured cellular immune function in animal models of HSV infection and have evaluated cellular immunity in human herpetic disease.

Cellular immune defenses to herpesvirus could protect the host in at least three different ways: 1) Transformation of host lymphocytes into blast cells by viral antigens could lead to the production of inteferon (40). 2) Viral infection of host cells could lead to macrophage activation and increased virucidal capacity. 3) Viral antigens on the surface of cells could be recognized by sensitized lymphocytes which could attack and destroy the cell (32).

Cell-mediated immune responses in animals can be measured in several different ways. Migration inhibition factor (MIF) is detectable 7 days after rabbits are infected with herpes intracorneally (89). Virus-specific cytolytic activity is maximum in lymphocytes taken from animals 11 days after inoculation. Specifically sensitized lymphocytes can also be detected by their ability to synthesize DNA and to incorporate tritiated thymidine in the presence of herpes antigen. This last response is increased in the presence of antiviral antibodies, which peak 11–21 days after infection, while the cytotoxic response is not. Virus-specific immunologic memory can also be demonstrated by lymphocyte transformation after rabbits are inoculated in the foot pads (54). This response is maximal in lymphocytes taken from lymph nodes draining the site of inoculation, suggesting that local immune responses may play a critical role in controlling herpes infections. Lymphocytes in peripheral blood, spleen, and distant lymph nodes also demonstrate specific immune responses but of a much smaller magnitude.

Certain animal models of herpes disciform keratitis require systemic sensitization of animals followed by intracorneal challenge with viral antigen (139, 166). Presensitization results in the development of disciform corneal edema which closely parallels the infiltration of the cornea by lymphocytes. This observation may represent a delayed hypersensitivity response analogous to the delayed skin test reaction which follows intracutaneous challenge. As with other cellular immune responses, it can be transferred with lymphoid cells but not with serum (78). Such cellular immune responses may be initiated by alteration of the host cell membranes through the incorporation of virus neoantigens (47). Recognition of these antigens by host lymphocytes may trigger a cytotoxic reaction directed against seemingly foreign host cells.

Cell-mediated immune responses in humans have also been studied. Patients with recurrent labial herpes have evidence of cell-mediated immunity to HSV antigens, as shown by lymphocyte transformation and positive skin tests (119). These responses can be abrogated by therapy with antilympocyte globulin. It has been suggested that recurrent herpes stomatitis is associated with impaired production of MIF and lymphocyte cytotoxins (168). Patients with herpes labialis have also been shown to have a slight depression of lymphocyte stimulation even though they are capable of producing lymphotoxin (118). Severe HSV infections are seen following kidney transplantation and are associated with a depression of both lymphocyte transformation and inteferon production (115). Deficient production of MIF and interferon are seen just before and during HSV-induced vesicular eruptions (105).

Some studies on ocular herpes infections have investigated the possible role of cellular immune mechanisms. Easty et al (32) have suggested that patients who develop severe stromal herpetic keratitis have diminished cellular immunity. Such patients demonstrate lower levels of blast transformation in response to herpes antigen than do subjects with epithelial disease only. The differences, however, were not statistically significant and Henley and his associates (46) were unable to demonstrate production of MIF in response to herpes antigen in patients with herpetic keratitis. MIF production was demonstrated when lymphocytes were cultured with corneal antigen, and it was suggested that chronic viral infection might alter host corneal cells so that they would be recognized as foreign. It is possible that herpetic infection could unmask or release certain host antigens from damaged corneal cells and thereby initiate an autoimmune type of response (88).

Interferon. Inteferon is produced by immune lymphocytes and macrophages (80) and can be detected in the circulation 2–6 weeks after active infection with HSV (116). Immune-specific interferon can inhibit HSV replication in infected cell monolayers (80). It has been suggested that the host's immunologic defense against HSV consists of two phases: an immunologically specific antigen recognition phase, and a nonspecific effector phase (80). During the first phase, antiviral antibody, complement, and immune leukocytes react with virus or virus-infected cells. This would generate a variety of mediators (C5a, lymphocyte-derived chemotactic factors, MIF) which could attract and hold inflammatory cells at the site of infection. In addition, a number of other mediators, including lymphotoxin and interferon, might be generated. During the second, nonspecific, phase, inflammatory cells and mediators act on infected and adjacent uninfected cells, breaking cell contacts and inhibiting viral replication. It may be during this nonspecific phase that viral replication and cell-to-cell spread of HSV could be inhibited by interferon. Interferon has not proved to be of importance in recovery from ocular HSV infection nor has it prevented recurrent infections (88).

Role of Macrophages. Macrophages appear to play a protective role, especially in the early phases of herpes infection (50, 175). Newborn mice develop a disseminated herpes infection from a dose of virus that will not affect adult mice, but if macrophages are transferred from the adult to the newborn, the newborn animals will be protected. Additionally, adult mice are rendered susceptible to disseminated infections when antimacrophage serum or reticuloendothelial blocking agents are administered.

Histopathology. The histopathologic changes in HSV infection have been described extensively. Intranuclear eosinophilic inclusions, probably representing byproducts of the virus, and multinucleated giant cells are frequently observable in infected tissues and can be helpful in making a proper diagnosis. Infiltration by lymphocytes, plasma cells, and histiocytes is seen in the viscera following systemic infection.

Histopathologic studies on corneas infected with HSV have also been carried out (86, 87, 90, 139). By use of immunohistopathologic techniques, herpes antigen, host antibody, and complement (C3) could be demonstrated in experimental animals with stromal keratitis (90). Complement could not be demonstrated in epithelial keratitis, a stage of the disease in which antiviral antibody is also absent.

The cellular infiltrate found in herpetic corneal infections depends a good deal on the model being studied. A predominantly mononuclear cell infiltrate (with some neutrophils) accompanies the disciform edema produced by corneal inoculation of herpesvirus in the rabbit (124). In other models, plasma cells and lymphocytes are seen at the limbus, while neutrophils, lymphocytes, and macrophages predominate in the central cornea (87). The corneal rings, often seen clinically in herpetic keratitis, contain large numbers of neutrophils as well as viral antigen, host antibody, and complement (88). In experimental models of delayed hypersensitivity to herpes antigen in the guinea pig cornea (139), the ocular response is one of delayed-onset edema with lymphocytic infiltration at the corneal limbus.

Rabbit corneas infected with the RE strain of HSV develop a severe necrotizing keratitis which leads eventually to complete opacification and vascularization (86). Accompanying the disciform edema, numerous lymphocytes, plasma cells, macrophages, and neutrophils are seen 14–21 days after corneal inoculation. Lymphocytes are found in close contact with keratocytes in various stages of degeneration, and viral antigens can be demonstrated by immunofluorescence in keratocytes of the anterior and midstroma. Similar lymphocyte contact with degenerating keratocytes can be demonstrated in human corneal buttons removed at the time of keratoplasty. The presence of viral antigen and the intimate contact between keratocytes and lymphocytes suggests to the authors of the study the possibility that cell-mediated cytotoxicity is occurring (86).

Latency. Herpesvirus persists in nerve ganglia during periods between clinical attacks. In experimental herpes in the rabbit, the trigeminal ganglion acts as a reservoir for latent HSV infection, with its axons functioning as conduits that in some way transmit the virus to the peripheral ocular tissues (99). Infected rabbits, like man, display periodic shedding of virus in the tear film whether or not there is clinically recognizable disease (63, 100). Autonomic ganglia may also harbor latent herpesvirus (83). Virus shedding could be increased by the topical application of epinephrine, but not corticosteroids, to the eye in one experimental model (65). In another model (83) topical epinephrine and systemic cyclophosphamide did not produce chronic viral shedding. In a large percentage of general human autopsies, HSV can be recovered from the trigeminal and sacral ganglia (7, 8).

HLA Typing. In a recent study of 46 patients with recurrent corneal HSV infections, the HLA-B5 antigen was significantly more common (26%) than in controls (10.6%). This may suggest a possible relationship between herpes simplex keratitis and a genetically linked abnormal immune reactivity (173).

Clinical Features

Primary Infection. In the newborn, initial contact with HSV can produce a blepharoconjunctivitis with typical herpetic vesicles on the lid margins (13, 98). Occasionally, a diffuse chorioretinitis and associated encephalitis can develop. In children and adults, primary infection often begins as a conjunctivitis, but this may be accompanied by a blepharitis with vesicles on the lid margins and with extensive lid edema (Fig. 5-10). The conjunctivitis is follicular or, less often, pseudomembranous. Typically there is a tender preauricular node. The conjunctivitis persists for 2–3 weeks and, since it is self-limited, therapy is not necessary. If a pseudomembrane develops, it may leave a fine, linear scar.

Recurrent Infection. Recurrent herpetic infections may take the form of several different types of epithelial disease. The most common manifestation of recurrent herpes infection in

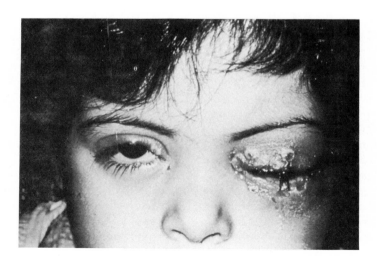

FIG. 5-10. Primary herpetic blepharitis in a child. Note vesicular lid lesions and extensive lid edema.

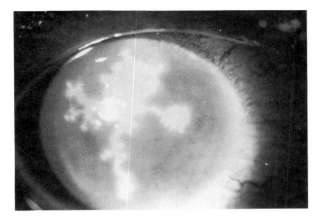

FIG. 5-11. Large dendritic ulcer in patient with herpes simplex keratitis.

the eye is the **dendritic ulcer** (Fig. 5-11). The ulcers are epithelial, frequently multiple, and often unilateral. They are usually accompanied by complete or partial loss of corneal sensation. The dendritic lesions are associated with replicating virus, and their linear nature is probably due to a sliding in of the corneal epithelium to cover the defect created by virus proliferating at the edge of the ulcer (28). Most dendritic ulcers last 7–14 days although some may persist longer. Sensory loss can be detected a day or two after onset of the attack.

Geographic ulcers are larger epithelial herpetic lesions which are also associated with replicating virus. They may form from smaller dendritic lesions and present with a broad area of epithelial ulceration with maplike borders (Fig. 5-12). Their clinical course is more prolonged than that of the dendritic lesions and they may take weeks or even months to heal. They may follow steroid treatment of dendritic ulcers or sloughing of a large area of devitalized epithelium.

Marginal keratitis, or epithelial herpetic lesions located near the limbus, tends to run a prolonged course and is more resistant to antiviral therapy than are other herpetic lesions (134, 148). It may sometimes be mistaken for catarrhal infiltrates associated with bacterial infections.

Persistent epithelial ulcerations may follow treatment of geographic ulcers or stromal

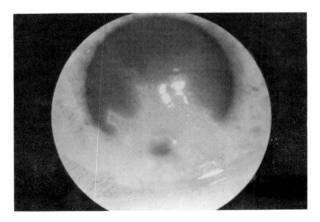

FIG. 5-12. Geographic herpetic ulcer with maplike borders.

keratitis. Such ulcers are not due to persistent viral infection but rather to a failure of the epithelium to attach to the underlying Bowman's membrane. These lesions are also known as trophic ulcers or metaherpetic keratitis (45). It has been suggested that these ulcerations are perpetuated by collagenases and proteases secreted by diseased epithelium (11). Antiviral medications, because of their toxicity, may contribute to the continued failure of the epithelium to cover the defect (154).

Persistent stromal disease may occur, as well as persistent epithelial lesions. Superficial keratitis, causing faint opacities in the anterior corneal stroma, may persist for several months after an epithelial lesion has healed. These opacities usually resolve in 6 months to 1 year, leaving no residual opacity in most cases. Long-standing opacities (known as ghost or phantom lesions) are sometimes seen after treatment of dendritic keratitis with antiviral agents (154).

Disciform keratitis consists of a round area of stromal edema with a variable amount of opacification and swelling (Fig. 5-13). Disciform lesions were first described after vaccinial infections and have also been seen following herpes zoster, mumps, and varicella. A disciform lesion may follow an epithelial lesion but may also appear long after the original epithelial lesion has healed. Disciform keratitis is associated with marked corneal an-esthesia, and keratic precipitates are often present. An uncomplicated disciform lesion will usually heal within a few weeks to a few months after onset. Severe cases, especially those complicated by superinfection or corticosteroid therapy, progress to permanent scarring (152).

In stromal keratitis, virus is rarely if ever cultured from the lesion. Therefore, it is assumed that the lesion is not directly attributable to viral proliferation but rather to a response to persistent viral antigen (28). It has been suggested that the corneal stroma acts as an immunologic "blotter," retaining viral antigens that diffuse in from the corneal epithelium (59), and that an antigen–antibody reaction in the corneal stroma attracts numerous inflammatory cells. Virus particles have been demonstrated in all layers of the corneal stroma in human corneas removed at the time of keratoplasty (27), and antigens associated with these virus particles might be capable of stimulating corneal inflammation similar to that produced by foreign antigens injected into the corneal stroma of immunized animals (108).

Deep stromal keratitis may also occur. Dense infiltration of the corneal stroma may be localized or diffuse. Necrosis and ingrowth of blood vessels frequently accompanies this type of lesion. Such a lesion is sometimes seen after the prolonged use of corticosteroids and

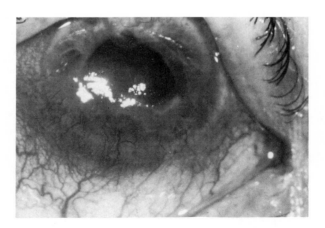

FIG. 5-13. Stromal involvement in patient with long-standing herpetic keratitis. Note edema encroaching on central cornea, and peripheral vascularization.

usually runs a prolonged course. Progression of deep stromal keratitis leads to corneal thinning and occasionally to perforation. The inflammation is felt to be secondary either to the presence of viral antigens or to replication of the virus within stromal cells. Such lesions are difficult to treat and are the most visually disabling type of herpetic lesion.

Uveitis accompanying herpes simplex keratitis may be of two general types. A few cells and a modest amount of flare may accompany the epithelial form of herpetic disease; this response is felt to be associated with an axon reflex from the cornea (103). A more profound uveal inflammation is associated with long-standing stromal disease. This is accompanied by photophobia, posterior synechia formation, and secondary glaucoma. The iris is heavily infiltrated by lymphocytes and plasma cells, and the trabecular meshwork is infiltrated by neutrophils (66). Spontaneous hemorrhage into the anterior chamber is more frequent than in other types of uveitis.

It is unclear whether herpetic uveitis is due to direct infection of the uveal tract with virus or whether hypersensitivity mechanisms are responsible (103). Alteration of host tissues by the virus could provoke an autoimmune response; this might help to explain the recurrent bouts of inflammation observed in some patients.

Treatment

The major aim of treatment in herpetic ocular disease is to preserve vision and reduce the morbidity caused by recurrent inflammation. It should be kept in mind that in most instances herpes simplex keratitis is a self-limited disease and except in rare instances it will resolve within a few months. A major theme of management should be "do no harm," since certain modes of therapy may lead to complications which are ultimately more visually disabling than the disease itself.

Dendritic ulcers can be effectively treated by epithelial debridement. A drop of 4% cocaine is instilled into the eye to induce anesthesia and to loosen the diseased corneal epithelium. A dry, sterile cotton swab is then used to wipe away loose epithelium. The edges of the lesion can be evened with a platinum spatula. A cycloplegic drug is instilled and the eye is patched for 48–72 h (106). This method is as effective as the use of antiviral drugs, and the corneal epithelium heals just as rapidly (110, 164). Debridement should be repeated after 4 days if the branching lesions persist.

Dendritic ulcers in man also respond to treatment with the antiviral agents idoxuridine (IDU), vidarabine (adenine arabinoside, ARA-A), and trifluorothymidine (TFT) (64, 163). All of these drugs appear to be useful in the treatment of epithelial disease but have little effect on stromal disease, iritis, or skin lesions. However, intravenously administered ARA-A has been shown to be effective in the treatment of herpetic iritis and deep stromal disease (62). This drug apparently does not suppress humoral or cell-mediated immunity when administered systemically to rabbits (172).

Significant ocular toxicity has been demonstrated with prolonged topical application of antiviral agents (60). IDU has a direct toxic effect on the corneal epithelium and can produce a toxic follicular conjunctivitis, conjunctival scarring, and contact dermatitis of the eyelids (28). Stenosis of the lacrimal puncta and superficial corneal vascularization are sometimes seen. Toxicity due to TFT resembles that of IDU, and a punctate keratopathy has been observed with ARA-A (60).

It has been stated that prior to the introduction of corticosteroids in 1952, herpes simplex keratitis was a self-limited disease which rarely lasted longer than a few months and that corneal perforation was almost unheard of (150). It is clear that many cases of herpes simplex keratitis currently last longer than a few months and that the incidence of opportunistic superinfection and corneal perforations has increased in recent years. This is not surprising in view of the fact that glucocorticoids are potent inhibitors of the immune system (22) and also potentiate the action of collagenase (15). The adverse effects of glucocorticoids on herpetic disease have been adequately documented in the literature (67, 104, 141). Not only may steroids worsen the clinical course of herpes simplex keratitis, but they also enhance viral replication and viral shedding (31, 104) and inhibit antibody-dependent cell-mediated cytotoxicity against HSV-infected fibroblasts (22). Although topical corticosteroids will quiet an inflamed eye and reduce stromal inflammation, side effects such as glaucoma, cataract formation, worsening of recurrent epithelial keratitis, melting of the corneal stroma, and superinfection make the routine use of steroids hazardous in the treatment of herpetic keratitis. If treatment with topical steroids is already under way, they should be tapered and discontinued as rapidly as possible. If the keratitis persists or increases with the reduction of steroid dosage, the drug should be increased to a high enough level to obtain a clinical response before its progressive reduction is begun again (28). Most stromal keratitis responds well to simple patching and dilation of the pupil early in the course of the disease.

Soft contact lenses may be useful in the treatment of large epithelial defects, particularly poorly healing trophic ulcers. Patching the eye can accomplish the same purpose when this therapy is appropriate.

Immunopotentiators may be of benefit in herpetic infections, since cellular immunity is important in the recovery from HSV infections. A number of drugs which enhance cellular immune responses have been evaluated clinically and experimentally. Levamisole, which nonspecifically enhances cellular immunity and stimulates phagocytic function, has had beneficial effects on the treatment of recurrent corneal ulcers, recurrent herpes labialis, and recurrent herpes genitalis (68, 140). Levamisole has also proved effective in the treatment of a rabbit model of chronic herpes simplex keratitis (39, 130). The efficacy of this drug remains controversial (85), and further studies are required to investigate its antiviral effects. Other drugs which enhance immune responses have also been investigated. Transfer factor and bacillus Calmette–Guérin (BCG) vaccine have proved unrewarding (128, 131). *Corynebacterium parvum* and a leukocyte extract used in the treatment of a rabbit model of herpes simplex keratitis appear to be more promising (132).

Interferon has also been studied. Recent reports (61, 138) have been encouraging in their demonstration of the therapeutic effects of human leukocyte interferon in the treatment of epithelial herpetic disease. Currently interferon is not widely available and further trials must be awaited.

Surgical procedures such as tarsorrhaphy, production of a conjunctival flap, and lamellar or penetrating keratoplasty are useful and often necessary adjuncts to the medical treatment of herpes simplex keratitis. While the results of corneal transplantation are relatively favorable (37, 109) it should be remembered that recurrence of herpetic disease in a graft is quite common (37).

Recurrent herpetic episodes can sometimes be prevented by recognizing that certain conditions can trigger a herpetic episode. The common triggers are fever, ultraviolet light, emotional stress, the onset of menstruation, and trauma. Aspirin can be taken to lower body temperature and can also be used at the beginning of menstruation (106). Patients should be cautioned to use sun screens and wear dark glasses and protective clothing when exposed to direct sunlight.

Vaccination is one possible method of obtaining the goal of prophylaxis in recurrent herpetic disease. To date, the efforts to develop a suitable herpes vaccine with proven efficacy have been unsuccessful (170). While experimental studies are currently under way with inactivated viral preparations, the possible association of HSV with carcinogenesis has prevented an enthusiastic effort to develop such a vaccine.

ADENOVIRUS INFECTIONS

Adenoviruses are responsible for a large number of sporadic cases of keratoconjunctivitis and for outbreaks of conjunctivitis in hospitals, schools, and factories. The virus has a predilection for the upper respiratory tract and the eye.

Immunopathology

Serologic typing has identified adenovirus 8 as the most common cause of epidemic keratoconjunctivitis (EKC) (57). Several other types of adenovirus, including type 19, have been associated with EKC (49). Adenovirus 3 and 7 are the most common causes of pharyngoconjunctival fever (PCF), an acute and highly infectious illness characterized by fever and a nonpurulent conjunctivitis.

The incubation period for adenovirus keratoconjunctivitis is usually 7–9 days but ranges from 2–14 days. Transmission is usually by finger to eye contact. EKC may occur in epidemics in shipyards, swimming pools, or eye clinics.

Viral culture for isolation of adenovirus is rather slow and requires 1–8 weeks for detection and identification of the virus (33). The complement-fixation test is a standard and useful serologic test for detection of adenovirus group antibody. A fourfold rise in the antibody titer of acute and of convalescent serum is significant for the diagnosis of adenovirus keratoconjunctivitis (33). Hemagglutination-inhibition tests for antibody measurements are fast, accurate, and more sensitive than other serologic tests (69). Patients with low antibody titers measured by this method develop a more severe keratitis than those with high titers. This suggests that high serum antibody may afford some protection of the cornea in EKC. (The role of cellular immunity in recovery from EKC has not been studied.) Another method for the rapid diagnosis of acute adenoviral keratoconjunctivitis is direct and indirect immunofluorescent staining for adenoviral antigens in epithelial cells obtained from conjunctival scrapings (52, 158). The immunofluorescence test detects group-reactive adenoviral antigen in the cytoplasm of infected epithelial cells using fluorescein-labeled antiserum to adenovirus.

Clinical Features

Epidemic Keratoconjunctivitis. EKC is usually bilateral but often affects only one eye at the onset. The first eye is usually more severely affected than the second. The patient complains of tearing, redness, and photophobia, and examination reveals a follicular conjunctivitis, conjunctival hyperemia, and edema of the eyelids. Subconjunctival hemorrhages may be present and a pseudomembrane is occasionally seen. A large tender preauricular node is characteristic of EKC. From 5 to 14 days after the onset of the conjunctivitis, epithelial and subepithelial opacities may appear in the central cornea (Fig. 5-14). They may persist for several months but generally heal without residual scarring. The conjunctivitis lasts 3–4 weeks at the most but is self-limited and does not require treatment. Pseudomembranes may occasionally be followed by flat scars or symblepharon formation. EKC in adults is confined to the external eye but children may have systemic symptoms such as fever, sore throat, and diarrhea. A conjunctival scraping reveals a predominance of mononuclear cells, and if a pseudomembrane is present, neutrophils may be seen in large numbers.

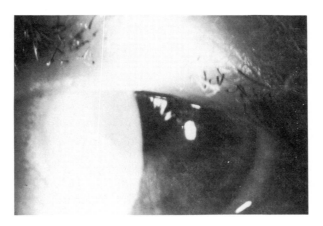

FIG. 5-14. Epidemic keratoconjunctivitis. Note epithelial and subepithelial corneal opacities.

Pharyngoconjunctival Fever. Pharyngoconjunctival fever (PCF) presents with fever, sore throat, and a follicular conjunctivitis that usually involves both eyes. Conjunctival injections and tearing are typically seen and there may be a transient superficial epithelial keratitis and occasionally subepithelial opacities. A nontender preauricular node is characteristically seen. A conjunctival scraping reveals mainly mononuclear cells. The condition is more common in children than in adults and may be transmitted in swimming pools. The disease is self-limited, lasting about 10 days, and does not require specific treatment.

Treatment

Adenoviral keratoconjunctivitis is self-limited, as was stated, and rarely produces any significant morbidity. Supportive treatment with cool compresses and astringents may be useful (76). Topical corticosteroids are sometimes used when symptoms are severe, but in general they are not necessary. Steroids will inhibit the appearance of subepithelial corneal infiltrates but when they are withdrawn the infiltrates often reappear. Antiviral drugs such as IDU or ARA-A have been ineffective in treating adenoviral keratoconjunctivitis (111). Recent reports suggest that topically applied human leukocyte interferon and amantadine may have a role in prophylaxis or treatment of adenoviral keratoconjunctivitis (1).

ACUTE HEMORRHAGIC CONJUNCTIVITIS

An unusual epidemic of acute conjunctivitis occurred in Ghana in June, 1969 (18). Because it appeared at about the time of the Apollo 11 moon landing it was nicknamed "Apollo 11 disease." Three years later a similar disease reached Japan, where it was termed "acute hemorrhagic conjunctivitis" because the incubation period was short, the clinical course was rapid, and subconjunctival hemorrhages were a prominent and characteristic feature (70). Since then, all the continents (except North and South America) and most islands of the world have had major epidemics. The causative virus was eventually isolated and

found to be enterovirus type 70. The virus can be isolated from the conjunctiva if cultures are taken within the first 3 days of the disease, but after this, neutralizing antibody in the serum is a useful diagnostic test.

The disease has a short incubation period of 8–48 h and a short course of 5–7 days. Patients present with pain, photophobia, foreign body sensation, copious tearing, redness, lid edema, and subconjunctival hemorrhages. The subconjunctival hemorrhages may be punctate at the outset and later diffuse. Conjunctival follicles, preauricular lymphadenopathy, and epithelial keratitis may be seen. Generalized myalgias are observed in 25% of patients and a motor paralysis of the lower extremities may appear after the conjunctivitis subsides (44). Resolution of the conjunctivitis is seen in 5–7 days and treatment is not necessary (165). Corticosteroids are not recommended because of the short duration and self-limited nature of the disease.

FUNGAL INFECTIONS

Immunopathology

During the past 25 years the number of fungal infections involving the eye has increased dramatically (122). This increase is generally attributed to the use of immunosuppressive and antineoplastic drugs, the increased longevity of debilitated patients, and a greater awareness on the part of physicians of the clinical manifestations of fungal disease. Fungi normally are found in the intestine and on mucous membranes but cause little or no disease under ordinary circumstances. When the natural defenses of the host are compromised either by drugs or by disease, these ordinarily harmless organisms can produce morbidity. Cellular immunity appears to be the most important immunologic factor in resistance to fungal infections, although humoral antibody almost certainly plays a role. Evidence of the importance of cellular immune reactions includes the following: 1) Fungal infections are most frequently associated with depressed cellular immunity (82), and 2) tissues infected with fungi show intense mononuclear and granulomatous reactions.

Fungal disease is common in a number of clinical situations where cellular immune responses are depressed. Patients with mucocutaneous candidiasis (77, 123) have an inherited defect in cell-mediated immunity and are unable to mount normal host responses to *Candida* (see Candidiasis, Ch. 6). Patients with chronic diseases, including diabetes mellitus, chronic liver disease, and widespread malignancy, are also particularly susceptible to fungal infections. A major complication of immunosuppressive drug regimens used in organ transplant recipients or in individuals with widespread malignancies is an increased susceptibility to opportunistic infections (5). Although bacterial infections are most frequent, fungal infections, particularly aspergillosis, are common and may lead to a fatal outcome. Mixed infections from bacteria and fungi are also of great importance. Patients receiving broad-spectrum antibiotics are at risk of developing fungal infections since one function of the normal bacterial flora is to prevent accelerated growth of fungi.

The recent dramatic increase in the incidence of fungal infections in the eye has been attributed to therapy with antibiotics, corticosteroids, or antiviral agents and to the use of contaminated solutions and ointments (29, 38, 153). It has been stated that keratomycosis is a preventable disease if immunosuppressive drugs are avoided in the treatment of corneal injuries or infections (153). The development of ocular fungal infection following the use of immunosuppressive drugs is well documented (34, 117, 125).

Other conditions which predispose to fungal infections of the eye are intravenous hyperalimentation and drug addiction. In the former category, candidal sepsis is frequently associated with the presence of indwelling venous catheters, and in the latter, drugs are frequently filtered through cotton contaminated with *Candida* (122). Another group of patients, those with chronic inflammatory disease such as sarcoidosis and collagen vascular diseases, may have accompanying defects in cell-mediated immune defenses. Since these patients are frequently treated with systemic corticosteroids, they are at increased risk of developing all kinds of opportunistic infections.

Clinical Features

Fungal infections of the cornea usually present as indolent ulcers with a whitish yellow surface, raised edges, and fingerlike processes extending into the stroma (Fig. 5-15). There may be satellite lesions and a hypopyon. The diagnosis can be confirmed by microscopic study of corneal scrapings and by culture. Intraocular fungal infections frequently present as whitish yellow chorioretinal lesions with an overlying vitreous haze. Hemorrhages, edema, and perivascular sheathing may be present. The morphology of the ocular lesions differs markedly depending on their location and severity.

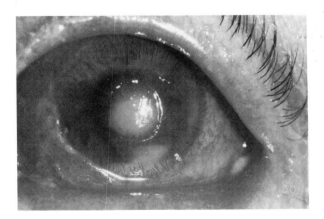

FIG. 5-15. Fungal corneal ulcer following tree branch injury.

Treatment

Therapy for ocular fungal infections is often disappointing. Few antifungal drugs are available and these may be associated with significant toxicity. Amphotericin B, pimaricin, and flucytosine may be useful topically in certain infections. A newer drug, miconazole, is a broad-spectrum antifungal agent with little toxicity and may prove useful in the treatment of ocular fungal disease. A guiding principle in the treatment of fungal disease is to treat the underlying disease and remove the cause of immunosuppression.

REFERENCES

1. Abel R: Adenovirus keratoconjunctivitis and new approaches to prophylaxis. Ann Ophthalmol 9: 1977
2. Alexander JJ: Effect of infection with the meningopneumonitis agent on deoxyribonucleic acid and protein synthesis by its L-cell host. J Bacteriol 97:653, 1969
3. Allen JH: Staphylococcic conjunctivitis. Am J Ophthalmol 21:1025, 1937
4. Allison AC: Immunity and immunopathology of virus infections. Ann Inst Pasteur 123:585, 1972
5. Anderson RJ, Schafer LA, Olin DB, Eickhoff TC: Infection risk factors in the immunosuppressed host. Am J Med 54:453, 1973
6. Aston DL, Cohen A, Spindler MA: Herpesvirus hominis infection in patients with myeloproliferative and lymphoproliferative disorders. Br Med J 4:462, 1972
7. Baringer JR: Recovery of herpes simplex virus from human sacral ganglions. N Engl J Med 291:828, 1974
8. Baringer JR, Swoveland P: Recovery of herpes simplex virus from human trigeminal ganglions. N Engl J Med 288:648, 1973
9. Baum J: Current concepts in ophthalmology. Ocular infections. N Engl J Med 299:28, 1978
10. Bellanti JA, Hurtado RC: Immunology and resistance to infection. In Remington JS, Klein JO (eds): Infectious Diseases of the Fetus and Newborn. Philadelphia, Saunders, 1976, p 35
11. Berman M, Kerza-Kwiatecki AP, Davison PF: Characterization of human corneal collagenase. Exp Eye Res 15:367, 1973
12. Bigley NJ: Immunologic Fundamentals. Chicago, Year Book Medical, 1975, p 10
13. Bobo CB, Antine B, Manos JP: Neonatal herpes simplex infection limited to the cornea. Arch Ophthalmol 84:697, 1970
14. Breese BB: Beta-hemolytic streptococcus. Its bacteriologic culture and character. Am J Dis Child 132:502, 1978
15. Brown SI, Weller CA, Vidrick AM: Effect of corticosteroids on corneal collagenase of rabbits. Am J Ophthalmol 70:744, 1970
16. Byrne GI: Requirements for ingestion of *Chlamydia psittaci* by mouse fibroblasts (L cells). Infect Immun 14:645, 1976
17. Centifanto YM, Kaufman HE: The development of tear antibodies and herpes simplex keratitis. In Dayton DH Jr., Small PA Jr., Chanock RM, Kaufman HE, Tomasi TB Jr, et al (Eds): The Secretory Immunologic System. Bethesda, US Department of Health, Education and Welfare, Public Health Service, NIH, 1969, p 331
18. Chatterjee S, Quarcoopome CO, Apenteng A: Unusual type of epidemic conjunctivitis in Ghana. Br J Ophthalmol 54:628, 1970
19. Cline MJ: The White Cell. Cambridge, Harvard University Press, 1975
20. Collier LH: The present status of trachoma vaccination studies. Bull WHO 34:233, 1966
21. Collier LH, Blyth WA: Immunogenicity of experimental trachoma vaccine in baboons. J Hyg 64:513, 1966
22. Cooper JAD Jr, Daniels CA, Trofatter KF Jr: The effect of prednisolone on antibody-dependent cell-mediated cytotoxicity and the growth of type I herpes simplex virus in human cells. Invest Ophthalmol Vis Sci 17:381, 1978
23. Cooperman EW, Friedman AH: Exogenous *Moraxella liquefaciens* endophthalmitis. Ophthalmologica 171:177, 1975
24. Davis SD, Sarff LD, Hyndiuk RA: Topical tobramycin therapy of experimental pseudomonas keratitis. Arch Ophthalmol 96:123, 1978
25. Dawson CR: Epidemic Koch-Weeks conjunctivitis and trachoma in the Coachella Valley of California. Am J Ophthalmol 49:801, 1960
26. Dawson CR: Lids, conjunctiva and lacrimal apparatus. Eye infections with Chlamydia. Arch Ophthalmol 93:854, 1975
27. Dawson CR, Moore T, Togni B: Structural changes in chronic herpetic keratitis studies by light and electron microscopy. Arch Ophthalmol 79:740, 1968
28. Dawson CR, Togni B: Herpes simplex eye infections: clinical manifestations, pathogenesis and management. Surv Ophthalmol 21:121, 1976
29. DeVoe AG, Silva-Hutner M: Fungal infection of the eye. In Locatcher-Khorazo D, Seegal BC (eds): Microbiology of the Eye. St Louis, Mosby, 1972, p 208
30. Dillon AC: Streptococcus skin infection and acute glomerular nephritis. Postgrad Med J 46:641, 1973
31. Easterbrook M, Wilkie J, Coleman V, Dawson CR: The effect of topical cortico-steroids on the susceptibility of immune animals to reinoculation with herpes simplex. Invest Ophthalmol 12:181, 1973
32. Easty DL, Maini RN, Jones BR: Cellular im-

munity in herpes simplex keratitis. Trans Ophthalmol Soc UK 93:171, 1973

33. Editorial: Adenovirus keratoconjunctivitis. Br J Ophthalmol 61:73, 1977

34. Editorial: Fungal infections of the eye. Br Med J 1:667, 1977

35. Elliott RH: Tropical Ophthalmology. London, Oxford University Press, 1920, pp 451–454

36. Fedukowicz H, Horwich H: The Gram-negative diplobacillus in hypopyon keratitis. Arch Ophthalmol 49:202, 1953

37. Fine M, Cignetti FE: Penetrating keratoplasty in herpes simplex keratitis. Recurrence in grafts. Arch Ophthalmol 95:613, 1977

38. François J, Rysselaere M: Oculomycoses. Springfield, IL, Thomas, 1972, p 59

39. Friedlaender MH, Smolin G, Okumoto M: Treatment of herpetic reinfection with levamisole. Am J Ophthalmol 86:245, 1978

40. Glasgow LA: Interrelationships of interferon and immunity during viral infections. J Gen Physiol 56:2125, 1970

41. Gordon RC: *In vitro* susceptibility of *Haemophilus influenzae* to eight antibiotics. Antimicrob Agents Chemother 6:114, 1974

42. Grayston JT, Wang S-P: New knowledge of chlamydiae and the diseases they cause. J Infect Dis 132:87, 1975

43. Grayston JT, Wang S-P, Woodridge RL et al: Prevention of trachoma with vaccine. Arch Environ Health 8:518, 1964

44. Green IJ, Hung T-P, Sung S-M: Neurologic complications with elevated antibody titer after acute hemorrhagic conjunctivitis. Am J Ophthalmol 80:832, 1975

45. Gunderson T: Herpes corneae. With special reference to its treatment with strong solutions of iodine. Arch Ophthalmol 15:225, 1936

46. Henley WL, Shore B, Leopold IH: Inhibition of leukocyte migration by corneal antigens in chronic viral keratitis. Nature 223:115, 1971

47. Henson D, Helmsen R, Becker KE et al: Ultrastructural localization of herpes simplex virus antigens on rabbit corneal cells using sheep antihuman IgG antihorse ferritin hybrid antibodies. Invest Ophthalmol 13:819, 1974

48. Hess MW, Keller HU, Schädeli J et al: Defense mechanisms against infectious diseases. Monog Allergy, Vol 9, Basel, Karger, 1975, pp 1–12

49. Hierholzer JC, Guyer B, O'Day D, Shaffner W: Adenovirus type 19 keratoconjunctivitis. N Engl J Med 290:1436, 1974

50. Hirsch MS, Zisman B, Allison AC: Macrophages and age-dependent resistance to herpes simplex virus in mice. J Immunol 104:1160, 1970

51. Hoffan MD, Roizman B: The isolation and properties of a variant of herpes simplex producing multinucleated giant cells in monolayer cultures in the presence of antibody. Am J Hyg 70:208, 1959

52. Imre G, Korchmaros I, Geck P et al: Antigenic specificity of inclusion bodies in epidemic keratoconjunctivitis. Ophthalmologica 148:7, 1964

53. Isa AM: The antibody response to chlamydial agents. In Nichols RL (ed): Trachoma and Related Disorders Caused by Chlamydial Agents. London, Excerpta Medica International Congress Series 223, 1971, pp 196–205

54. Jacobs RP, Aurelian L, Cole GA: Cell-mediated immune response to herpes simplex virus: type-specific lymphoproliferative responses in lymph nodes draining the site of primary infection. J Immunol 116:1520, 1976

55. Jawetz E: Chemotherapy of chlamydial infections. Adv Pharmacol Chemother 7:253, 1969

56. Jawetz E, Coleman V, Allende MR: Studies on herpes simplex virus. II. A soluble antigen of herpes virus possessing skin-reactive properties. J Immunol 67:197, 1951

57. Jawetz E, Thygeson P, Hanna L et al: The etiology of epidemic keratoconjunctivitis. Am J Ophthalmol 43:79, 1957

58. Jeffrey MP: Ocular diseases caused by nematodes. Am J Ophthalmol 40:41, 1955

59. Jones BR: The clinical features of viral keratitis and a concept of their pathogenesis. Proc Soc Med 51:917, 1958

60. Jones BR: Rational regimen of administration of antivirals. Trans Am Acad Ophthalmol Otolaryngol 79:104, 1974

61. Jones BR, Coster DJ, Falcon MG, Cantell K: Topical therapy of ulcerative herpetic keratitis with human interferon. Lancet 2:128, 1976

62. Kaufman HE: Systemic therapy of ocular herpes. Int Ophthalmol Clin 15:163, 1975

63. Kaufman HE, Brown DC, Ellison EM: Recurrent herpes in rabbit and man. Science 156:1628, 1967

64. Kaufman HE, Nesburn AB, Maloney ED: IDU therapy of herpes simplex. Arch Ophthalmol 67:583, 1962

65. Kibrick S, Takahashi GH, Leibowitz HW et al: Local corticosteroid therapy and reactivation of herpetic keratitis. Arch Ophthalmol 86:694, 1971

66. Kimura SJ: Herpes simplex uveitis: a clinical and experimental study. Trans Am Ophthalmol Soc 60:440, 1962

67. Kimura SJ, Okumoto M: The effect of corticosteroids on experimental herpes simplex keratoconjunctivitis in the rabbit. Am J Ophthalmol 43:131, 1957

68. Kint A, Verlinden L: Levamisole for recurrent herpes labialis. N Engl J Med 291:308, 1974

69. Knopf HLS, Hierholzer JC: Clinical and immunologic responses in patients with viral keratoconjunctivitis. Am J Ophthalmol 80:661, 1975

70. Kono R, Sasagawa A, Ishii K et al: Pandemic of new type of conjunctivitis. Lancet 1:1191, 1972

71. Kordova N, Wilt JC, Sadiq M: Lysosomes in L

cells infected with *Chlamydia psittaci* 6BC strain. Can J Microbiol 17:955, 1971

72. Korsager B, Spencer ES, Mordhorst CH, Anderson HK: Herpesvirus hominis infections in renal transplant recipients. Scand J Infect Dis 7:11, 1975

73. Kreger AS, Gray LD: Purification of *Pseudomonas aeruginosa* proteases and microscopic characterization of pseudomonal protease-induced rabbit corneal damage. Infect Immun 19:630, 1978

74. Kuo CC, Wang S-P, Grayston JT: Studies on delayed hypersensitivity with trachoma organism. I. Induction of delayed hypersensitivity in guinea pigs and characterization of trachoma allergens. In Nichols RL (ed): Trachoma and Related Disorders Caused by Chlamydial Agents. London, Excerpta Medica International Congress series 223, 1971, pp 158–167

75. Kupka K, Nizetic B, Reinhards J: Sampling studies on the epidemiology and control of trachoma in southern Morocco. Bull WHO 39:547, 1968

76. Laibson PR: Adenoviral keratoconjunctivitis. Int. Ophthalmol Clin 15:187, 1975

77. Landau JW: Chronic mucocutaneous candidiasis-associated immunologic abnormalities. Pediatrics 42:227, 1968

78. Lausch RN, Swyers JS, Kaufman HE: Delayed hypersensitivity to herpes simplex virus in the guinea pig. J Immunol 96:981, 1966

79. Lodmell DL, Niwa A, Hayashi K, Notkins AL: Prevention of cell to cell spread of herpes simplex virus by leukocytes. J Exp Med 137:706, 1973

80. Lodmell DL, Notkins AL: Cellular immunity to herpes simplex virus mediated by interferon. J Exp Med 140:764, 1974

81. Londer L, Nelson DL: Orbital cellulitis due to *Haemophilus influenzae.* Arch Ophthalmol 91:89, 1974

82. Lurie HI, Duma RJ: Opportunistic infections of the lungs. Hum Pathol 1:233, 1970

83. Martin HG, Dawson CR, Jones P et al: Herpesvirus in sensory and autonomic ganglia after eye infection. Absence of chronic viral shedding. Arch Ophthalmol 95:2053, 1977

84. McComb DE, Nichols RL: Antibodies to trachoma in eye secretions of Saudi Arab children. Am J Epidemiol 90:278, 1969

85. Mehr KA, Albano L: Failure of levamisole in herpes simplex. Lancet 2:773, 1977

86. Metcalf JE, Kaufman HE: Herpetic stromal keratitis—evidence for cell-mediated immunopathogenesis. Am J Ophthalmol 82:827, 1976

87. Metcalf JF, McNeill JI, Kaufman HE: Experimental disciform edema and necrotizing keratitis in the rabbit. Invest Ophthalmol 15:979, 1976

88. Meyers RL: Immunology of herpes simplex virus infection. Int Ophthalmol Clin 15:37, 1975

89. Meyers RL, Chitjian PA: Cell-mediated immunity in herpes simplex virus infection in vitro. Studies of lymphocytes from rabbits with herpes keratitis. Fed Proc 33:788, 1974

90. Meyers RL, Pettit TH: Corneal immune response to herpes simplex virus antigens. J Immunol 110:1575, 1973

91. Modabber F, Bear SE, Cerny J: The effect of cyclophosphamide on the recovery from a local chlamydial infection. Immunology 30:929, 1976

92. Mondino BJ, Rabin BS, Kessler E et al: Corneal rings with Gram-negative bacteria. Arch Ophthalmol 95:2222, 1977

93. Montgomerie JZ, Becroft DMO, Croxon MC et al: Herpes-simplex-virus infection after renal transplantation. Lancet 2:867, 1969

94. Muller SA, Herrmann EC, Winkelman RK: Herpes simplex infections in hematologic malignancies. Am J Med 52:102, 1972

95. Murray ES, Charbonnet LT, MacDonald AB: Immunity to chlamydial infections of the eye. J Immunol 110:1518, 1973

96. Musher DM, McKenzie SO: Infections due to *Staphylococcus aureus.* Medicine 56:383, 1977

97. Nahmias A, Dowdle W, Josey W et al: Newborn infection with Herpesvirus hominis Type 1 and 2. J Pediatr 75:1194, 1969

98. Nahmias AJ, Visintine AM, Caldwell DR, Wilson LA: Eye infections with herpes simplex virus in neonates. Surv Ophthalmol 21:100, 1976

99. Nesburn AB, Dickinson R, Radnoti M: The effect of trigeminal nerve and ganglion manipulation on recurrence of ocular herpes simplex in rabbits. Invest Ophthalmol 15:726, 1976

100. Nesburn AB, Elliott JM, Leibowitz HM: Spontaneous reactivation of experimental herpes simplex keratitis in rabbits. Arch Ophthalmol 78:523, 1967

101. Newman EW: *Diplococcus pneumoniae* and *Streptococcus viridans* in ocular disease. Arch Ophthalmol 19:95, 1938

102. Notkins AL: Immune mechanisms by which the spread of viral infections is stopped. Cell Immunol 11:478, 1974

103. O'Connor GR: Recurrent herpes simplex uveitis in humans. Surv Ophthalmol 21:165, 1976

104. Oh JO: Enhancement of virus multiplication and interferon production by cortisone in ocular herpesvirus infection. J Immunol 104:1359, 1970

105. O'Reilly RJ, Chibbaro A, Anger E, Lopez C: Cell-mediated immune responses in patients with recurrent herpes simplex infections. II. Infection-associated deficiency of lymphokine production in patients with recurrent herpes labialis or herpes progenitalis. J Immunol 118:1095, 1977

106. Ostler HB: The management of ocular herpes-virus infections. Surv Ophthalmol 21:136, 1976

107. Ostler HB, Lanier JD: Phlyctenular kerato-conjunctivitis with special reference to the staphylococcal type. Trans Pac Coast Otoophthalmol Soc 55:237, 1974

108. Parks JJ, Leibowitz HM, Maumenee AE: A transient stage of suspected delayed sensitivity during the early induction phase of immediate corneal sensitivity. J Exp Med 115:867, 1962

109. Patten JT, Cavanagh HD, Pavan-Langston D: Penetrating keratoplasty in acute herpetic corneal perforations. Ann Ophthalmol 8:287, 1976

110. Patterson A, Jones BR: The management of ocular herpes. Trans Ophthalmol Soc UK 87:59, 1967

111. Pavan-Langston D, Dohlman CH: A double-blind clinical study of adenine arabinoside therapy of viral keratoconjunctivitis. Am J Ophthalmol 74:81, 1972

112. Perkins HR, Allison AC: Cell-wall constituents of rickettsiae and psittacosis-lymphogranuloma organisms. J Gen Microbiol 30:469, 1963

113. Rager-Zisman B, Bloom BR: Immunological destruction of herpes simplex virus I infected cells. Nature 251:542, 1974

114. Rake GW: Chlamydoaceae Rake. In Bergey's Manual of Determinative Bacteriology, 7th ed. Baltimore, Williams and Wilkins, 1948

115. Rand KH, Rasmussen LE, Pollard RB et al: Cellular immunity and herpesvirus infections in cardiac-transplant patients. N Engl J Med 296:1372, 1976

116. Rasmussen LE, Jordan GW, Stevens DA, Merigan TC: Lymphocyte interferon production and transformation after herpes simplex infections in humans. J Immunol 112:728, 1974

117. Rodrigues MM, MacLeod D: Exogenous fungal endophthalmitis caused by Paecilomyces. Am J Ophthalmol 79:687, 1975

118. Rosenberg GL, Snyderman R, Notkins AL: Production of chemotactic factor and lymphotoxin by human leukocytes stimulated with herpes simplex virus. Infect Immun 10:111, 1974

119. Russell AS: Cell-mediated immunity to herpes simplex virus in man. J Infect Dis 129:142, 1974

120. Schachter J: Chlamydiae. In Rose NR, Friedman H: Manual of Clinical Immunology. Washington DC, American Society for Microbiology, 1976, pp. 494–499

121. Schachter J: Chlamydial infections. N Engl J Med 298:428–435, 490–495, 540–549, 1978

122. Schlaegel TF, O'Connor GR: Fungal uveitis. Int Ophthalmol Clin 17:121, 1977

123. Schulkind ML, Adler WH III, Altemeier WA, Ayoub EM: Transfer factor in the treatment of a case of chronic mucocutaneous candidiasis. Cell Immunol 3:606, 1972

124. Sery TW, Nagy RM: Cellular reaction in experimental herpetic disciform keratitis. Am J Ophthalmol 84:675, 1977

125. Sher NA, Hill CW, Eifrig DE: Bilateral intraocular Nocardia asteroides infection. Arch Ophthalmol 95:1415, 1977

126. Shore SL, Nahmias AJ, Starr SE et al: Detection of cell-dependent cytotoxic antibody to cells infected with herpes simplex virus. Nature 251:350, 1974

127. Smith BG, Johnson HM: The effect of staphylococcal enterotoxins on the primary in vitro immune response. Immunology 115:575, 1975

128. Smolin G, Okumoto M: Human transfer factor in the treatment of guinea pig keratitis. Ann Ophthalmol 8:427, 1976

129. Smolin G, Okumoto M: Staphylococcal blepharitis. Arch Ophthalmol 95:812, 1977

130. Smolin G, Okumoto M, Friedlaender MH: The treatment of herpes simplex keratitis with levamisole. Arch Ophthalmol 96:1078, 1978

131. Smolin G, Okumoto M, Meyer R, Belfort R Jr: Effect of immunization with attenuated Mycobacterium bovis (BCG) on experimental herpetic keratitis. Can J Ophthalmol 10:385, 1975

132. Smolin G, Tabbara K, Okumoto M: Guinea pigs herpes simplex keratitis treated with a lymphocyte extract. Am J Ophthalmol 78:921, 1974

133. Soldati M, Verini MA, Isetta AM et al: Immunization researches in the field of trachoma: some laboratory and clinical contributions. In Nichols RL (ed): Trachoma and Related Disorders Caused by Chlamydial Agents. London, Excerpta Medica International Congress Series 223, 1971, pp 407–419

134. Sood NN, Marmion VJ: Superficial herpetic keratitis treated with 5-iodo-2-deoxyuridine. Br J Ophthalmol 48:609, 1964

135. Stevens JG, Cook ML: Maintenance of latent herpetic infection: an apparent role for antiviral IgG. J Immunol 113:1685, 1974

136. St Geme JW, Prince JT, Burke BA et al: Impaired cellular resistance to herpes simplex virus in Wiskott-Aldrich syndrome. N Engl J Med 273:299, 1965

137. Stossel TP: Phagocytosis. N Engl J Med 290:719, 1974

138. Sundmacher R, Neumann-Haefelin D, Cantell K: Successful treatment of dendritic keratitis with human leukocyte interferon. Albrecht von Graefes Arch Klin Ophthalmol 201:39, 1976

139. Swyers JS, Lausch RN, Kaufman HE: Corneal hypersensitivity to herpes simplex. Br J Ophthalmol 51:843, 1967

140. Symoens J, Brugman J: Treatment of recurrent aphthous stomatitis and herpes with levamisole. Br Med J 4:592, 1974

141. Takahashi GH, Leibowitz HM, Kibrick S: Topically applied steroids in active herpes

simplex keratitis. Arch Ophthalmol 85:350, 1971

142. Thatcher RW: Treatment of acute gonococcal conjunctivitis. Ann Ophthalmol 10:445, 1978

143. Thomas CI: The Cornea. Springfield, IL, CC Thomas, 1955

144. Thygeson P: Bacterial factors in chronic catarrhal conjunctivitis. Arch Ophthalmol 18:373, 1937

145. Thygeson P: Marginal corneal infiltrates and ulcers. Arch Ophthalmol 39:432, 1948

146. Thygeson P: Acute central (hypopyon) ulcers of the cornea. Calif Med 59:18, 1948

147. Thygeson P: Observations on nontuberculous phlyctenular keratoconjunctivitis. Trans Am Acad Ophthalmol Otolaryngol 58:128, 1954

148. Thygeson P: Marginal herpes simplex keratitis simulating catarrhal ulcer. Invest Ophthalmol 10:1006, 1971

149. Thygeson P: Historical review of oculogenital disease. Am J Ophthalmol 71:975, 1971

150. Thygeson P: Historical observations on herpetic keratitis. Surv Ophthalmol 21:82, 1976

151. Thygeson P, Dawson CR: Trachoma and follicular conjunctivitis in children. Arch Ophthalmol 75:3, 1966

152. Thygeson P, Kimura S: Deep forms of herpetic keratitis. Am J Ophthalmol 43:109, 1957

153. Thygeson P, Okumoto M: Keratomycosis: a preventable disease. Trans Am Acad Ophthalmol Otolaryngol 78:433, 1974

154. Thygeson P, Sexton R, Corwin M: Observations on the IUDR therapy of herpetic keratitis. Trans Pac Coast Otoophthalmol Soc 45:81, 1963

155. Thygeson P, Stone W: Epidemiology of inclusion conjunctivitis. Arch Ophthalmol 27:91, 1942

156. Tokamuru T: A possible role of γ A immunoglobulin in herpes simplex virus infection in man. J Immunol 97:248, 1966

157. Valenton M, Okumoto M: Toxin-producing strains of *Staphylococcus epidermidis.* Arch Ophthalmol 89:186, 1973

158. Vastine DW, Schwartz HS, Yamashiroya HM et al: Cytologic diagnosis of adenoviral epidemic keratoconjunctivitis by direct immunofluorescence. Invest Ophthalmol Vis Sci 16:195, 1977

159. Vaughan D: The contamination of fluorescein solutions. Am J Ophthalmol 39:55, 1955

160. Wang S-P, Grayston JT: Pannus with experimental trachoma and inclusion conjunctivitis agent infection of Taiwan monkeys. Am J Ophthalmol [Suppl] 63:1133, 1967

161. Wang S-P, Grayston JT: Local and systemic antibody response to trachoma eye infection in monkeys. In Nichols RL (ed): Trachoma and Related Disorders Caused by Chlamydial Agents. London, Excerpta Medica International Congress Series 223, 1971, pp 217–232

162. Watson RR, Mull JD, MacDonald AB et al: Immunity to chlamydial infections of the eye. II. Studies of passively transferred serum antibody in resistance to infection with guinea pig inclusion conjunctivitis. Infect Immun 7:597, 1973

163. Wellings PC, Awdry PN, Bors FH, Jones BR: Clinical evaluation of trifluoro-thymidine in the treatment of herpes simplex corneal ulcers. Am J Ophthalmol 73:932, 1972

164. Whitcher JP, Dawson CR, Hoshiwara I et al: Herpes simplex keratitis in a developing country. Natural history and treatment of dendritic and geographic ulcers in Tunisia. Arch Ophthalmol 94:587, 1976

165. Whitcher JP, Schmidt NJ, Mabrouk R et al: Acute hemorrhagic conjunctivitis in Tunisia. Report of viral isolations. Arch Ophthalmol 94:51, 1976

166. Williams LE, Nesburn AB, Kaufman HE: Experimental induction of disciform keratitis. Arch Ophthalmol 73:112, 1965

167. Wilson LA, Ahearn DG: Pseudomonas-induced corneal ulcers associated with contaminated eye mascaras. Am J Ophthalmol 84:112, 1977

168. Wilton JMA, Ivanyi L, Lehner T: Cell-mediated immunity in herpes virus hominis infections. Br Med J 1:723, 1972

169. Wing EJ, Remington JS: Cell mediated immunity and its role in resistance to infection (Medical Progress). West J Med 126:14, 1977

170. Wise TG, Pavan PR, Ennis FA: Herpes simplex virus vaccines. J Infect Dis 136:706, 1977

171. Wood RE: Pseudomonas: the compromised host. Hosp Pract 11:91, 1976

172. Zam ZS, Centifanto YM, Kaufman HE: Failure of systemically administered adenine arabinoside to affect humoral and cell-mediated immunity. Am J Ophthalmol 81:502, 1976

173. Zimmerman TJ, McNeill JI, Richman A et al: HLA types and recurrent corneal herpes simplex infection. Invest Ophthalmol Vis Sci 16:756, 1977

174. Zinkernagel RM: Major transplantation antigens in host responses to infection. Hosp Pract, 13:83, 1978

175. Zisman B, Hirsch MS, Allison AC: Selective effects of antimacrophages. I. An analysis of cell-virus interaction. J Exp Med 113:19, 1971

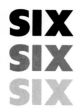

SIX
SIX
SIX the eye and systemic infections

Infectious diseases are intimately associated with the functions of the immune system. Much of our knowledge about basic mechanisms in immunology was derived from the study of host interactions with infectious agents. Immune mechanisms probably evolved in order to protect the individual from the destructive effects of invading organisms and their products. If these protective mechanisms are successful, they will eliminate the infectious agent. Under certain conditions, however, immune mechanisms can behave as pathogenic forms of hypersensitivity. The eye may be involved in direct infection (see Immunology of Ocular Infections, Ch. 5) or in a variety of systemic infections. It may also be the focus of hypersensitivity reactions to a number of infectious agents.

BACTERIAL DISEASES

TUBERCULOSIS

Mycobacterium tuberculosis is a facultative intracellular aerobic acid-fast bacillus which is pathogenic mainly for man. While the disease that it produces primarily involves lung tissue, many extrapulmonary sites, including the eye, may be affected. Tuberculosis is a disease in which cellular immunity rather than humoral immune mechanisms is decisive in recovery from infection. Likewise, in the diagnosis of tuberculosis, the tuberculin skin test, a manifestation of cellular immunity, is useful, rather than measurement of serum antibody.

Immunopathology

M. tuberculosis has the ability to survive and proliferate within phagocytic cells. It may evade the bactericidal activity of macrophages by preventing the fusion of enzyme-containing lysosomes with phagosomes containing the organism. The organism produces no known toxins, but the host's respose to the tubercle bacillus is influenced by certain constituents of the organism. High-molecular-weight lipids and waxes comprise up to 60% of the cell wall of the bacillus. These substances may be responsible for the tissue reaction to the microorganism and possibly for its impermeability to tissue stains. Wax D and tuberculoproteins may be responsible for the induction of hypersensitivity and the skin test reaction. A substance known as cord factor is responsible for the serpentine cordlike growth of the tubercle bacillus and may inhibit the migration of leukocytes and stimulate granuloma formation.

Cellular immunity is the mechanism by which the individual deals with *M. tuberculosis*, as demonstrated by the following: Macrophages ingest the organism in the course of the cell-mediated immune response. Cell-mediated immunity to tuberculin may be transferred passively in experimental animals by living lymphoid cells, but not by serum. Such immunity may also be transferred by a leukocyte extract known as transfer factor. Patients with agammaglobulinemia produce no demonstrable antibodies, yet are capable of developing delayed-type hypersensitivity and normal resistance to tuberculosis. Patients with defects in delayed hypersensitivity, however, are more susceptible to the disease.

Apparently, immunity and tuberculin hypersensitivity are not inextricably linked. Skin test reactivity to tuberculin does not always correlate with protection against infection. Strongly positive reactors to tuberculin may in fact experience reactivation of the disease. On the other hand, persons vaccinated with bacillus Calmette–Guèrin (BCG) vaccine are often resistant even after skin test responses wane. Moreover, wax D may produce tuberculin hypersensitivity without conferring immunity against infection. On the other hand, animals immunized with a complex consisting of mycobacterial RNA and protein will have increased resistance without positive skin reactions. This suggests that the nonspecific factors of inflammation may be less important than specific lymphocyte-mediated immune responses in recovery from infection.

Clinical Features

General. The first infection with tuberculosis produces few if any clinical signs or symptoms, and may go unrecognized. A localized infection in the periphery of the lung develops after inhalation of the organism. The inflammatory response is exudative and composed mainly of neutrophils and monocytes. Mild fever and malaise may develop; however, the primary infection is generally well tolerated. Local spread to the hilar lymph nodes results in the formation of the classic Ghon complex, which later calcifies. Virulent bacilli may persist in these lesions for many years.

Secondary infection with tuberculosis results in a distinct disease process associated with tissue destruction. This process may result from exogenous reinfection, but more commonly it is the result of reactivation of an old infection. It may be precipitated by a depression of the individual's immune system due to advanced age, debilitating illness, or the use of immunosuppressive drugs. Reinfection tuberculosis is associated with cavitation in the apical or subapical pulmonary segments. Caseating granulomas form and tissue destruction may be profound. Hematogenous

dissemination may result in involvement of other organs such as the kidney, central nervous system, bones, or eye.

Ocular Findings. The first description of ocular tuberculosis was that of Maitre Jan (64) in 1740. During the early nineteenth century, a number of cases of probable ocular tuberculosis were reported. Jaeger (53), in 1855, described the clinical manifestations of ocular tuberculosis. In 1858 Manz (66) described tuberculosis involving the choroid, and in 1869 Gradenigo (37) described tuberculous iritis. Corneal tuberculosis was reported in 1885 by Roy and Alvarez (93) and subsequently scleral involvement was recognized. Much of our understanding about the pathogenesis of ocular tuberculosis is owed to Woods (123 124). He classified ocular tuberculosis into three types: 1) the juvenile type, which produces extensive, fulminating anterior and posterior segment lesions; 2) the adolescent type, which causes marked inflammatory lesions such as a sclerokeratitis or chronic choroiditis in a previously infected individual; and 3) the adult type, which develops in older individuals with declining immunity and runs a prolonged, chronic course. Typical lesions of the last-named type include corneal infiltrates, chronic uveitis, and disseminated choroiditis.

Tuberculosis may affect nearly all ocular tissues. Eyelid involvement may be either primary or secondary. Both types of infection are rare. The most common form of secondary infection is known as **lupus vulgaris.** This is a chronic and slowly progressive infection characterized by soft, "apple jelly" tubercles. These lesions may spread slowly and may produce ulceration and scarring which can result in ectropion and exposure keratitis.

Rarely, tuberculosis may affect the conjunctiva in either primary or secondary infection. The primary form is generally unilateral and occurs in young people. It may follow minor trauma and is characterized by edema, lacrimation, and mucoid discharge. Large follicles may form, and these tend to ulcerate and scar. In secondary tuberculous conjunctivitis, infection is found to spread from neighboring tuberculous foci. It may take either a nodular or an ulcerative form. A chronic course with

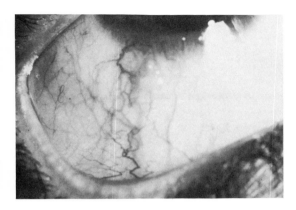

FIG. 6-1. Phlyctenule at the limbus. (Courtesy of F. I. Proctor Foundation)

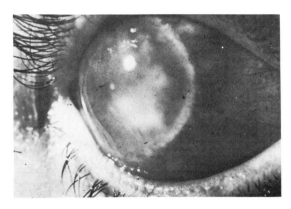

FIG. 6-3. Corneal involvement in tuberculosis. (Courtesy of F. I. Proctor Foundation)

scarring and involvement of the globe may occur.

Phlyctenular keratoconjunctivitis (Figs. 6-1 and 6-2) was frequently associated with tuberculosis at one time and use to be a major cause of corneal blindness. Now this entity is more commonly associated with staphylococcal disease. It is thought to be due to a delayed hypersensitivity reaction involving the cornea and conjunctiva. It is not due to direct infection of the tissues, and tubercle bacilli are not found in these lesions. The first phlyctenule generally occurs at the limbus. Subsequent attacks may involve either the conjunctiva or the cornea. The phlyctenules are vascularized and are usually associated with marked photophobia and lacrimation. They run a self-limited

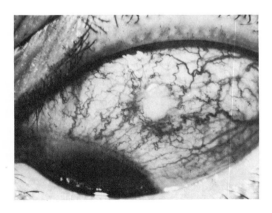

FIG. 6-2. Phlyctenule of the conjunctiva. (Courtesy of F. I. Proctor Foundation)

course of 10-14 days. Lesions may become necrotic and then epithelialize.

Tuberculosis of the cornea (Fig. 6-3) develops secondary to infection of adjacent parts of the eye, such as the sclera, conjunctiva, or uveal tract. It may take the form of a sclerokeratitis, interstitial keratitis, a deep central keratitis, or multiple infiltrates of the peripheral or central cornea (27). The interstitial keratitis is felt to be allergic in origin, and may be similar clinically to syphilitic interstitial keratitis. Frequently the keratitis is sector like and may consist of nodular corneal lesions. Scleral tuberculosis may occur as a superficial episcleral inflammation or as a deep scleritis. The former is thought to have an immune basis (27), while the latter is generally due to direct infection of ocular tissues (10).

The most important form of ocular tuberculosis is that which affects the uveal tract. Uveal tuberculosis may be divided into two main types: 1) proliferative tuberculous lesions due to direct infection of uveal tissues, and 2) diffuse hypersensitivity states which occur in previously infected individuals having immunity to the organism. Uveitis due to tuberculosis is a granulomatous type of inflammation characterized by "mutton-fat" keratic precipitates and a chronic course. Involvement may be primarily anterior, in which case there may be extensive posterior synechiae, Koeppe nodules, and vitreous opacities. Other forms of anterior uveitis have also been described. One of rather short duration may occur during the course of treatment and is probably due to an allergic mechanism. A nodular form has been described in young people with low resistance and miliary tuberculosis. A conglomerate tubercle of the iris may form by the coalescence of several miliary tubercles. This progresses rapidly and is associated with pain and secondary glaucoma.

Posterior tuberculous uveitis may present as a solitary tubercle of the choroid or as a tuberculoma of the posterior uvea. The former first appears as a grayish white raised mass which leaves an atrophic scar in the fundus. It occurs in adults and frequently involves the macular region. The tuberculoma of the choroid usually occurs in adults with low resistance and is characterized by multiple lesions throughout the fundus, vitreous opacities, and atrophy and gliosis of the choroid and retina.

Frequently a diagnosis of tuberculosis is entertained in the presence of a diffuse posterior choroiditis of uncertain etiology. Patients with such findings will often have a strongly positive tuberculin test but no sign of active systemic disease. In some instances, empiric treatment of these patients with isoniazid has resulted in clinical improvement.

Hematogenous spread of tuberculosis in patients with no evidence of active disease may occasionally result in acute tuberculous panophthalmitis (24). Such cases may be associated with mutton-fat keratic precipitates and Koeppe nodules. A tuberculoma of the orbit can produce an orbital apex syndrome and proptosis (76).

Retinal tuberculosis has been described; it generally is thought to occur secondary to choroidal tuberculosis. Originally, the retinitis described by Eales (28) (see Retinal Vasculitis, Ch. 7) was considered to be a manifestation of tuberculosis. It is doubtful, however, that most cases of Eales' disease are related to tuberculosis. An exudative retinitis, however, consisting of multiple well-defined exudative patches, has been described in adults with tuberculin hypersensitivity.

Diagnosis

In most cases of ocular tuberculosis, no evidence of active pulmonary disease can be detected but frequently patients will show evidence of old, healed pulmonary lesions. A tuberculin skin test may be helpful in making a diagnosis. The commonly used antigenic preparations include old tuberculin, which is prepared by concentrating a heat-inactivated filtrate of culture broth in which tubercle bacilli have been grown, and purified protein derivatives of tuberculin (PPD), which are prepared by ammonium sulfate precipitation of culture filtrates of *M. tuberculosis*. First-strength and intermediate-strength PPD are customarily used in routine skin testing. If these tests are negative, and tuberculosis is still suspected, a second strength PPD test is then administered. A positive skin test response consists of 10 mm or more of erythema or induration. The test site is examined 48 and 72 h after the skin test substance is applied.

False-negative tests for tuberculin may occur in disseminated tuberculosis, measles, sarcoidosis, and lymphoma, or in other conditions which depress cellular immunity. In addition, the administration of immunosuppressive drugs, such as corticosteroids, may reduce or abolish tuberculin skin test reactivity. False-positive tests are encountered much less often but may occur with infection caused by atypical mycobacteria. Individuals who have received prophylactic BCG vaccine will also have positive tuberculin skin test reactions for up to 15 years following vaccination.

Treatment

Isoniazid (INH) is the most commonly used antituberculosis drug and has many advantages. It penetrates tissues well and crosses the blood–brain barrier. It is relatively nontoxic and is tolerated well by patients. It occasionally causes a peripheral neuritis or hepatic dysfunction. Isoniazid hepatitis usually develops in individuals over the age of 35 during the first several months of therapy. Ethambutol is often used in combination with INH. It is also well tolerated and has few toxic side effects. Optic nerve toxicity may occur with ethambutol and monitoring of vision is suggested. Rifampin is a very effective drug, but when it is used alone resistance can develop rapidly. It is also associated with little toxicity, especially when used in combination with INH. Rifampin has been shown to produce immunosuppression. Streptomycin was the first effective chemotherapeutic agent used in tuberculosis. It is associated with eighth nerve toxicity and is less desirable for routine use than the above-mentioned drugs. Aminosalicylic acid (PAS) is an effective drug for tuberculosis but is generally not used because of gastrointestinal side effects.

In addition to the systemic form of treatment just described, subconjunctival or topical treatment with streptomycin has been used in scleral tuberculosis (10). In cases of uveitis in which a tuberculous etiology is suspected, a course of isoniazid may be used on empiric grounds. Pyridoxine (vitamin B$_6$) should be administered with this drug to prevent peripheral neuropathy.

LEPROSY

Leprosy is a chronic infectious disease caused by *Mycobacterium leprae*, an obligate intracellular acid-fast bacillus (Fig. 6–4). This organism has the ability to invade nerves and skin, giving rise to widespread clinical manifestations. Three main types of clinical disease are recognized: 1) Lepromatous (nodular) leprosy is characterized by a marked deficiency in cellular immunity and extensive infiltration of tissues with *M. leprae*. 2) Tuberculoid leprosy is distinguished by the preservation of immune responses and an absence of demonstrable bacilli in tissues. 3) Intermediate or borderline leprosy has features of both the lepromatous and tuberculoid types. Some 90% of lepromatous leprosy cases have ocular manifestations and nearly one-third of these show significant visual loss.

Immunopathology

Leprosy patients have a number of immunologic defects involving both the humoral and cellular immune systems. Patients with lepromatous leprosy have impaired cell-mediated immunity against *M. leprae* organisms. They demonstrate skin anergy to the lepromin skin test antigen, while normal persons often have a positive delayed hypersensitivity reaction.

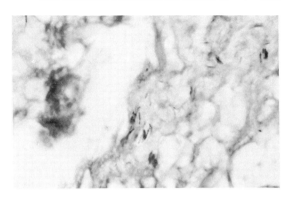

FIG. 6-4. *Mycobacterium leprae*. (Courtesy of M. Okumoto)

These patients also may fail to develop contact hypersensitivity to dinitrochlorobenzene (DNCB) and other contact sensitizers (118). They also have depressed delayed hypersensitivity reactions to common bacterial antigens (16) and demonstrate prolonged skin allograft survival.

Patients with lepromatous leprosy have significantly lower than normal levels of circulating T and B lymphocytes and marked depletion of T cells in the paracortical regions of their lymph nodes (70). The peripheral lymphocytes of these patients show diminished blast transformation in the presence of the mitogen phytohemagglutinin. The development of the infection is apparently related to the survival of the bacillus within macrophages. Recent electron microscopic studies have demonstrated that the organism is capable of escaping from the phagosome and remaining free in the macrophage cytoplasm. Laboratory studies have demonstrated that mice thymectomized at birth, and therefore lacking in cellular immunity, develop widespread infections with *M. leprae* (90).

In contrast to the deficits in cellular immunity, patients with lepromatous leprosy have normal or hyperactive antibody production and may produce excessive autoantibodies. These patients have an increase in γ-globulin and a significant increase in the levels of cryoproteins. In addition, thyroglobulin antibodies and rheumatoid factor are found in 50% of patients with lepromatous leprosy, and

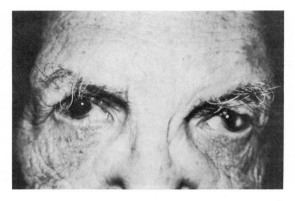

FIG. 6-5. Lepromatous leprosy. (Courtesy of Dr. J. Wolfe)

false-positive VDRL (Venereal Disease Research Laboratory) tests are present in about 10%. Occasionally LE cells can be found in leprosy patients. Anti–basement-membrane antibodies and anti–intercellular-substance antibodies have been demonstrated in the skin of patients with lepromatous leprosy (86). The similarity between leprosy and the collagen vascular diseases, particularly lupus erythematosus, has been pointed out by some authors. Both may have similar clinical manifestations, including butterfly facial rashes and arthritis, as well as depressed cellular immunity and autoantibody production.

In contrast to the usual findings of depressed cellular immunity and autoantibody formation, Rea *et al* (89) have reported that patients with lepromatous leprosy have normal immunologic responses to antigens other than lepromin. These patients could be sensitized to DNFB (dinitrofluorobenzene) or DNCB, and had normal percentages of T and B lymphocytes, normal responses to mitogens, and no excessive autoantibody production. Thus, lepromatous leprosy may not always be associated with these well-documented immunologic abnormalities. (This same group of investigators had previously demonstrated anti–basement-membrane antibodies and anti–intercellular-substance antibodies in the skin of lepromatous leprosy patients.) Whether these immune defects are predisposing factors in the development of leprosy or are consequences of the infection still remains debatable.

Clinical Features

Lepromatous Leprosy. This form of the disease is distinguished by widespread invasion by leprosy bacilli, which infiltrate the skin, mucous membranes, and nerves extensively. The nose particularly may be affected. Nerve destruction occurs late in the course of this disease. The end stage of the disease leads to the leonine facies so characteristic of leprosy (Fig. 6-5).

The supraciliary ridges are thickened and there is loss of the eyebrows, beginning temporally during the early stages of the disease. Nodules, which histologically resemble xanthomas, appear on the face and lids. These contain multinucleated giant cells (**lepra cells**) and many bacilli. The lids become infiltrated by granulomatous inflammation and the cellular infiltrate extends through the tarsal plate and onto the conjunctival surface. Lashes may show poliosis, and in the later stages of the disease there may be a marked loss of cilia and eyebrows, and disfiguration of brows, nose, and lips. A hyperemic keratoconjunctivitis may occur, followed by symblepharon formation and lid deformities. Nodules may develop on the cornea, usually beginning at the limbus; interstitial keratitis may be seen as well (Fig. 6-6). An acute inflammatory iridocyclitis or a slow and nodular granulomatous cyclitis may develop (97). Chorioretinitis has also been reported. Involvement of the lacrimal sac and duct is rare.

Tuberculoid Leprosy. This form of leprosy is in general less severe than the lepromatous form. There may be only a few well-demarcated skin lesions which are erythematous and raised, and possess an anesthetic, atrophic center. Palpable nerve trunks may be present in the area of the skin lesions. This type of leprosy has a predilection for nervous tissue. However, acid-fast bacilli may only rarely be demonstrated histologically.

Skin lesions may affect the lids and the brow. This leads to loss of the eyebrows and cilia, and to degenerative changes involving the brows and lid margins. The muscles of the eyelids and iris are particularly affected in tuberculoid leprosy. Seventh nerve involvement

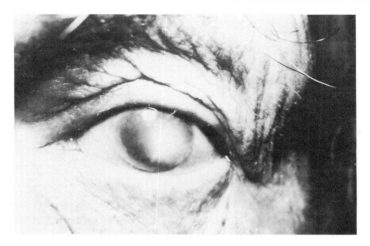

FIG. 6-6. Corneal opacification in patient with leprosy. (Courtesy of Dr. J. Wolfe)

may lead to a decrease in blinking, lid dysfunction, and exposure keratitis. The third, fourth, and sixth cranial nerves are less frequently involved and therefore extraocular muscle paresis is unusual.

Borderline Leprosy. This form of leprosy is intermediate between the lepromatous and tuberculoid types and may have features of either or both. Those cases more nearly resembling lepromatous leprosy have more numerous skin lesions and greater defects in cellular immunity. Those cases resembling tuberculoid leprosy have fewer skin lesions, more skin anesthesia, and a more intact cellular immunity.

Immunologic Diagnosis

The lepromin skin test, introduced by Mitsuda, is performed with extracts of skin nodules from leprosy patients. A positive intradermal test leads to a tuberculin-type skin reaction at 24–48 h and a later nodular reaction (the Mitsuda reaction) appearing at about 7 days and reaching a maximum at 3–4 weeks. The only value of this test is in differentiating the type of leprosy in patients already known to have the disease. A positive lepromin skin test is diagnostic of tuberculoid or near-tuberculoid disease, whereas a negative skin test indicates progression to lepromatous leprosy.

Positive skin tests are common in the normal population, owing to cross reactivity with other mycobacterial antigens and foreign skin proteins.

Treatment

The mainstay of treatment in leprosy is dapsone (4,4′-diaminodiphenyl sulfone). Other medications include rifampin, which is bactericidal for *M. leprae*, and clofazimine, a phenazine dye which stimulates macrophage bactericidal activity and also has direct anticomplement activity. Leprosy patients are said to tolerate surgery better than might be expected, and plastic repair of lid changes can be undertaken successfully although results may not be permanent.

Recently, transfer factor has been used to restore cellular immunity in patients with leprosy (44). Patients with lepromatous leprosy have shown a marked decrease in the bacillus population of the skin following weekly injections with transfer factor over a 3-month period. However, no definite clinical improvement has been obtained.

Immunologic Complications

There are five basic immunologic complications which are seen in leprosy:

1. "Antigen overload" due to lack of cellu-

lar immunity: Large numbers of *M. leprae* may accumulate in the skin, blood, and nasal secretions. The presence of this large load of a foreign antigen stimulates massive antibody production and consequent hypergammaglobulinemia, cryoglobulinemia, and autoantibody production. Rheumatoid factor and false-positive serologic tests for syphilis are frequently obtained.

2. Erythema nodosum leprosum: When large numbers of circulating immune complexes are present in patients with leprosy, they will be deposited in the blood vessels, joints, and kidneys. This produces an Arthus-type immune reaction with complement fixation, and results in a vasculitis and panniculitis. Clinically, this results in the appearance of hundreds of tender, erythematous skin lesions over the entire body, associated with severe systemic symptoms. Nearly 50% of lepromatous leprosy patients acquire erythema nodosum during the course of the disease. Erythema nodosum may be treated with thalidomide or clofazimine.

3. Lucio phenomenon (erythema necroticans): This is a necrotizing vasculitis which may be a variant of erythema nodosum. It is characterized by ulceration and sloughing of large areas of skin.

4. Reversal and downgrading reactions: These immunologic complications represent sudden shifts in cell-mediated immunity. In the downgrading reaction, granulomas dissolve and lymphocytes become sparse. In the reversal reaction, an inactive area may become rapidly populated with lymphocytes. In either of these reactions, inactive skin lesions may become tender and red. Treatment involves the use of corticosteroids.

5. Amyloidosis: Amyloid deposition may lead to renal failure and death in patients with advanced leprosy. It is seen more commonly in Caucasians than in other racial groups.

SYPHILIS

Syphilis is caused by the spirochete *Treponema pallidum*, a motile, highly infectious agent which functions predominantly as an extracellular pathogen. It occurs naturally only in man and is most easily transmitted by sexual contact. Both humoral and cellular immunity are important in the host's defense against syphilis. Three stages of syphilis are identifiable clinically. The eye may be involved at any stage of the disease. While severe destructive syphilitic lesions have become far less common since the advent of penicillin, the disease must be kept in mind in the differential diagnosis of many clinical problems.

Immunopathology

Immunity to *T. pallidum* depends on a complex interaction between humoral and cellular factors. Several lines of evidence suggest the importance of antibody in this infection. A partial immunity to the organism develops in the rabbit following passive transfer of serum from immune animals. It is also possible to demonstrate immobilizing antibodies against treponemes in the serum of patients who have syphilis. These antibodies are found with increased frequency in the later stages of syphilis. A number of nonspecific, or reaginic, antibodies are found in the serum of patients who have syphilis; these form the basis for many of the serologic tests for syphilis. Antibodies which develop during the course of syphilitic infection are at best only partially protective. Syphilis progresses through the primary and secondary stages in spite of the presence of antibodies which immobilize treponemes.

Immune complex deposition may play a role in the nephropathy associated with secondary syphilis in adults, and IgG may be deposited along the glomerular basement membrane in patients with the glomerulopathy of congenital syphilis (57).

Although *T. pallidum* functions as an extracellular pathogen, cellular immunity is felt to be important in the body's control of this organism. Delayed hypersensitivity directed against treponemal antigens develops late in secondary syphilis but is absent in primary and early secondary disease. It is regularly found in latent and tertiary syphilis. Immunization with live microorganisms is capable of stimulating immunity to treponemes, but killed microorganisms will not.

The reason for the long delay in the development of immunity to *T. pallidum* is unknown. The organism may be unusually resistant to phagocytosis because of a possible antiphagocytic factor. This may result in "antigen overload" and secondary immunosuppression. Alternatively, infection with *T. pallidum* may lead to the generation of blocking antibodies which attach to antigenic sites and inhibit the cellular immune response.

Histologically, the typical lesion of syphilis is a granulomatous inflammation. Granulomas are characterized by the presence of reticuloendothelial cells, including epithelioid and giant cells. Granulomas are considered to represent a cell-mediated immune response to poorly soluble substances, including foreign bodies, insoluble antigens, and microorganisms that cannot easily be eliminated. Granulomatous reactions are clearly different from typical delayed-type hypersensitivity reactions. For example the onset is much slower in granulomatous reactions, which require weeks or even months to develop. Many granulomatous lesions are accompanied by a vasculitis, suggesting the possibility of an associated immune complex disease.

Clinical Features

General. Primary syphilis is characterized by the appearance of a chancre, a painless indurated ulcer. This usually occurs on the genitalia but may develop on the lip, rectal area, or eyelid. The chancre appears 5 days to 3 months after infection but generally is seen within 2–3 weeks. The chancre typically lasts for 10–14 days and then heals spontaneously.

The hallmark of secondary syphilis is the appearance of a mucocutaneous rash. Typically, the palms and the soles of the feet are involved. The skin lesions are quite varied but may be macular, papular, or mixed in character. Lid involvement may occur during this stage. Aside from the skin rash, there may be no other manifestations of systemic disease at this stage. Sometimes, however, headache, low-grade fever, and diffuse lymphadenopathy may occur. Spontaneous resolution of the skin rash occurs with or without treatment. In 25% of untreated patients, repeated episodes of infection may occur.

A latent period develops after the resolution of secondary syphilis. The first 4 years are referred to as early latency, and beyond 4 years, as late latency. Although there is no outward disease at this time, local infection is presumably taking place at various sites in the body.

Fifteen percent of patients with untreated latent syphilis will eventually develop tertiary syphilis. This is the most devastating form of the disease. The most severe forms affect the aorta, the central nervous system, and the eye. Other sites of involvement include the skin, larynx, testes, liver, and bones. Many patients will reach the stage of tertiary syphilis without definite evidence of primary and secondary infection.

Early congenital syphilis may present with skin lesions like those of secondary syphilis and, in addition, with bullous skin lesions which are characteristic for this stage of the disease. A catarrhal discharge from the nose and a progressive wasting or marasmus are also characteristic. In late congenital syphilis, Hutchinson's triad of notched and narrow-edged incisors, eighth nerve deafness, and interstitial keratitis may be seen. Other stigmata of late congenital syphilis include mulberry molars, osteitis, saddle deformity of the nose, fissures or cracks in the skin (rhagades), frontal bossing, and scaphoid scapula. Interstitial keratitis (Fig. 6-7 and 6-8), the most common finding in congenital syphilis, occurs in approximately 50% of the patients.

Ocular Findings. A primary extragenital chancre may occasionally develop on the lid or conjunctiva. It may result from genital or finger contact or be transmitted from an infected mouth lesion. The primary chancre appears as a purple nonulcerated patch, as an indurated subcutaneous nodule, or most commonly as an indurated ulcer. A conjunctivitis may accompany a lid chancre. Lid edema and regional adenopathy also may be present. Pain is usually absent and resolution occurs in 5–6 weeks with little scarring.

The eyelids may be affected in secondary syphilis. Pinkish irregular macules or acnelike papules may develop on the lids as elsewhere. Ulcerative blepharitis leads to scarring and

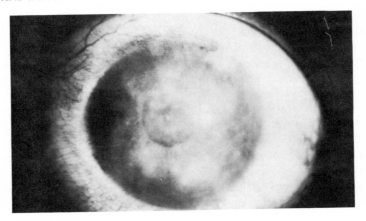

FIG. 6-7. Syphilis: Interstitial keratitis. (Courtesy of Dr. R. S. Weinberg)

loss of cilia. Lid edema and temporary loss of eyebrows may also be seen.

During secondary syphilis, the uveal tract may be involved. Roseola of the iris, consisting of engorged vascular loops in the middle third of the iris, may last for a few days. Iridocyclitis is not uncommon in the early secondary stages of syphilis (126). It is usually unilateral and acute, and is accompanied by a rash in three-fourths of the cases. The second eye may be affected in 45% of patients but both eyes are not usually involved simultaneously. Although well described, iridocyclitis associated with secondary syphilis is rarely seen in uveitis clinics (81).

Syphilitic iridocyclitis may be seen rarely with recurrent syphilis. A skin rash is usually absent. The inflammation may be severe, and secondary glaucoma can develop. An acute iritis may develop following treatment of syphilis with penicillin. This is due to the Jarisch–Herxheimer reaction and occurs 10–16 h after the first injection of penicillin. It is thought to be due to liberation of endotoxin following the death of a large number of organisms.

Chorioretinitis associated with syphilis occurs in the late secondary and tertiary stages of the disease. Lesions are circumscribed, and may be disseminated or localized. The lesions are usually bilateral and may be accompanied by a vasculitis and proliferation of retinal pigment. Choroidal lesions may vary in size, shape, and location. Recurrences develop at variable time intervals: uveitis may accompany tertiary syphilis 20 years or more after the original infection. Inflammation ranges from mild to severe and the entire uveal tract may be involved. A nodular iritis is typical and broad synechiae may develop. Choroiditis is generally present in such cases. Tertiary syphilis may be accompanied by central nervous system lesions; the Argyll Robertson pupil is a well-known ocular accompaniment of neurosyphilis.

Severe ischemic retinopathy, rubeosis iridis, and secondary glaucoma may also develop (96). Hemorrhages and sheathing of vessels may be seen in this condition. New vessels may form on the optic disc in association with rubeosis iridis.

The **gumma** (a soft gummy tumor of tuberculous origin) is a characteristic destructive lesion of late syphilis. It probably represents a hypersensitivity process (73). An obliterative endarteritis resulting in inflammatory and necrotic changes may also be responsible for the lesions of late syphilis.

Interstitial keratitis is a widespread infiltrative inflammation of the corneal stroma that is usually bilateral. It is more frequently associated with congenital syphilis than with acquired disease. It generally appears after the age of 5 and usually before the age of 20. Rarely, it appears at birth or during early infancy. Spontaneous remissions occur in 10% of cases. Clinically, interstitial keratitis develops in three stages. The initial stage consists of a

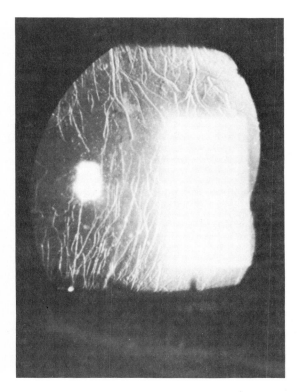

FIG. 6-8. Syphilis: Interstitial keratitis. (Courtesy of Dr. G. Mintsioulis)

rapid onset of diffuse corneal edema. Descemet's folds and keratic precipitates are seen. The second stage consists of the ingrowth of limbal blood vessels extending into all parts of the cornea. This stage lasts for several weeks before the third stage of gradual clearing ensues. The cornea is left with ghost vessels and areas of clearing throughout the cornea. Thinning of the cornea, high myopia, and corneal guttata may occur as complications. Because interstitial keratitis is thought by some to be a hypersensitivity phenomenon, it is generally treated with topical corticosteroids. The disease, however, is self limited when left untreated, and penicillin does not modify its course.

Other ocular features of congenital syphilis include an acute iridocyclitis, a chorioretinitis with a "salt-and-pepper" mottling of the fundus, and malformations of the optic disc.

A nonsyphilitic interstitial keratitis with vestibuloauditory symptoms has been described by Cogan (22). Patients with this disorder may have an increased incidence of the histocompatibility antigen HLA-Bw17 and increased cell-mediated immunity against normal allogeneic corneal antigens (19).

Diagnosis

During primary and secondary syphilis, the spirochete can be demonstrated by darkfield microscopic examination. Serologic tests do not become positive until 14–21 days after the initial infection. Since spirochetes are difficult to demonstrate in the later stages of syphilis, serologic tests are extremely important. Two categories of serologic tests are available: tests for reaginic antibodies and tests for treponemal antibodies. Although the antibodies are called "reaginic," they bear no relationship to IgE reaginic antibody. Rather, they are antibodies directed against a tissue-derived substance, known as cardiolipin, which is thought to be a component of mitochondrial membranes. Beef heart is used as a source of cardiolipin in many of these tests. Examples of tests for reaginic antibody include the Venereal Disease Research Laboratory (VDRL), Hinton, and Kahn tests.

A so-called biologic false-positive (BFP) reaction in serologic tests occurs in other diseases, including systemic lupus erythematosus, leprosy, infectious mononucleosis, and hepatitis. This is due to the prevalence of mitochondrial membranes in many tissues and microorganisms.

Tests for treponemal antibodies include the *Treponema pallidum* immobilization (TPI) test and the fluorescent treponemal antibody (FTA) test. The former test detects specific antibodies against the spirochete. The latter utilizes spirochetes from infected rabbit testes which are overlaid with serum from the patient being tested. If an antigen–antibody reaction takes place, the bound antibody can be detected with fluoresceinated antibody to human γ-globulin. Other nonpathogenic treponemes are usually absorbed from the serum, in which case the test is referred to as the FTA-ABS test.

The FTA-ABS test is positive in 80% of primary syphilis cases. The VDRL test is positive in 50%. In secondary syphilis both tests are positive in nearly 100% of cases. The VDRL test tends to decline after treatment of syphilis, while the FTA-ABS test usually remains positive for many years. While false-positive results are common with VDRL tests, they are rarely encountered with the FTA-ABS test, except, possibly, in systemic lupus erythematosus. In latent syphilis, the VDRL test is negative in up to one-third of patients.

The VDRL and FTA-ABS tests should be performed in cases of diffuse choroiditis of uncertain etiology. Treponemes may sometimes be detected in the aqueous humor of uveitis patients (102). These may, however, be nonpathogenic organisms such as **T. microdentium.** Aqueous humor aspiration may be productive in a search for treponemes using a fluorescent antibody technique.

Treatment

The drug of choice for syphilis is penicillin. The current regimen for early syphilis (primary, secondary, or latent syphilis of less than 1 year's duration) is benzathine penicillin G 2.4 million units at one time, or aqueous procaine penicillin G 600,000 units daily for 8 days. Patients allergic to penicillin may be given either tetracycline or erythromycin, 500 mg four times a day orally for 15 days. In syphilis of more than 1 year's duration, treatment consists of benzathine penicillin G 2.4 million units IM weekly for 3 consecutive weeks, or aqueous procaine penicillin G 600,-000 units IM daily for 15 days (116). Cerebrospinal fluid (CSF) examination is mandatory in patients with suspected neurosyphilis, and serial monitoring of the blood and CSF by serologic testing should be done at 4-month intervals during therapy. Penicillin should be continued if the VDRL test remains positive or if the CSF contains inflammatory cells.

Infants with congenital syphilis should receive a CSF examination before treatment. If the CSF is abnormal, aqueous crystalline penicillin G should be given, 50,000 units/kg of body weight IM or IV daily in two divided doses for a minimum of 10 days. Alternatively, aqueous procaine penicillin G 50,000 units/kg IM can be given daily for a minimum of 10 days. In infants with a normal CSF, benzathine penicillin G 50,000 units/kg IM can be given as a single dose.

Treatment for interstitial keratitis usually involves the use of topical corticosteroids and dilating agents; penicillin therapy should also be given for the systemic syphilitic disease.

TULAREMIA

Francisella tularensis, the causative organism of tularemia, is a pleomorphic gram-negative coccobacillus. It requires special culture media for isolation. As small a dose as 50 organisms of the more virulent type A can produce an infection in man. Type B produces a milder disease. Infection is transmitted by rodents and other hosts, especially the rabbit. A substantial number of cases have also been reported in association with exposure to ticks. Other vectors include squirrels, cats, foxes, and raccoons. Tularemia is an occupational hazard for sheep herders, mink ranchers, hunters, and butchers, all of whom may handle infected tissues. Recent studies have shown a steadily decreasing incidence of tularemia; however, epidemics of this highly infectious disease are still occurring (46). It is not solely a rural disease and its incidence in animals has remained essentially unchanged in recent years.

Immunopathology

Host defenses are not fully understood in tularemia; however, cell-mediated immunity appears to be important. Immunity is associated with the appearance of a delayed hypersensitivity skin test response to tularemia skin test antigen, and the enhanced ability of rabbit macrophages to kill *F. tularensis. In vitro* correlates of cell-mediated immunity are present in sensitized individuals. Inactivated vaccines have no protective benefit, but a live attenuated strain can afford protection in both man and animals. There is no evidence that antibody formation is protective in tularemia.

Clinical Features

General. Tularemia may present as four distinct clinical syndromes. The most common is the ulceroglandular form, which accounts for 80%–90% of all cases. This form begins with a papule, followed by ulcer formation, fever, and regional lymphadenopathy. The pneumonic form is the most serious type of tularemia. It accounts for 20%–30% of the cases, and may be associated with other forms of the disease. Pulmonary infiltrates and pleural effusions occur in the pneumonic type. A typhoidal form of tularemia, which accounts for 15% of cases, may be indistinguishable from enteric fever. The fourth clinical syndrome (Fig. 6-9) involves the eye and is known as the oculoglandular form.

Ocular Findings. The oculoglandular form of tularemia is produced by accidental inoculation of organisms into the conjunctival sac. A conjunctivitis that is teeming with organisms may result. This has been described by Vail as looking like "a turkey red calico dress with yellow polka dots" (114). A typical Parinaud's syndrome may develop, with granulomatous or ulcerative conjunctivitis (Fig. 6-10), regional lymphadenitis, and signs of systemic involvement. The palpebral conjunctiva is most commonly affected. The ocular disease has been reported 10 days after accidental inoculation with blood from an infected tick (40).

Diagnosis and Treatment

Diagnosis is based on isolation of the organism and a rise in agglutinating antibodies. Titers usually rise after the first 2 weeks of illness but may take much longer. In most cases there is a fourfold or greater rise in antibody titer. A skin test using lyophilized, ether-extracted bacterial antigen may be useful but is not routinely available.

Systemic antibiotic treatment with streptomycin, chloramphenicol, gentamicin, or tetracycline is effective.

BRUCELLOSIS

Brucellosis is an infection acquired by man through contact with infected tissues of cattle, pigs, sheep, and goats, or by ingestion of raw milk or milk byproducts. It is one of the most prevalent zoonoses in the United States. It is

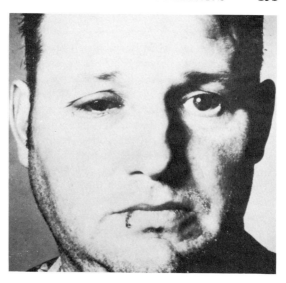

FIG. 6-9. Parinaud's oculoglandular syndrome in tularemia. (Courtesy of Dr. J. U. Dy-Liacco)

caused by several species of a small gram-negative bacillus, including *Brucella abortus, B. melitensis, B. suis,* and, rarely, *B. canis.* Veterinarians and abattoir workers are frequent intermediate hosts. The organism is transmitted from infected tissues to man through cuts in the skin, or by conjunctival contact, ingestion of uncooked meat, or inhalation of organisms.

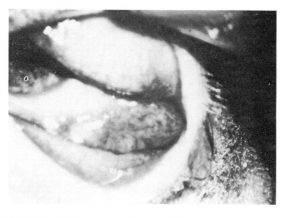

FIG. 6-10. Conjunctival granuloma in Parinaud's syndrome. (Courtesy of Dr. J. U. Dy-Liacco)

Immunopathology

The brucella organism has a proclivity for the reticuloendothelial system. Once ingested, the organisms are rapidly taken up by neutrophils and transported to histiocytic cells of the liver, spleen, and lymph nodes. There they enter a period of prolonged intracellular residence. They may remain intracellular for several weeks (or rarely, for months), during which time phagocytes containing the organisms form noncaseating granulomas. Clinical symptoms occur when organisms are released from infected reticuloendothelial cells.

Immunity to *Brucella* appears to be a manifestation of cell-mediated immunity. Delayed hypersensitivity develops during experimental infection with *Brucella*. A skin test was developed but was found to lack specificity and its routine use has been discontinued in the United States.

Antibody measurement is useful in the diagnosis of brucella infection; however, these antibodies are not protective. Agglutinating and complement-fixing antibodies can be measured. An IgA antibody can act as a blocking factor and produce spuriously low agglutinin levels. Interference by this factor can be avoided by using a Coombs test. Antibody measurement is important in the diagnosis of brucellosis, since the organism is fastidious and culture is difficult.

Clinical Features

General. Brucellosis is difficult to diagnose in man. It has no pathognomonic signs or symptoms. Its onset may be abrupt or insidious. Subclinical cases are quite common. Its most characteristic features are chronic recurrent fevers and weakness, producing the syndrome of undulant fever.

Ocular Findings. Ocular disease is rare, occurring in about 2% of patients with brucellosis. Blurring of vision or ocular pain may be the presenting complaint. A history of febrile illness may or may not be present. Examination reveals ocular inflammation which may take the form of a nummular keratitis, chronic anterior uveitis, or optic neuritis with papil-

litis, papilledema, papillary congestion, or atrophy (105). Scleritis and an extraocular muscle palsy have been described. Optic nerve involvement is four times as frequent as involvement of other parts of the eye. None of the ocular findings, however, are specific for brucellosis. No organisms have been cultured from a human eye, but in cases of optic neuritis with meningitis the organism has been isolated from cerebrospinal fluid.

Treatment

Treatment of brucellosis involves administration of tetracycline for long periods of time. This is often used in combination with streptomycin to minimize the chance of relapse: the relapse rate with this regimen is less than 1%. An attenuated strain of *B. abortus* has been used to immunize cattle; however, because it produces infection and transient bacteremia, it is not used in humans.

VIRAL DISEASES

VARICELLA-ZOSTER

The varicella-zoster (V-Z) virus is the etiologic agent in varicella (chickenpox) and in herpes zoster. Chickenpox, the common contagious disease of childhood, is the most common clinical manifestation of the virus. Herpes zoster and herpes zoster ophthalmicus are more common in the middle-aged and older population. Herpes zoster may occur in apparently healthy individuals with no obvious precipitating cause, in which case it is referred to as "primary" or "spontaneous." Many of these patients may have an underlying condition which leads to an immunosuppressed state. "Secondary" or "symptomatic" herpes zoster develops in individuals who have some impairment of natural immunity. This may be related to old age, malignancy, immunosuppressive therapy, chronic illness, or trauma.

Immunopathology

The V-Z virus is neurotropic and produces a skin rash in a dermatome distribution. Most herpes zoster infections are caused by a reactivation of latent V-Z virus residing in the dorsal root ganglia. This generally occurs at a time when the immunity of the host is compromised in some way. The reactivated virus can travel down the nerve axon and produces the characteristic vesicular lesions of the skin along the nerve distribution. A second mode of infection involves the host's reexposure to the virus by contact with a patient having either chickenpox or herpes zoster. In both cases, the affected individual does not have an adequate immune response to ward off the viral infection.

It has been demonstrated that varicella can be prevented by passive immunization with antibody to V-Z virus. The role of antibody in prevention of herpes zoster, however, and in the eventual recovery from zoster and varicella, is somewhat less clear. It has been suggested that antibody plays a protective role in preventing active V-Z virus disease. Hope-Simpson (47) has suggested that a critical antibody level may exist, above which an individual is protected from latent virus in neuronal tissues. This titer may be maintained at an adequate level by endogenous or exogenous stimulation from viral antigens.

Complement-fixing antibody generally appears early in the course of varicella-zoster infection. There has been some speculation that patients lacking detectable complement-fixing antibody early in the course of herpes zoster are more likely to have a disseminated zoster infection. While some patients with disseminated zoster do not synthesize detectable levels of complement-fixing antibodies until 2–3 weeks after the disease begins, some of these patients have been shown to have V-Z antibody when tested by a newer, more sensitive immunofluorescence method. This newer method detects antibodies to membrane antigens of cells infected with the virus. Using this method it has been shown that a prompt rise in specific IgA, IgG, and IgM could be detected both in localized and generalized zoster (15). Dissemination may occur even in the presence of high levels of serum antibody. Thus, a brisk serum antibody response to V-Z virus does not necessarily alter the course of the disease.

It has long been suspected that cellular immunity is important in the recovery from in-fection with V-Z virus (75). Patients with deficiencies in cell-mediated immunity prove to be more prone to zoster infection than are patients with humoral immune deficiencies. Depression of cellular immunity due to malignancy or treatment with immunosuppressive drugs also predisposes to the development of herpes zoster. *In vitro* studies have demonstrated that leukocytes from persons immune to varicella are more efficient in inactivating V-Z virus than are leukocytes from persons susceptible to varicella (36). Leukocytes from the latter patients produce no decrease in V-Z virus titer. Thus, individuals who recover from V-Z virus infection have specific cell-mediated immunity against the virus. In addition to cell-mediated immunity, local levels of interferon also appear to correlate with recovery from herpes zoster.

Clinical Features

Varicella. The skin lesions of varicella appear as clumps of erythematous papules. They undergo healing within 2 weeks and scarring rarely occurs. While the disease is more common in children, it is the adult form which is more severe. Intense itching may occur. The skin lesions go through a macular, then a papular, and finally a vesicular stage. They undergo crusting and usually heal within 2 weeks. Skin lesions may affect the lids and lid margins.

Occasionally, vesicular lesions appear on the conjunctiva. These may occur at the limbus and resemble a phlyctenule (Fig. 6-11). Conjunctival lesions may heal without ulceration but more often they do ulcerate and produce considerable pain and inflammation. A mild catarrhal conjunctivitis may also be seen. The limbal lesions may in some instances involve the cornea and lead to adjacent infiltration and vascularization. Rarely, an epithelial keratitis with opacities in the midstroma may develop, or an epithelial and disciform keratitis may occur. Iridocyclitis of variable severity may rarely be seen during the convalescent period. Fine keratic precipitates, fibrinous exudates, and iris atrophy have also been described. Secondary glaucoma may sometimes be associated with iridocyclitis. A focal

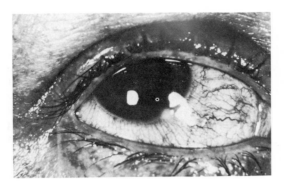

FIG. 6-11. Limbal lesion in varicella. (Courtesy of F. I. Proctor Foundation)

chorioretinitis has been described as well as optic neuritis, optic atrophy, and cranial nerve palsies.

Herpes Zoster. The highest incidence of herpes zoster occurs between ages 50 and 80. While the disease may occur in children, the course is much shorter and the likelihood of complications is far less. The thoracic dermatomes are the most likely to be involved, with cranial dermatomes next in frequency (Fig. 6-12). Involvement of the first division (ophthalmic) of the trigeminal nerve leads to herpes zoster ophthalmicus. Any of the three branches of the ophthalmic division may be involved. The frontal nerve is most often affected; however, the nasociliary branch is most

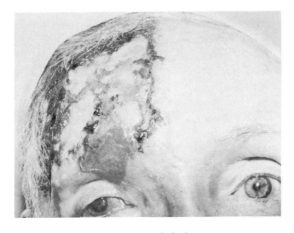

FIG. 6-12. Herpes zoster ophthalmicus.

important to the ophthalmologist since it is the main sensory nerve to the eye. If the nasociliary nerve is involved, it is likely that ocular complications will develop. In one series, 85% of patients with nasociliary involvement had one or more ocular complications.

The prodromal symptoms of herpes zoster include malaise, fever and chills, and pain along the dermatome distribution. Vesicles appear on the skin in a linear distribution, and may be accompanied by neuralgic pain. This varies from tingling and numbness to severe persistent pain. The skin eruption may last for several months while the postherpetic neuralgia can last for several years. Herpes zoster, unlike herpes simplex, affects the dermis in addition to the epidermis and may cause permanent scarring where vesicles have healed.

Ophthalmic Herpes Zoster. In herpes zoster ophthalmicus, the severity of the disease depends on the age and physical condition of the patient. While usually the disease is self-limited, severe ocular complications may develop in some patients with poor immunologic defenses. The skin lesions of herpes zoster may involve the lids or lid margins and may lead to permanent scarring. Cicatricial lid retraction or entropion with trichiasis may result. Permanent loss of lashes and poliosis may occur. Rarely, dacryoadenitis and canaliculitis may occur. The conjunctiva may be hyperemic and infiltrated by inflammatory cells. A papillary reaction is generally seen; however, pseudomembranes, follicles, transitory vesicles, and ulceration may rarely be present (58).

Corneal and uveal tract involvement are especially likely if the nasociliary branch is involved, as indicated by a skin lesion on the tip of the nose (Hutchinson's sign). A dendritic keratitis may involve the epithelium in some cases. These dendrites differ from the ones seen in herpes simplex keratitis in that they are elevated, stain poorly, and do not have the knoblike endings seen in simplex dendrites. A coarse, punctate epithelial keratitis may be seen and is almost always accompanied by stromal lesions and uveitis unlike herpes simplex keratitis. The stromal lesions may be round and nummular or a disciform keratitis with a round central opacity may occur (Fig.

6-13). Corneal vascularization may develop. Corneal anesthesia often occurs but generally resolves 6–12 months after the acute disease subsides; occasionally, sensation may be permanently lost. The anesthesia may be highly localized and limited to a sector of interstitial keratitis. A neuroparalytic keratitis with ulceration may occur owing to impairment of lid function or cicatrization.

An iridocyclitis is another common ocular complication of herpes zoster. Inflammation may be mild or severe. Photophobia, a ciliary flush, and keratic precipitates may be present. The iris may be edematous and hyperemic. Later, sector atrophy and anterior and posterior synechiae may be present. Hypopyon and hemorrhage into the anterior chamber have also been reported. There may be some color change in the iris due to atrophy of the pigment layers. Secondary glaucoma is not uncommon in ophthalmic zoster and may be related to synechia formation or to inflammation of the trabecular meshwork.

The posterior pole may be affected and a focal choroiditis or hemorrhagic retinitis is occasionally seen. Various neurologic disturbances are associated with herpes zoster, including pupillary abnormalities such as the Argyll Robertson pupil, ptosis, and other cranial nerve palsies. Proptosis, anterior segment ischemia, and scleritis, although rare, may occur. Ischemia of the retinal vessels associated with edema and exudates, and even retinal detachments, have occasionally been reported.

Patients with trigeminal zoster are among the most likely to develop postherpetic neuralgia. Age appears to be a factor in the occurrence of this complication since neuralgia is uncommon in patients below the age of 50. Among patients aged 70 or older, as many as 50% may be affected.

Treatment

The treatment of the ocular manifestations of chickenpox should be supportive since the disease is self-limited. Good hygiene should be practiced, and cold compresses may be used. Low illumination will diminish the photophobia experienced by these patients. My-

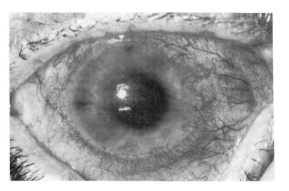

FIG. 6-13. Herpes zoster ophthalmicus with stromal keratitis.

driatics may be used to prevent synechiae if iritis is severe. Topical antibiotics are also worthwhile if significant corneal or conjunctival erosion has occurred. Steroids in general are contraindicated in the treatment of varicella. However, if a late interstitial keratitis develops, judicious use of topical steroids is said to be beneficial. Antiviral agents have no proven value in this disease. Cyproheptadine (Periactin) may be used to help control the itching of widespread varicella.

The skin lesions of ophthalmic herpes zoster should be treated with supportive therapy. If bacterial superinfection occurs, topical antibiotics are indicated. Antihistamines may be of value in reducing the itching which sometimes occurs. Idoxuridine given topically as a 40% solution in dimethyl sulfoxide (DMSO) has been claimed to be of value in Great Britain; however, this preparation is not available in the United States. Intravenous cytarabine has been reported as being useful in the treatment of steroid-resistant zoster ophthalmicus. Other studies, however, claim that this antiviral agent has no value and may actually prolong the course of disseminated zoster in the severely compromised host.

Conjunctivitis rarely occurs in herpes zoster; however, when it does, treatment should be supportive. Secondary bacterial infections are best treated with appropriate antibiotics. The treatment of zoster keratouveitis is somewhat controversial. Often the disease is mild and self-limited, in which case no treatment is required. At other times, dilating drops constitute adequate therapy in preventing the formation of posterior synechiae. In a patient who is compromised immunologically, keratouveitis may be severe and may lead to visual loss. Topical corticosteroids can suppress the inflammation dramatically but probably prolong the course of the disease. It may also be difficult to decrease the strength or frequency of topical steroids once the patient has been using these medications for some time. When a significant uveitis is present, dilating drops should be employed to prevent the formation of posterior synechiae. Short-acting dilating agents, which keep the pupil moving, are preferable to long-acting cycloplegics.

The use of systemic corticosteroids in the treatment of herpes zoster is also a subject of controversy. Many reports have been favorable toward their use and claim a reduction in the incidence and severity of keratitis, uveitis, and secondary glaucoma. Some investigators have even claimed a reduction in the incidence of postherpetic neuralgia when treatment with systemic steroids was begun early in the course of the disease. Other investigators, however, report no success in reducing the incidence of postherpetic neuralgia. It should be kept in mind that patients who develop herpes zoster are immunologically compromised to begin with. The use of steroids, which further depress the immune system, may lead to dissemination of zoster and severe iatrogenic disease. Thygeson (111) has pointed out the worsening of zoster keratitis during the past 20 years and the increased frequency of opportunistic superinfections in zoster patients. He feels that this worsening of zoster may be due in part to the increasing age of the population, but that to a large extent it is a result of immunosuppressive antiinflammatory medication, particularly systemic and topical corticosteroids. These drugs depress cellular immunity, which may be deficient to begin with in these patients. Methods of restoring cellular immunity, such as the use of transfer factor and levamisole, are more logical ways of controlling this disease, and may be useful in the future.

Some time ago, Gunderson used convalescent serum for the treatment of herpes zoster

ophthalmicus which involved the uveal tract and cornea (41). He felt that if this preparation were given very early in the course of the disease, further spread of the lesions, especially to the eye, could be prevented. In view of the recent findings of immune deficiencies in patients developing zoster, this type of immune therapy has some rationale.

Patients who are at special risk of developing varicella or herpes zoster may be given varicella-zoster hyperimmune globulin. There is evidence that this treatment will prevent or significantly modify the disease if given within 72 h of exposure.

Recent findings of defects in cellular immunity rather than in antibody response in patients with zoster have suggested that theoretically the administration of antibody to these patients would be unlikely to be of benefit (113). Still, the extensive clinical experience of physicians who use zoster immune globulin cannot be ignored.

The secondary glaucoma which sometimes develops in herpes zoster ophthalmicus may be extremely difficult to control. Topical cycloplegics and carbonic anhydrase inhibitors are useful. When these fail to control the disease some clinicians feel that a short course of topical steroids may be warranted. Scleritis may also occur with herpes zoster but is a rare complication. Steroids are sometimes recommended for the treatment of herpetic scleritis, but their benefit is questionable. Optic neuritis and cranial nerve palsies have been treated with systemic antiviral agents such as vidarabine (ara-A) or cytarabine (ara-C). Again, these are immunosuppressive drugs which are toxic and their value is unproven.

Postherpetic neuralgia is a painful and difficult complication to treat. Chlorprothixene (Taractan) 50 mg three or four times a day for 5 days has recently been used with good results. Carbamazepine (Tegretol) has also been used successfully. Occasionally, mild analgesics will be effective in controlling pain.

VACCINIA

Vaccinia inoculation for immunization against smallpox was first reported by Edward Jenner in 1798. The vaccinia virus has low pathogenicity for man and affords protection against infection with smallpox virus because of cross reactivity between the two viruses. Ocular vaccinia may occur after vaccination if the eye is accidentally inoculated. Generalized vaccinia can develop after vaccination in immunodeficient patients and individuals with widespread dermatoses, especially those with atopic dermatitis.

Immunopathology

Dermal inoculation with vaccinia virus induces a delayed-type hypersensitivity reaction at the skin site approximately 8 days later (117). The vaccinia virus contains antigens which cross react with smallpox virus and therefore its use protects the vaccinated individual against smallpox. Vaccination of normal individuals produces no systemic disease but generalized vaccinia can occur if the patient is a compromised host.

The immune response to vaccinia virus appears to involve an interaction between antibody, cell-mediated responses, and interferon. A normal, immunocompetent person responds to intradermal vaccination with a "primary take," in which the person's immune defenses localize and eradicate the virus at the site of inoculation. Subsequent revaccination in the same individual produces a milder skin reaction. This reaction, which reaches a maximum in 4–5 days, is probably due mainly to cell-mediated immune responses to the virus. Patients with a severe defect in cellular immunity almost always have a fatal response to smallpox vaccination. Individuals with defective antibody responses may develop a severe necrotic skin reaction (**vaccinia gangrenosum**), but this may be successfully treated with vaccinia immune globulin (VIG) or the drug thiosemicarbazone. These drugs are ineffective, however, in preventing a fatal response to smallpox vaccination in patients with severe T cell defects. These observations have led to the impression that both humoral and cellular immunity are important in the control of vaccinia virus infection. It may be that antibody is involved in reducing the antigen load (*i.e.*, the mass of virus particles), and failure of the humoral immune system to do this may result in

temporary immune paralysis of the T cell system. With the lack of an immunocompetent T cell system, even in the presence of antibody, the individual is apparently not effective in eliminating the virus.

Immunization of rabbits with vaccinia virus vaccine by the intranasal route results in the appearance of IgA antibody activity in tears (61). If vaccination is given intradermally, however, the antiviral activity of tears is associated with IgG. IgG is also the predominant serum immunoglobulin found in immunized animals. Antibody titers in both tears and serum can be enhanced by the interferon inducer, polyinosinic-polycytidilic acid (poly I:C). Vaccination by either the intradermal or intranasal route results in decreased shedding of the virus and a decrease in clinical disease in the rabbit (60). While high levels of neutralizing antibody in the serum can be correlated with mild illness, tear antibody has no apparent relationship to illness or virus shedding. The lack of protection by neutralizing antibody in tears may suggest a role for a cellular immune mechanism in vaccinia virus infection.

Following inoculation of the rabbit cornea with vaccinia, the cells within the deep layers of the epithelium are the first to manifest infection and to undergo degeneration (68). Viral replication is thought to occur within the stromal keratocytes (74).

Clinical Features

General. Following initial inoculation of the skin with vaccinia, there is an incubation period of approximately 8–10 days, after which time vesicles erupt. In patients with eczema, vaccination may lead to dissemination of skin lesions and constitutional symptoms. Other predisposing dermatoses include dermatitis herpetiformis, pemphigus, herpes simplex, and varicella. The skin lesions appear approximately 10 days after inoculation, become vesicular, then purulent, and then heal with punctate scarring. Fever and regional lymphadenopathy may be present.

Vaccinia gangrenosum may occur in four immunologic settings: 1) in generalized hypogammaglobulinemia with normal T cell func-

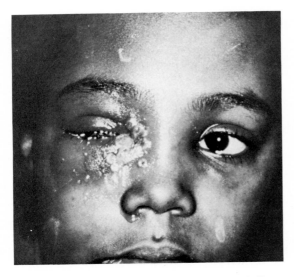

FIG. 6-14. Ocular vaccinia. (Courtesy of F. I. Proctor Foundation)

tion (Bruton's agammaglobulinemia), 2) in patients with a selective defect in antibody formation against vaccinia virus, 3) in patients with combined antibody and T cell defects (Swiss and Gitlin types of agammaglobulinemia), and 4) in patients having defective T cell function with normal antibody formation (DiGeorge and cartilage–hair syndromes).

Ocular Findings. Inadvertent inoculation of the eye is a hazard of vaccination (Fig. 6-14). The extent of the ocular disease depends on the immune status of the host. In an individual who has been vaccinated previously and has well-established immunity, only an acute, purulent blepharoconjunctivitis will occur. Usually one of two types of lesions will be seen clinically: a vaccinial pustule at the site of inoculation on the outer surface of the lid, or vaccinial blepharitis.

In the unimmunized or weakly immune patient, a severe ocular reaction can occur. After approximately a 3-day incubation period, the lids and conjunctiva show marked edema and erythema. A purulent discharge with a yellowish gray inflammatory membrane may be present. Regional lymphadenopathy, fever, and malaise may also be seen. Multifocal conjunctival ulcers may occur and may lead to scarring, loss of eyelashes, and symblepharon formation.

Corneal involvement is said to occur in approximately 30% of cases. Corneal findings range from a mild superficial punctate keratitis to a severe, disciform stromal keratitis. The latter may undergo necrosis and even perforation. Punctate subepithelial opacities similar to those of epidemic keratoconjunctivitis may develop and undergo gradual clearing over several months or years. This results eventually in a variable amount of scarring and vascularization. The deep stromal keratitis may resemble that caused by herpes simplex and may persist for several months. An anterior uveitis may develop and corneal vascularization and scarring may follow.

Treatment

Vaccinia immune globulin (VIG) may be useful in the treatment of generalized vaccinia, disseminated skin lesions associated with dermatoses, or ocular vaccinia. In ocular involvement, topical VIG applied every 2 h has been recommended if the cornea is not yet involved (84). Topical vidarabine or idoxuridine ointment may be applied every 4 h [in experimental vaccinia keratitis in the rabbit, vidarabine was found to be more effective and less toxic than idoxuridine (50)]. Topical antibiotics can be given for bacterial superinfection.

RUBELLA

The teratogenic potential of the rubella virus was first recognized by the Australian ophthalmologist, Sir Norman Gregg (39). Infection during early pregnancy leads to fetal malformations involving the eye, heart, and ear. Ocular findings in congenital rubella syndrome include cataract, microphthalmia, nystagmus, retinopathy, and transient corneal clouding. Ocular defects are seen in 30%–60% of infants exposed fetally to rubella, the most frequent being cataracts and retinopathy.

Immunopathology

The fetus is most susceptible to the effects of the rubella virus during the 20th to 40th day of gestation. The mechanism of malformation is not completely understood. It is believed that death of the infected cells, or a change in rate of cell growth, or perhaps both mechanisms, is important. The reason for the persistence of the virus in the fetus is not understood. Endogenous IgM antibodies and maternal IgG antibodies are present in the infant at birth and antibody responses are felt to be intact. Cellular immunity is depressed, however, and this may be a factor in the inability to clear virus from the fetal tissues.

In postnatal rubella infection, antibodies to the virus increase rapidly, reaching maximum titers in 7–10 days. IgM antibody can be detected for approximately 1 month while IgG antibody persists for many years (88). Antibodies to rubella virus can be assayed by various techniques, including hemagglutination inhibition, neutralization of virus infectivity, complement fixation, indirect immunofluorescence, and immunoprecipitation. All assay methods except complement fixation yield similar results, with titers reaching their peak within 2 weeks after detection and then gradually decreasing. Antibodies usually remain detectable for life. Individuals with antibodies in their serum are felt to be immune from reinfection with rubella virus.

A defect in cellular immunity is suggested in situations where virus persists (26, 87), since lymphocytes from some infants with congenital rubella do not show a blastogenic response to phytohemagglutinin (67, 120), and rubella virus, when added to lymphocytes from normal individuals, will suppress the blastogenic response to phytohemagglutinin (83). However, it remains uncertain whether viral persistence is due to a defect in the immune mechanism or to a prolonged survival of clones of infected cells.

Clinical Features

General. The most characteristic findings in congenital rubella are the triad of heart lesions, cataracts, and deafness. Congenital heart disease occurs in nearly 70% of patients with congenital rubella. Patent ductus arteriosus is the most common lesion. Peripheral pulmonary artery stenosis, aortic stenosis, coarctation of the aorta, and ventricular septal defects also occur. A permanent mild or severe sensorineural hearing loss may be unilateral or bilateral. Vestibular function may also be impaired. Other abnormalities are common and virtually any organ can be involved. Failure of growth and development, bone lesions, hepatitis, and hemolytic anemia are other manifestations of congenital rubella.

Ocular Findings. Ocular defects occur in 30%–60% of infants exposed to rubella. Cataracts can be unilateral or bilateral and may be associated with microphthalmia. Cataracts are usually present at birth, but may not be detectable until the infant is several weeks old (Fig. 6-15). They result from direct viral infection of the lens, and progress rapidly. Microphthalmia is usually not severe and may be difficult to detect. A corneal diameter of less than 10 mm is indicative of microphthalmia.

A retinopathy characterized by discrete patchy black pigmentation interspersed with areas of patchy depigmentation is commonly observed. usually these findings are most prominent in the perimacular area. Congenital glaucoma, myopia, iris hyperplasia, strabismus, and nystagmus have also been observed.

Treatment

A live attenuated vaccine is now available for rubella. It is given after the first year of life. It is contraindicated during pregnancy, and women should not become pregnant for 2 months after immunization.

Variable results have been reported after surgery for cataracts in patients with rubella syndrome (11, 127). An incidence of phthisis bulbi following cataract surgery may range from 5% to 24%. It has been suggested that an increased incidence of complications may result from local cellular immune reactions to rubella virus antigen in patients having multiple procedures (11). For this reason, discission and aspiration in a one-stage procedure has been recommended (11).

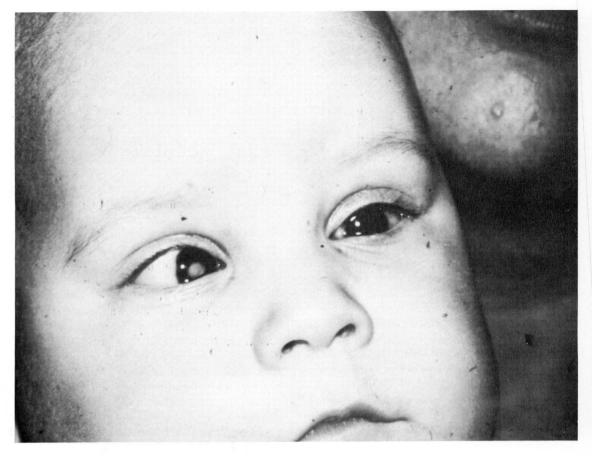

FIG. 6-15. Congenital rubella syndrome. (Courtesy of Dr. I. Wong)

CYTOMEGALOVIRUS

Cytomegalovirus infection has become recognized in recent years as a significant form of congenital disease in newborns and an acquired infection in immunosuppressed adults. The virus is not easily eliminated and persists in host tissues for months, years, or a lifetime. It produces a chronic infection with a variable incubation period, outcome, and course. It may produce a chorioretinitis, optic atrophy, mental or motor retardation, and involvement of various other organ systems.

Immunopathology

The virus (Fig. 6-16) infects the fetus, which *in utero* has an incompletely developed immune system. It also infects adults with malignan-

cies, particularly of the hematopoietic or reticuloendothelial systems. Cytomegalovirus infection is especially common in kidney transplant patients who are undergoing treatment with immunosuppressive agents. It has been detected in up to 90% of kidney transplant patients (1, 42). In renal transplant recipients, cytomegalovirus infection may lead to bacterial superinfection and transplant rejection (49). High antibody titers are felt to afford protection against the virus infection.

Cytomegalovirus infection is associated with abnormal serum globulins and depressed cellular immunity (56). Cytomegalovirus causes suppression of primary and secondary immune responses to sheep red blood cells in mice (49). The degree of immune suppression is directly related to the size of the virus inoculum. Cytomegalovirus also causes de-

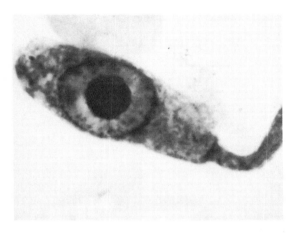

FIG. 6-16. Cytomegalovirus inclusion body in a tissue cultured cell. (Courtesy of F I. Proctor Foundation)

pression of cell-mediated immunity, as reflected by prolonged skin graft survival and inhibition of lymphocyte responsiveness to phytohemagglutinin (48).

Human cytomegalovirus also causes alterations of the humoral immune system. Abnormal immunoglobulins, including rheumatoid factor, cryoglobulins, cold agglutinins, and antinuclear antibodies, as well as positive Coombs tests, have been detected after cytomegalovirus infection (56). Apparently, cytomegalovirus causes depression of the immune response only during the acute phase of the infection. The mechanism by which cytomegalovirus causes immunosuppression is not fully understood. It has been suggested that infection with cytomegalovirus may inhibit antibody responses to other antigens. A more likely explanation, however, is that infection of potential antibody-producing cells by virus may divert lymphoid cells away from their normal immune function and toward producing more virus (48).

Several different tests are available for the detection of antibodies to human cytomegalovirus. A complement-fixation test is commonly used; however, a sensitive fluorescent antibody test may prove more useful in the future (8). Since IgM of maternal origin does not pass the intact placenta, demonstration of IgM antibody in the infant's serum is indica-

tive of congenital infection. Neutralizing antibodies are also present in the adult disease. The appearance of complement-fixing antibody or a fourfold rise in titer, or both, in association with the characteristic clinical features in a kidney transplant recipient, are usually diagnostic. Diagnosis is also possible by histopathologic examination of biopsy material or by exfoliative cytology. The characteristic cytomegalic cells may be seen in the sedimented urine. The virus can also be cultured in human fibroblasts, where they produce characteristic plaques and cellular inclusion bodies.

Clinical Features

General. Clinically, the manifestations of cytomegalovirus infection are related to the age at which infection occurs. The infection occurring *in utero* results in fetal death or the clinical syndrome of cytomegalic inclusion disease. The syndrome consists of prematurity, jaundice, hepatosplenomegaly, thrombocytopenic purpura, pneumonitis, and central nervous system damage with microcephaly, periventricular calcification, choroiditis, optic atrophy, and mental or motor retardation. Acquired cytomegalovirus infection in children produces subacute or chronic hepatitis, interstitial pneumonitis, or hemolytic anemia. An infectious-mononucleosislike syndrome due to cytomegalovirus has been reported in adults and children after transfusion of whole fresh blood (55). In the adult, infection occurs locally in the gastrointestinal tract, lung, and elsewhere.

As mentioned, a high incidence of cytomegalovirus infection has been reported in association with malignancies, and in kidney transplant patients under treatment with immunosuppressive agents. Whether these represent a primary infection or reactivation of latent virus is unknown. The frequency of acquired infection increases with age, so that 80% of the population over age 35 have positive complement-fixation titers to cytomegalovirus (92).

Ocular Findings. Ocular involvement is characterized by chorioretinitis which may be difficult to distinguish from toxoplasmosis. Both peripheral and central focal necrotizing lesions have been described. Peripheral lesions may be accompanied by vitreous haze resembling the "snowbank" of chronic cyclitis (17) (see Chronic Cyclitis, Ch. 7). Healing of chorioretinal lesions may lead to hyperplastic, heavily pigmented retinal scars. While some authors feel that cytomegalovirus lesions may at times be indistinguishable from toxoplasmosis, the features of the acute disease are typical. Retinal lesions first appear as scattered white spots or patches with some irregular sheathing of adjacent retinal vessels. Later, these spots coalesce and are accompanied by intraretinal hemorrhage. Subsequently, the white spots lose their granular appearance and become grayish brown, and are associated with marked atrophy of the retina and pigment epithelium. Ultimately, a pale scar with little pigment proliferation may be seen. A clustering of new whitish granular lesions may be seen to go through the same evolution at the margin of the larger lesion.

The anterior chamber may contain inflammatory cells or even a hypopyon. Cytomegalovirus has been cultured from the anterior chamber (17, 21). Fine keratic precipitates may be present. Other ocular lesions associated with cytomegalovirus infection include optic nerve hypoplasia, partial coloboma, and complete coloboma associated with microphthalmia (43).

Treatment

Treatment with antiviral agents such as cytarabine and vidarabine has not been of definite clinical benefit (85), although some encouraging results have recently been obtained in treating infected renal transplant recipients with systemic vidarabine. Because there are no effective alternatives, these agents are sometimes employed. They may be less effective in immunosuppressed patients (20). It is clear that immunosuppression is a significant factor in potentiating cytomegalovirus infection. If corticosteroids or immunosuppressive agents can be reduced or eliminated, amelioration of the disease can usually be expected.

RUBEOLA (MEASLES)

Rubeola, or measles, is an acute febrile disease of childhood. It is caused by a paramyxovirus and clinically manifests as a maculopapular rash and catarrhal inflammation of the eye and respiratory tract.

Immunopathology

Vaccination with measles virus results in augmentation of delayed hypersensitivity to the virus. Inactivated virus also causes elevation of serum IgG antibody titers, which then wane. Upon natural reexposure to measles, a hyperacute atypical measles syndrome may develop. This is characterized by fever, pneumonia with pleural effusion and a severe hemorrhagic rash. This atypical measles may reflect immune-complex deposition: antibody complexing with antigen causes a precipitate which induces an Arthus-type response in the skin and respiratory tract.

Subacute sclerosing panencephalitis (SSPE) is a fatal degenerative disease which occurs during the first and second decades of life. It is characterized by personality change, progressive dementia, seizures, and myoclonus. An inflammatory demyelination of white matter occurs, and inclusion bodies, which are probably viral particles, have been demonstrated in brain tissue. Measles virus antigen has been demonstrated in infected brain material by fluorescent antibody staining, and complete, infective measles virus has been recovered from the brain of a few patients. Half of these patients had contracted measles before the age of 2. Antibodies to measles virus are found in the cerebrospinal fluid of patients with SSPE. The fact that large amounts of antibody are present in spite of continued infection has led to the feeling that these patients may have a defect in cellular immunity. Several studies have suggested a specific defect in cellular immunity towards measles virus. Other studies have shown no such defects. Some patients with SSPE have a blocking factor, possibly antibody, in the cerebrospinal fluid and blood, which appears to block the destruction of measles-infected cells by leukocytes.

Clinical Features

The incubation period for measles is approximately 10 days to 2 weeks. During the prodromal period, fever and conjunctivitis occur, as well as photophobia which results from an epithelial keratitis. Epithelial keratitis may be seen early in children and later in adults. The enanthem of measles often precedes the skin eruption. The conjunctiva has a glassy appearance and there may be swelling of the semilunar fold. A mucopurulent discharge and catarrhal conjunctivitis develop several days before the skin eruption. At the time of the skin eruption, Koplik's spots may appear on the conjunctiva and caruncle, especially in the region of the semilunar fold. A maculopapular blotchy or confluent rash appears on the forehead and progressively involves the face and neck, trunk, and limbs. A desquamation may develop as the rash progresses. By this time the conjunctivitis usually has subsided. A secondary bacterial infection due to pneumococci, *Haemophilus influenzae*, or other organisms may develop. This is often associated with a severe pseudomembranous conjunctivitis. Other ocular findings include strabismus, cellulitis, retinal edema, dacryocystitis, and dacryoadenitis.

Complications are rare but may occur in immunodeficient patients or in localities where malnourishment is a problem. Neurologic complications, which may occur in approximately 1 out of 700 cases, include diffuse cerebral involvement, multiple focal or diffuse lesions, a single focal lesion, cerebellar syndrome, spinal syndrome, and optic neuritis. In the last-named, congestion of the optic disc may be present and may be associated with increased intracranial pressure and retrobulbar neuritis. Vascular constriction simulating a central retinal artery occlusion may be seen during the acute stage of retinal involvement. Retinal veins may be dilated, and pigmentary retinopathy may be seen.

Subacute sclerosing panencephalitis may present with cerebral signs, convulsive disorders, coma, opisthotonos, or mutism. In a series of 20 cases of SSPE, 75% had some ocular abnormality (38). The most frequent findings were pigmentary macular changes and temporal pallor or edema of the optic disc. Other ocular manifestations included optic atrophy, cortical blindness, and papilledema.

Treatment

No effective treatment is presently available for measles or SSPE. Only supportive measures are indicated unless secondary infection intervenes. A live attenuated vaccine affords permanent protection and may prevent natural disease if given less than 48 h after exposure.

FUNGAL DISEASES

HISTOPLASMOSIS

Histoplasmosis is an intracellular mycotic infection caused by the dimorphic fungus *Histoplasma capsulatum*. This organism is capable of producing acute or chronic pulmonary disease. A large body of epidemiologic, clinical, and experimental evidence strongly supports the etiologic role of *H. capsulatum* in the ocular condition known as **presumed ocular histoplasmosis.** This clinical entity consists of hemorrhagic or nonhemorrhagic macular disciform lesions, peripheral and peripapillary choroidal atrophic scars, and a positive histoplasmin skin test.

Immunopathology

Infection with *H. capsulatum* induces both humoral and cellular immune responses. While the measurement of antibody is useful in the diagnosis and prognosis of the infection, it is the host's cellular immunity which is critical in the body's defense against the organism. In addition, the inflammatory and necrotic lesions which accompany the systemic disease may be a manifestation of cell-mediated hypersensitivity.

Following primary infection with *H. capsulatum*, cellular immunity develops rapidly. The immunizing constituent is thought to be a glycoprotein complex. Its components can confer delayed histoplasmin skin test reactivity and specific lymphocyte migration inhibition factor (MIF) activity on animals. Lymphocytes taken from patients with positive histoplasmin skin tests become activated in the presence of histoplasmin antigens. The granuloma formation and the pulmonary tissue destruction seen in histoplasmosis are generally attributed to vigorous cell-mediated immune responses to the infection. While aspects of cell-mediated immunity are present in both acute and chronic infections, cell-mediated immunity may fail in disseminated histoplasmosis. This implies a failure of macrophage activation and other normal host immune responses in dealing with the organism. Humoral immune responses, however, remain intact.

Humoral immune responses also develop readily in histoplasmosis, and may indicate a recent infection. Neutrophils are unable to kill the fungi. Antibodies are not protective in histoplasmosis, but, rather, indicate progressive disease. Thus, high titers of antibody suggest progressive infection rather than improvement. Antibody titers fall when the disease regresses and increase with dissemination of the infection. An antibody known as the H antibody correlates with active and progressive infection and may persist for as long as two years after recovery.

Cellular immune responses may play an important role in the pathogenesis of presumed ocular histoplasmosis. Although individuals with disseminated histoplasmosis may have a defect in cellular immunity against the fungus, patients with ocular histoplasmosis are felt to have intact cellular immunity (107). Patients with macular disciform lesions have a high incidence of healed pulmonary lesions. Males have a higher frequency of both unilateral and bilateral ocular involvement than do females (98a) and also a greater mean induration response to histoplasmin skin testing. Patients with ocular histoplasmosis are hyperreactive to a number of skin test antigens (119). This includes a markedly positive histoplasmin skin test, especially in patients with inactive disciform scars, as well as a positive intermediate-strength tuberculin test (32). Patients with disciform lesions also have greater *in vitro* spontaneous lymphocyte transformation in 5- and 7-day cell cultures. Their lymphocytes demonstrate enhanced activation with mitogens, with antigens derived from *H. capsulatum*, and with various other microbial

antigens as compared with lymphocytes from control patients (33). Patients with disciform lesions are thus considered to be basically hyperreactive in terms of their lymphocyte responses.

A flareup of macular disease may occur following a skin test with histoplasmin (62, 65). This phenomenon has been noted in 7% of ocular histoplasmosis cases (99). An *in vitro* enhanced response to histoplasmin antigen has been reported in the lymphocytes cultured from individuals sensitized to *H. capsulatum* (34). Perhaps a heightened cellular immune response is responsible for the flareups of macular lesions observed following skin testing. A similar flareup may be seen with histoplasmin desensitization therapy (65, 99). The reported success of corticosteroids and azathioprine in the treatment of acute macular lesions supports the idea that flareups of these lesions may have an immunologic basis (77, 98).

The immunopathogenesis of the disciform macular lesion is unknown. Local hypersensitivity responses of the choroid, secondary to either histoplasmin antigen or antigen–antibody complexes, has been suggested (33). Alternatively, cross-reacting fungal antigens or antigenic alteration of normal ocular tissue may be a factor. The lack of active systemic disease in patients with presumed ocular histoplasmosis suggests that local hypersensitivity or reinfection contributes to the disciform lesion. Recently, viable lymphocytes have been found in clinically inactive scars in pathologic specimens from two patients (25). It has been suggested that these lymphocytes are T cells which become activated upon reintroduction of antigen.

Animal Models

Several animal models of *Histoplasma* chorioretinitis have been developed (104, 122). Focal choroidopathy can be produced in the eyes of rabbits by intravenous or intracarotid injection of *H. capsulatum* organisms. In general, these models have not completely simulated the human disease. Although focal choroidal lesions can be produced in the rabbit, they may be associated with acute inflammation, and they require spores rather than yeast forms and hematogenous rather than pulmonary inoculation. Additionally, the rabbit lacks a macula and has a different retinal vascular pattern than man, so that it does not develop the peripapillary or neovascular changes seen in man.

Clinical Features

General. Histoplasmosis occurs in all races and age groups. The incidence of primary infection is highest in childhood; however, chronic pulmonary histoplasmosis is more common over the age of 40. Often, infection is inapparent: asymptomatic infections account for more than 99% of human histoplasma infections. In areas where histoplasmosis is endemic, such as the eastern and central United States, 60%–90% of residents may have positive histoplasmin skin tests.

Acute pulmonary histoplasmosis is the most common symptomatic form of the disease. It usually presents as an influenza-like syndrome consisting of cough, dyspnea, pleuritic chest pain, and occasionally hemoptysis. Frequently there is a history of exposure to chicken houses, caves, or other soil where organisms may be deposited. Occasionally, there may be arthralgias, myalgias, anorexia, and weight loss. Erythema nodosum and erythema multiforme may be associated with the acute form of the disease, especially in young Caucasian women. Fungi proliferate in the lung and are disseminated by the blood stream to many organs. In most cases the disease is self-limited and resolves leaving characteristic "buckshot" calcifications visible on a chest x-ray (Fig. 6-17). As the primary and metastatic lesions resolve, cell-mediated immunity to histoplasmin develops.

Occasionally, acute disseminated histoplasmosis will develop in patients who cannot contain the initial infection. This occurs most frequently in young children and is characterized by hepatosplenomegaly, fever, anemia, and leukopenia. The disease may be fatal if not treated immediately.

Acute reactivation of histoplasmosis occurs in individuals who have previously been exposed to the fungus and who subsequently

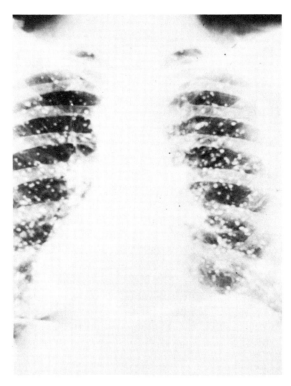

FIG. 6-17. Histoplasmosis: "Buckshot" calcifications on chest x-ray (Courtesy of F. I. Proctor Foundation)

undergo massive exposure to the organism. An intense hypersensitivity response can occur in pulmonary tissue. Antiinflammatory drugs as well as antifungal drugs are important in treatment. Acute reactivation of histoplasmosis is generally but not always self-limited.

Chronic pulmonary histoplasmosis, the common form of the disease encountered in hospitalized patients, has some similarities with chronic tuberculosis. It is most common in Caucasian men over the age of 40 and is probably due to endogenous reinfection. Symptoms include cough, purulent sputum, fever, night sweats, weight loss, and hemoptysis. The process usually involves the upper lobes of the lungs, and cavitating granulomas indistinguishable from those of tuberculosis may be seen on chest x-ray. Without treatment, patients develop respiratory insufficiency and bacterial secondary infection. Cellular immunity is basically intact in these patients. The disease seems to persist because of underlying abnormal pulmonary anatomy.

Chronic disseminated histoplasmosis occurs in patients with defective cell-mediated immunity. Common antecedent conditions include lymphomas, carcinoma, tuberculosis, diabetes mellitus, and therapy with steroids or immunosuppressive agents. Although pulmonary infiltrates occur in this phase of the disease, the most important aspects are secondary to a generalized invasion of the reticuloendothelial system by histoplasma organisms. Clinical findings include fever, anemia, leukocytopenia, hepatosplenomegaly, lymphadenopathy, and wasting. Ulcerative mucous membrane lesions are common. Gastrointestinal, cardiac, and central nervous system involvement may develop and adrenal destruction may be seen many years after diagnosis and treatment. The mortality rate in untreated chronic disseminated histoplasmosis is 80%; however, many patients can be expected to improve or be cured with appropriate treatment.

Ocular Findings. The typical features of presumed ocular histoplasmosis include peripheral atrophic scars, peripapillary choroidal scars, and macular disciform lesions (125). Anterior segment inflammation is absent. Pulmonary histoplasmosis is not generally associated with ocular lesions of histoplasmic choroiditis. However, it is generally accepted that the ocular disease is associated with histoplasmosis. Histoplasmin skin tests are positive in 93% of patients with the ocular syndrome (115), and these patients frequently show radiographic evidence consistent with previous systemic histoplasmosis infection. *H. capsulatum* has been demonstrated in a human eye with endophthalmitis (45) and has also been demonstrated histologically in granulomatous choroiditis occurring in disseminated histoplasmosis (59). In this latter case, the patient was compromised immunologically. Organisms compatible with *H. capsulatum* were also demonstrated in one of five cases of presumed ocular histoplasmosis at the Armed Forces Institute of Pathology (95).

Peripheral atrophic scars (Fig. 6-18) are present in 1%–3% of the normal population in areas of endemic histoplasmosis. The scars are bilateral in 62% of patients and a mean of 7.8 scars has been quantitated, with a range of 1 to 70 (103). The peripheral lesions are choroidal and measure 0.3 to 0.7 disc diameters. They are inactive and are located posterior to the equator. They have irregular borders, and are depigmented but often contain a clump of pigment. These peripheral atrophic scars are thought to be secondary to hematogenous dis-

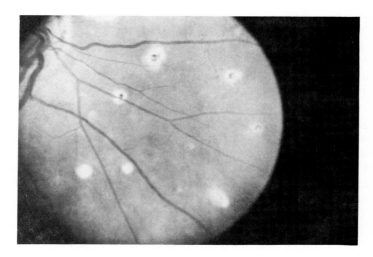

FIG. 6-18. Histoplasmosis: Peripheral atrophic scars. (Courtesy of Dr. G. Mintsioulis)

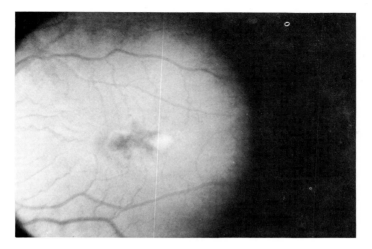

FIG. 6-19. Histoplasmosis: Hemorrhagic disciform macular lesion. (Courtesy of Dr. G. Mintsioulis)

semination of organisms. It is not clear when these lesions develop; however, the choroiditis must be so mild that lesions are almost never recognized in their active stage. Fluorescein angiography of these scars shows only a loss of pigment epithelium and choriocapillaris, and no evidence of leakage suggesting active inflammation.

Circumpapillary choroiditis is another typical feature of presumed ocular histoplasmosis. It is observed in 70%–85% of cases and is usually bilateral. Peripapillary changes are more common in patients with macular lesions than in those with only peripheral scars. Fluorescein angiography of the posterior pole reveals a patchy loss of choriocapillaris and pigment epithelium around the disc. Typically, the circumpapillary changes are separated from the disc by a rim of pigment.

Hemorrhagic macular disciform lesions are the most serious ocular complication of presumed ocular histoplasmosis (Fig. 6-19). They occur mainly in patients between the ages of 20 and 50 and may develop 10 to 20 years after the peripheral atrophic scars. Approximately 5% of persons with peripheral fungal lesions will eventually develop macular disease.

The exact pathogenesis of the macular lesion is not known. Presumably, focal areas of choroiditis develop after primary infection in the periphery. This may in some way sensitize

the uveal tract immunologically. When histoplasma antigen is released at a later stage, an inflammatory reaction develops at or near the fovea, which is predisposed anatomically to serous or hemorrhagic changes (125). Alternatively, seeding of organisms may take place in the macular region, which becomes a site of chronic choroidal vascular decompensation. There is a tendency for serum and blood to leak into this region, with development of typical disciform lesions. When Bruch's membrane is damaged, new vessels can proliferate from the choriocapillaris and spread beneath the retina. Perhaps a combination of a hypersensitivity reaction in the macular region and a compromised vasculature may lead to the disciform macular lesion.

Clinically, the patient first notices metamorphopsia. Gradually a central or paracentral scotoma and blurring of vision develop. Exacerbations may be encountered after physical or emotional stress or even after skin testing with histoplasmin. A localized serous detachment of the retina may be seen, often adjacent to an old parafoveal scar. This leakage of fluid is secondary to highly permeable new blood vessels which grow through a damaged Bruch's membrane. Recurrent hemorrhages may develop and give rise to fibrous scars. Fluorescein angiography shows leakage of these new vessels and serous detachment of the macula. A pigment ring beneath a localized disciform detachment of the sensory retina is typical of presumed ocular histoplasmosis. This pigment ring measures about one-third disc diameter and results from a defect in the pigment epithelium.

The macula of the second eye may be involved from 1 month to 28 years after the initial diagnosis. Estimations of involvement of the second eye are variable, but the incidence seems to be far greater when old, healed scars are present in the macular region. If an old scar is present, the chances of a symptomatic attack are about 1 in 5 (98). If no scars are present, the chances are reduced to 1 in 50. Some authors believe that it is extremely rare to have macular involvement of a second eye in the absence of paramacular or peripapillary scarring (35).

Immunologic Diagnosis

Immunologic tests have little use in the diagnosis of systemic histoplasmosis. Skin tests are frequently positive in endemic areas and serologic titers may be falsely elevated due to previous skin testing. The elevation in the complement-fixation titer may last for several months. Histoplasmin complement-fixing antibodies are elevated in only about one-half of patients with disseminated histoplasmosis. Therefore, many infected patients may be missed with this test. Histoplasmin antigen also cross reacts serologically with blastomycin and coccidioidin.

Despite these pitfalls, both skin tests and serology have some value in the diagnosis of presumed ocular histoplasmosis. In a nonendemic area, a positive histoplasmin skin test may aid in making a proper diagnosis. The complement-fixation test for histoplasmosis can be of value in rare cases in which the skin test is falsely negative (about 11%). In all instances, serum should be drawn before a skin test is applied, and it should be kept in mind that only one-third of patients with presumed ocular histoplasmosis have elevated antibody titers. The histoplasmin skin test is of some use in evaluating a patient for skin-test anergy, in epidemiologic studies, and in assessing cellular immunity in mycologically confirmed histoplasmosis patients. The complement-fixation test may sometimes be useful in making a presumptive diagnosis in very ill patients pending culture results.

In summary, the histoplasmin skin test and complement-fixation titers have limited usefulness in the diagnosis of histoplasmosis. In the systemic disease, culture of the fungus is the best method for making the diagnosis. In presumed ocular histoplasmosis, the characteristic clinical features of the disease provide the major diagnostic clues.

Treatment

The mainstay of treatment for systemic histoplasmosis is amphotericin B. This agent is relatively toxic and must be administered intravenously over a fairly long period of time. Idiosyncratic reactions, which are rare, include anaphylaxis, thrombocytopenia, acute liver failure, convulsions, and cardiac arrest. Predictable toxicity consists of phlebitis, fever, chills, nausea, vomiting, anorexia, headache, anemia, and nephrotoxicity. Amphotericin B is useful mainly in the chronic pulmonary and disseminated forms of histoplasmosis; it is not indicated in the presumed ocular histoplasmosis syndrome.

Various types of therapy have been recommended for management of ocular histoplasmosis. The peripheral choroidal scar and the peripapillary changes are asymptomatic and do not require treatment. The hemorrhagic disciform lesions have been treated in various ways. Schlaegel feels that high doses of corticosteroids should be given orally at the first sign of macular disease (98). Patients can be taught to use the Amsler grid at home and check their macular vision in each eye daily. They can often detect macular lesions before the ophthalmologist can. They are instructed to take 100 mg prednisone with each breakfast for 7 days beginning at the first sign of distortion, or the first moment they suspect a recurrence, and are told to see their ophthalmologist on the seventh day. Once the disease is established, Schlaegel uses prednisone 50–150 mg every other day with breakfast, and injections of a long-acting steroid, such as 40 mg methylprednisolone (Depo-Medrol), behind the equator. Injections may be repeated from three times a week to once every 3 weeks, depending on how the macula responds to therapy. Treatment is continued with reduced levels of steroids for weeks to months depending on the level of activity.

Photocoagulation has been used in an attempt to halt progression of the macular lesion. It is most useful when the process is one-quarter disc diameter or more away from the fovea, and is most useful in neovascular lesions diagnosed by fluorescein angiography. The argon laser with its small spot size is particularly useful for treating blood vessels and the pigment epithelium.

Histoplasmin desensitization has been used but is of questionable value. Aside from the unproven efficacy, it may conceivably reactivate dormant lesions.

CANDIDIASIS

Candida albicans (Fig. 6-20) is an opportunistic fungus which produces systemic disease in immunologically compromised patients and frequently causes ocular complications. Candidal infection may occur in patients with diabetes mellitus or neoplasms, and in patients receiving intravenous hyperalimentation therapy administered through indwelling venous catheters. Candidal infection may also be seen in debilitated patients and those addicted to narcotics. The ocular manifestations are generally part of a systemic disease and the patient requires systemic treatment as well as treatment for the sight-threatening ocular infection.

Immunopathology

Candida albicans grows on some culture media as a yeast (Fig. 6-21) and forms pseudomycelia on other media. The fungus has an affinity for mucous surfaces and may penetrate them under certain conditions. The growth of *Candida* organisms is controlled by certain local factors. A low pH favors the growth of *Candida* by causing transferrin to release iron, which *Candida* requires. *Candida* grows well in high concentrations of glucose; this is thought to be a factor in the susceptibility of diabetic patients to candidiasis. Broad-spectrum antibiotics eliminate normal bacterial flora which compete with *Candida* for glucose. If these bacteria are eliminated, more glucose is available for *Candida* organisms.

Humoral and cellular immunity collaborate to defend the host against candidal infection.

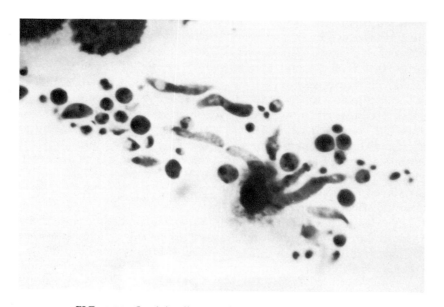

FIG. 6-20. *Candida albicans.* (Courtesy of M. Okumoto)

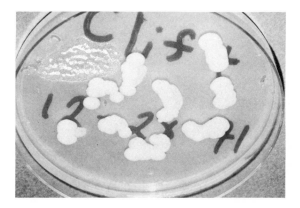

FIG. 6-21. *Candida albicans* on Sabouraud's medium. (Courtesy of M. Okumoto)

Anticandidal "clumping factors" in serum cause agglutination of *Candida* organisms and further uptake of the organisms by phagocytes. Neutrophils, monocytes, and macrophages are all capable of killing *Candida.*

Cellular immunity is extremely important in protecting the host against candidal infection. Patients with chronic mucocutaneous candidiasis have defects in cellular immunity which apparently lead to chronic candidal infection. This syndrome occurs in patients with various types of immunodeficiency. Such patients develop superficial candidal infections of the nails, skin, and mucous membranes. Patients are generally affected before the age of 2 and usually have widespread candidal infections. The syndrome is seen in various endocrine abnormalities, especially hypothyroidism and adrenal insufficiency. It is also seen in patients with Hodgkin's disease and thymomas, in children with severe combined immune deficiency, and in the DiGeorge and Nezelof syndromes. These patients have cutaneous anergy to candida skin test antigen. Sometimes they also have generalized defects in cellular immunity, including delayed allograft rejection and inability to become sensitized to dinitrochlorobenzene. They may have defects in lymphocyte transformation and production of migration inhibition factor. Often, however, these *in vitro* indicators of cellular immunity are normal.

Patients with mucocutaneous candidiasis have also been found to have a serum inhibitory factor which prevents lymphocytes from proliferating in response to antigenic challenge *in vitro.* They may also have a deficiency of IgA and a decreased capacity to produce anticandidal antibody. In addition they may have a defect in neutrophil and mononuclear chemotaxis. The main finding in these patients, however, appears to be related to the T lymphocyte system. While the prognosis is guarded, some success is obtained through treatment with immunologic reconstitution. Transfusion of normal homologous leukocytes, thymic transplantation, and administration of transfer factor and antifungal agents have all been used successfully in the treatment of this disease.

Candida albicans has a tendency to proliferate in patients who are receiving corticosteroids or immunosuppressive therapy. Steroids raise blood glucose levels and also impair neutrophil function and chemotaxis. These factors may permit *Candida* to overgrow superficially and gain access to the blood stream. Once in the blood stream, the organisms can spread in a metastatic fashion to a number of organs, including the eye. If a leukocytopenia is present, as may occur in cancer chemotherapy, the organism may disseminate dramatically. Granulocyte transfusions may be of some help in these situations.

Agglutinins and precipitins may be detectable in the serum of patients with candidiasis. However, since immunosuppressed patients do not make antibody very well, their detection cannot be relied on for making a diagnosis. In addition, these antibodies may be complexed with candida antigen and may therefore be undetectable. Detection of cellular constituents of *Candida* by gas–liquid chromatography may prove useful in diagnosis once this technique is perfected.

Clinical Features

Superficial infection with *Candida albicans* involves the skin and mucous membranes extensively. Infants may be infected with thrush. Some 25% of pregnant women have candidal vaginitis. As mentioned, candidal infection is also common among diabetics, patients with neoplasms, and those receiving immunosuppressives, broad-spectrum antibiotics, or intravenous hyperalimentation. Lesions may be seen in heroin users who filter the heroin through unsterile cotton pledgets. Once *Candida* enters the blood stream, the organism can disseminate to preferred target tissues including the eyes, meninges, myocardium, and kidneys.

Initial ocular complaints include floating spots and diminished visual acuity. Cottonlike whitish lesions are seen on the retina (Fig. 6-22). After a few days, cellular aggregates develop in the vitreous. These appear as puffballs which contain inflammatory cells and the fungal agent. Retinal hemorrhages and Roth's spots may occur. Later, a fully developed endophthalmitis may develop. Diagnosis can be made by obtaining a careful history, by looking for a predisposing factor, and by doing cultures of blood, or of a catheter tip in the case of patients receiving intravenous hyperalimentation. A vitreous biopsy may be useful in confirming the diagnosis.

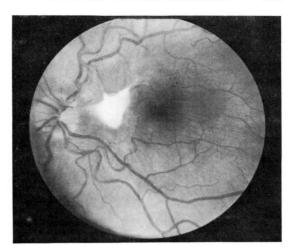

FIG. 6-22. *Candida albicans:* Retinal infiltrate. (Courtesy of Dr. G. Mintsioulis)

Treatment

Treatment of candidal endophthalmitis is currently less than satisfactory, although amphotericin B has been used successfully to treat the ocular as well as the systemic disease. Toxicity, consisting of blood urea nitrogen elevation and a decrease in hemoglobin, must be watched for. Amphotericin B may be combined with rifampin or flucytosine, with which it may act synergistically (7, 63).

Once the candidal infection has left the surface of the retina and invaded the vitreous, prognosis for complete cure is considerably diminished. Amphotericin B can be given by intravitreal injection. Recent studies have shown that up to 10μg amphotericin B can be injected intravitreally in rabbits without causing damage (5), although other studies have shown that localized retinal necrosis may occur with doses of only 1μg (106). Pars plana vitrectomy may be an effective therapeutic approach in patients with candidal endophthalmitis, both for the purpose of sampling the vitreous humor for microbial studies and for removing the site of infection. A combination of vitrectomy and intravitreal amphotericin B may be the best approach available at the present time.

COCCIDIOIDOMYCOSIS

This is a rare disease caused by the dimorphic fungus *Coccidioides immitis* (Fig. 6-23). It is an endemic mycosis in the southwestern United States, and in Central and South America. It causes pulmonary disease in the primary form but may involve virtually any organ. It is a rare cause of granulomatous conjunctivitis associated with a grossly visible preauricular node (**Parinaud's oculoglandular syndrome**).

The fungus exists either as mycelia or as endospores. The mycelia may disintegrate into clouds which can be inhaled, causing clinical outbreaks of coccidioidomycosis. The arthrospores convert to spherules within alveolar macrophages. These spherules enlarge, their outer wall thins, and they release endospores.

Immunopathology

Cellular immunity is important in the body's handling of the primary infection. In healthy individuals, the fungal spherules are ingested by macrophages, and granuloma formation takes place. The granulomas slowly decrease in size and become fibrotic. In the absence

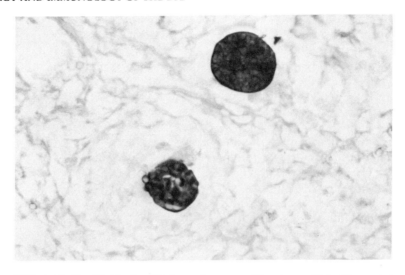

FIG. 6-23. *Coccidioides immitis* in optic nerve. (Courtesy of M. Okumoto)

of intact cellular immunity, progressive pulmonary disease occurs, with necrotizing pneumonia and widespread dissemination. Alternatively, a chronic coccidioidal granuloma may form, which contains viable spherules.

Endospores are chemotactic for neutrophils, which attempt to ingest and destroy the organisms. The neutrophils themselves are destroyed, however, and contribute to the massive pulmonary necrotic tissue. if the organism is successfully handled, the spherules are limited in their number of growth cycles. Over several weeks, the host develops delayed hypersensitivity to coccidioidin (mycelial antigen) or spherulin (spherule antigen). Positive skin reactions can be elicited in patients with pulmonary disease or mild active disseminated disease. More extensive involvement leads to anergy or reaction only to very concentrated antigen. In this case, positive tests may revert to negative with exacerbation of the disease, and negative tests turn positive with improvement. Coccidioidin is prepared from autolyzed mycelia but its exact composition is unknown. The 1:100 dilution is more specific than the 1:10 concentrate since the latter frequently cross reacts with other fungi, including *H. capsulatum.* Spherulin is a recently introduced alternative to coccidioidin skin test antigen. It is as specific as 1:100 coccidioidin and is considerably more sensitive, but in concentrated solutions it also shows cross reactivity to histoplasmin. Lymphocyte activation and production of migration inhibition factor have also been used to test immunologic responses.

Antibody does not play a protective role in this disease. Antibody assays can, however, be helpful in diagnosis of acute and chronic infection. Four serologic methods, including precipitin tests, complement fixation, immunodiffusion, and latex agglutination, are currently used. In acute infection, the precipitin test is positive within 2 weeks after the onset of symptoms. In over 90% of infections, this test reverts to negative within 6 months. The latex agglutination test may become positive earlier than the precipitin test but false-positive results occur in 10% of cases. When the precipitin antibody titer falls, the complement-fixation titer rises and remains positive in chronic disease. A titer of 1:2 or more is significant. The immunodiffusion test also remains positive in chronic disease. However, it is not quantitative and is used only for screening purposes. A decline in the complement-fixation titer indicates clinical improvement.

Clinical Features

General. Sixty percent of infected patients are asymptomatic. Of the remainder, most develop an influenzalike illness, with fever, malaise, cough, aches, pains, and night sweats. Pulmonary infiltrates and hilar adenopathy are common. Skin rashes occur in up to 50% of symptomatic individuals and are thought to represent a hypersensitivity phenomenon. Most rashes are of the erythema nodosum or erythema multiforme type. These hypersensitivity skin reactions are accompanied by eosinophilia and indicate a good prognosis. Arthralgias and arthritis occur in 25% of affected women and 10% of affected men. Like the skin rashes, they may also represent a hypersensitivity mechanism, probably one related to immune-complex deposition.

In progressive disease, walled-off cavities similar to those of tuberculosis may persist in the lungs for many years. In disseminated disease, the infection may involve the central nervous system, viscera, skin, lymph nodes, and bones. Transplacental infection can also occur. Meningitis is the most ominous form of the disease, and is fatal in 50% of cases even with vigorous therapy. Dissemination occurs with strikingly increased frequency among Filipinos and blacks. The reasons for this ethnic predisposition are unknown.

Ocular Findings. Ocular disease is usually manifested as a Parinaud's syndrome. Often there is a mucopurulent discharge, and a thin, transparent pseudomembrane may be present. Conjunctival granulomas are raised, erythematous lesions with small areas of necrosis. The ocular disease represents a metastatic focus of infection: primary ocular disease has not been recognized. Cutaneous involvement, which occurs in the disseminated form of the disease, may affect the skin of the eyelids. A granuloma may persist for decades and is associated with a low risk of spread to other sites.

Treatment

The only drug currently available for the treatment of coccidioidomycosis is amphoteri-cin B. This must be given intravenously for long periods of time, or intrathecally in the case of meningitis. However, miconazole may be an alternative drug in this disease. Recently, transfer factor has been used in desperately ill patients (108). Immunologic conversion and clinical improvement have been seen with this therapy. Such studies are encouraging but inconclusive at present because of the natural course of the disease and because concomitant therapy with amphotericin B was given.

CRYPTOCOCCOSIS

Cryptococcus neoformans is a yeastlike fungus which causes widespread infection in immunosuppressed individuals. Neurologic involvement is common, and papilledema and cranial nerve involvement are frequently seen. The organism is most frequently transmitted to humans through avian droppings, particularly those of pigeons and starlings. Pigeon breeders frequently have a positive skin test for cryptococcal antigen.

Immunopathology

Both antibody and cellular immunity collaborate in host defenses against *C. neoformans.* The organism possesses a capsular polysaccharide which impairs phagocytosis by neutrophils. Antibody and complement, however, potentiate phagocytosis of cryptococci. It has been suggested that the fungi "escape" to the central nervous system, thereby avoiding antibody- and complement-dependent opsonization. This mechanism, however, is speculative. Histologically, the inflammatory response is granulomatous and neutrophils are virtually absent. Individuals with hypogammaglobulinemia are not unusually susceptible, but Hodgkin's disease patients are more likely to be infected again suggesting a prominent role for cellular immunity in the host's defenses. The skin test response to cryptococcal antigen is of the delayed type. Lymphocyte activation and production of migration inhibition factor have been demonstrated in cultures of lymphocytes from healthy donors. Activated macrophages have an increased capacity to destroy the organism.

Clinical Features

Patients with depressed immunity, such as those receiving immunosuppressive medication, are more likely to be infected. Inhalation of the fungus may be followed by hematogenous dissemination with metastatic foci in the skin, mucous membranes, lymph nodes, bones, adrenals, prostate, kidney, spleen, liver, and other viscera. The most common site of the disease by far is the central nervous system. Patients may present with headaches, irritability, and personality changes.

About one-third of patients show papilledema and one-fifth have cranial nerve involvement. They may present with blurred vision, diplopia, facial numbness or weakness, and loss of hearing. Without treatment, this disease may be fatal because of the neurologic complications.

Diagnosis and Treatment

Diagnosis is best made by demonstration of the organism with an India ink preparation of cerebrospinal fluid. If this test is negative, diagnosis can be made by using a test which detects free cryptococcal polysaccharide. Anticryptococcal antibody adsorbed onto latex beads detects minute amounts of cryptococcal antigen. Tests for cellular immunity are of little help since patients are frequently anergic.

No effective vaccine has been developed for cryptococcosis. Amphotericin B is the mainstay of therapy and flucytosine may be given supplementally. Transfer factor has been used to augment the immune response, but its value has not yet been established.

PARASITIC DISEASES

TOXOPLASMOSIS

The protozoan parasite *Toxoplasma gondii* commonly produces infection in man and is a leading cause of posterior uveitis. Serologic surveys have demonstrated that up to 50% of the population in the United States has been infected with the organism. Most of the infections are asymptomatic and subclinical. Frequently the disease goes unrecognized. Most of the ocular disease associated with toxoplasmosis probably occurs because of reactivation of congenital infection. Factors which compromise the host's immunity appear to lead to reactivation of a dormant infection or dissemination of the infectious process.

Epidemiology

Toxoplasma gondii (Fig. 6-24) is an obligate intracellular parasite with almost universal geographic distribution. It can live in all cells except nonnucleated erythrocytes. Three forms of the organism are recognized. The trophozoite is a rapidly multiplying form of the organism that is often responsible for acute infections. The tissue cyst is usually present in chronic infections. The oocyst, the third major form of the organism, has been recognized in the feces of cats. It is the cat which is the definitive host for the *Toxoplasma* organism and it is in the cat intestine where sexual reproduction of the organism takes place. Oocysts are shed in cat feces and are highly resistant to environmental conditions. They may remain infectious for 3–6 weeks. Man and other animals can be infected by ingesting organisms from the soil or by eating uncooked meat from animals which have ingested the parasite.

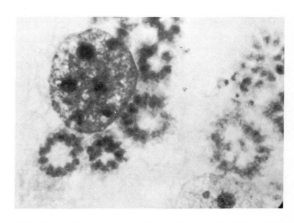

FIG. 6-24. *Toxoplasma gondii* in HeLa cells. (Courtesy of M. Okumoto)

Ingested oocysts release invasive organisms which encyst in most tissues of the animal. If raw or undercooked meat from such an animal is eaten by man, a systemic infection may result. Another mode of transmission is by the transplacental route. This occurs when the mother acquires the infection during pregnancy. Usually such an infection is subclinical or else the illness is misdiagnosed. Many cases of the ocular disease are felt to occur by this type of transmission. Another mode of infection is through human contact with cats. Close contact with cats (*e.g.*, changing their litter boxes) may be a way in which the infection is acquired.

Immunopathology

Infection with *Toxoplasma* results in the production of IgG and IgM antibodies which are detectable by various serologic techniques. The presence of antibody, however, is insufficient to protect the host from infection. Even in the presence of high levels of antibody, the parasite can persist. However, the ability of macrophages to destroy infective trophozoites is greatly enhanced if the *Toxoplasma* organisms are first exposed to antibody and complement. The organisms multiply within macrophages until the host's cells are destroyed. When this occurs, the extracellular parasite comes into contact with antibody and can be more efficiently destroyed.

Recent work in several laboratories has shown conclusively that resistance to toxoplasma infection is mediated by cellular immune mechanisms (12, 31, 54). The proliferation of *Toxoplasma* organisms is controlled by activated macrophages which are probably dependent upon sensitized T lymphocytes. These lymphocytes produce migration inhibition factor and other lymphokines early in the course of a toxoplasma infection. Interferon is also produced during infection with live organisms. The activated macrophages act in both a specific and non-specific fashion to inhibit multiplication of the parasite. Monocytes and macrophages from normal or chronically infected individuals are unable to destroy *Toxoplasma* organisms *in vitro*. However, when these leukocytes are in-

cubated with certain lymphokines (3), they gain the capability to kill the organism or inhibit its multiplication (2). The relationship of these properties to actual infection in man remains to be defined.

Owing to the importance of the lymphocyte–macrophage immune cell axis, drugs which suppress immunity, such as corticosteroids and cytotoxic agents, can induce reactivation of toxoplasmosis and lead to dissemination of the parasite. Transplant recipients may develop life-threatening infection with *Toxoplasma*, and patients with malignancies, particularly Hodgkin's disease, are unusually susceptible (72).

It is possible that certain modes of immunologic enhancement may prove valuable in the treatment of toxoplasma infections and supplement the use of drug therapy (94). Certain adjuvants, such as Freund's adjuvant, and preparations of various *Toxoplasma* antigens, may activate macrophages and confer resistance to toxoplasma infections.

The typical ocular lesion of toxoplasmosis is a necrotizing retinochoroiditis. It has been suggested that the initial ocular lesion of toxoplasmosis results from invasion of the retinal cells by rapidly multiplying organisms. After a phase of multiplication, the *Toxoplasma* organism enters a cystic phase, at which time the lesions become quiescent. It is the encysted form of the parasite that is usually found in subsiding inflammatory lesions of the retina. These encysted forms of the organism may be particulary difficult to eradicate with currently available chemotherapeutic agents. The recurrent chorioretinal lesion may be produced by rupture of cysts; however, the cause of such rupture is uncertain.

Recurrent uveitis may be due to a hypersensitivity phenomenon in the uvea and the retina (30). Some feel that both acute and recurrent types of necrotizing retinochoroiditis are due to multiplication of *Toxoplasma* organisms in the retina. Injection of soluble nonliving antigen into the suprachoroidal space of the rabbit eye does not produce the typical histopathologic lesions of ocular toxoplasmosis (79).

As in the systemic infection, antibody alone does not appear to prevent recurrences of ocular toxoplasmosis. It is the cellular immune system which seems to be important in protecting the host (80). Recently, however, it has been shown that antibody along with complement may influence the encystment of *Toxoplasma* organisms (101). It is believed that plasma cells and the specific antibody they produce at the site of infection may perpetuate the cystic stage.

Clinical Features

General. Toxoplasmosis may be either congenital or acquired. Congenital toxoplasmosis may be acute, subacute, or asymptomatic. The type of infection depends on the stage of pregnancy at which the infection occurs, the immune status of the mother, and the number of organisms passed to the fetus. Maternal infection between the second and sixth months of pregnancy probably results in the acute or subacute form of the disease. During the last trimester, infection produces a mild or asymptomatic disease in the fetus. It is estimated that even if infection occurs during pregnancy, more than half the offspring are completely free of infection.

The acute form of congenital infection may have disastrous consequences. Still birth, prematurity, or spontaneous abortion may result. If the infant survives, hydrocephalus, convulsions, retinitis, hepatosplenomegaly, and jaundice may be seen. Severe mental and physical retardation and often death ensue. The subacute form is less severe. Many of the acute manifestations may be present. Neurologic and ophthalmologic complications predominate, with approximately 10% of the infants having ocular involvement only. In the asymptomatic form, there is usually no evidence of toxoplasma infection at birth. Chorioretinitis later in life may be due to latent congenital infection.

Acquired toxoplasmosis in the immunocompetent host produces mild and frequently unrecognized disease. Fever, lymphadenopathy, myalgia, headache, and anorexia are commonly seen. The systemic disease may be confused with infectious mononucleosis, lymphoma, or sarcoidosis. A lymph node biopsy will reveal typical features of toxoplasmosis. These include a reactive hyperplasia of follicles, and irregular clusters of epithelioid cells and histiocytes in the cortical and paracortical zones. It is presumed that acquired infection results from the ingestion of oocysts from cat feces or ingestion of uncooked meat contaminated with the parasite.

Toxoplasmosis may occur as an opportunistic infection in patients with neoplastic or collagen vascular disease or in recipients of organ allografts (94). These patients, who are immunosuppressed as a result of systemic disease or therapy, may develop widespread and fatal disease. Manifestations include diffuse encephalopathy and meningoencephalitis.

Ocular Findings. The characteristic ocular lesion in toxoplasmosis is a focal necrotizing retinitis. Lesions in the acute or subacute stage are yellowish white cotton like patches. Solitary lesions about the size of the optic disc or smaller clusters of lesions may be seen. In the acute phase, lesions are whiter and have indistinct borders. Often there is an overlying vitreous reaction. In older lesions, the outline is sharper, the color is whitish gray, and choroidal pigment may be present (Fig. 6-25).

A deep punctate retinochoroiditis which does not cloud the vitreous has been associated with toxoplasmosis (29). These lesions, which resemble those of histoplasmosis and are located near the macula, may gradually change to more typical toxoplasmosis lesions. A punctate inner retinal lesion consisting of small single or multifocal gray areas of retinitis has also been described (29).

A vasculitis with sheathing of retinal blood vessels may be seen. This may be due to a local antigen–antibody reaction. Retinal edema which may involve the macula may also be seen, and may result in cystic changes in the fovea. The optic nerve may be affected primarily or secondarily. An optic nerve lesion initially may have the appearance of papilledema (Fig. 6-26) and later develop pallor and loss of substance or segmental atrophy. The latter finding may occur when the macula is involved, owing to retrograde degeneration of ganglion cells. Some cases of juxtapapillary chorioretinitis may be due to toxoplasmosis. Occasionally, peripheral lesions may be observed.

Anterior uveitis can occur in association with the posterior lesions. Occasionally, a reaction may be severe and may include formation of posterior synechiae, iris nodules, and large keratic precipitates. It is believed that anterior uveitis is due to hypersensitivity rather than to direct infection with *Toxoplasma* organisms. Proliferating toxoplasmas have never been demonstrated convincingly in the anterior uveal tract in man. Circulating antigen or antigen–antibody complexes might, however, trigger the reaction in the anterior uvea.

Scleritis may occasionally develop and is perhaps also an immunologic rather than a direct infectious phenomenon.

Diagnosis

Serologic methods are most commonly used in the diagnosis of toxoplasmosis. Since antibody may be detected in a high percentage of the normal population, however, the usefulness of these tests may be limited. It is important to remember that any titer of antibody is significant if the patient has an ocular lesion characteristic of toxoplasmosis. Patients with widespread ocular disease may have positive antibody tests only in undiluted serum. In addition, there seems to be no correlation between the level of the serologic titer and the activity of the ocular disease, as there is in systemic disease.

Several serologic tests are useful in the detection of *Toxoplasma* antibodies. The Sabin–Feldman dye test was the first reliable test to be developed and is a standard by which other newer tests are judged. It measures the capacity of immune serum to modify the cell wall of *Toxoplasma* and change its staining characteristics. Since live organisms are required, other tests have become increasingly popular. The indirect fluorescent antibody (IFA) test and the indirect hemagglutination (IHA) test are technically simple and utilize a killed antigen, thus posing no threat of infection to laboratory workers. The IFA test is the most widely used. It is as sensitive

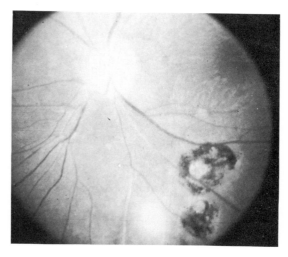

FIG. 6-25. Toxoplasma chorioretinitis. (Courtesy of Dr. G. Mintsioulis)

and specific as the dye test. With the IHA test, antibody appears about one week later than with the dye or IFA test, although titers frequently go as high and persist equally long with all three tests. The complement-fixation test detects antibodies which appear later in the disease, rise to a lower level than other antibodies, and usually disappear within 5 years.

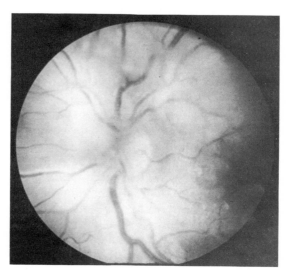

FIG. 6-26. Toxoplasmosis involving the optic disk. (Courtesy of Dr. G. Mintsioulis)

This test is useful in detecting a comparatively recent infection. An immune adherence hemagglutination (IAHA) test has been developed for the detection of surface antigens to *Toxoplasma* (100). This test, which utilizes human erythrocytes and inactivated *Toxoplasma* organisms, correlates well with the results of the dye test. A plate hemolysin test has also been developed for rapid screening of *Toxoplasma* antibodies (52). This test detects hemolytic antibodies directed against *Toxoplasma* antigens bound to red blood cells.

A recently developed test is the IgM-IFA test, which detects IgM antibodies to *Toxoplasma*. Since IgM antibodies appear early and fall after a short period of time, this test can detect acute infections. If the IgM-IFA titer is low or absent, an elevated IFA titer probably indicates chronic infection. In congenital toxoplasmosis, it is sometimes unclear whether the IgG antibodies are maternal or fetal in origin; IgM antibody demonstrated in cord or neonatal serum indicates intrauterine infection (91).

Treatment

Drug therapy of active toxoplasma retinochoroiditis is reserved for inflammatory lesions which threaten the macula or for massive vitreous inflammation. For lesions located in the periphery of the fundus, observation is usually preferable.

The drugs of choice for ocular toxoplasmosis are pyrimethamine (Daraprim) and triple sulfonamides. A loading dose of 100–150 mg pyrimethamine is given over 24–48 hours followed by 25–50 mg of the drug daily for a period of 4–6 weeks. Sulfonamides are administered as a 2-g loading dose followed by 1 g four times a day. The peripheral leukocyte count and platelet count are monitored once a week and if these are depressed, 3 mg folinic acid may be given two or three times a week. In patients who have severe vomiting or hematopoietic depression with pyrimethamine, sulfonamides may be used alone or chlortetracycline may be substituted. The average retinal lesion retains its inflammatory activity for 2 weeks to 2 months. Chronic elevated lesions seem to show little effect with treatment.

These lesions are thought to represent massive necrotic granulomas which chemotherapeutic agents probably cannot penetrate. Such lesions require 6–18 months to heal regardless of treatment.

Oral corticosteroids are sometimes administered when inflammation is so severe that damage to central vision seems imminent. They may be administered in doses equivalent to 80–120 mg prednisone and should be given with pyrimethamine and/or sulfonamides. It should be remembered that corticosteroids are a two-edged sword. Although they quiet the inflammation, which may be necessary to preserve macular vision, they also depress the cell-mediated defenses which are necessary for eliminating the *Toxoplasma* organism. Under no circumstances should corticosteroids be administered in toxoplasmosis without antimicrobial coverage. Both active and recurrent lesions may be associated with proliferating microorganisms, and corticosteroids alone will perpetuate this proliferation. Repository forms of corticosteroids are probably not indicated in ocular toxoplasmosis. Their administration in several cases has resulted in a precipitous downhill course with marked worsening of inflammation (78). The dangers of steroid treatment in toxoplasmosis and their suppressant effects on the immune system have been described by O'Connor and Frenkel (82).

Recently, clindamycin, a 7-chloro derivative of lincomycin, has been found to eradicate toxoplasma infection in mice (69). This drug also controls ocular lesions of toxoplasmosis in the rabbit (109). The drug is well tolerated and high levels can be established in the retina and choroid by periocular or systemic administration. The encysted form of the parasite, the form generally found in subsiding retinal lesions, is highly resistant to antimicrobial therapy, although there is some indication that sulfonamides reduce the number of viable cysts (9). Clindamycin has been shown to penetrate the cysts of infected mice except in the brain (3). The close relation between the brain and the eye makes the efficacy of clindamycin in human ocular toxoplasmosis uncertain. Clindamycin unfortunately has been associated with severe diarrheal symptoms and with pseudomembranous colitis (112).

An alternative to antimicrobial therapy in toxoplasmosis is the possibility of augmentation of the patient's own immune system. Enhancement of cell-mediated immunity may be a sounder approach to dealing with the parasite than antiparasitic chemotherapy. Transfer factor, BCG vaccine, and levamisole are drugs which can enhance the immune system. Levamisole has been used with some success in the treatment of chronic infection in immunologically depressed patients. BCG (bacillus Calmette–Guérin) vaccine provides nonspecific host resistance and can delay the onset of toxoplasma retinochoroiditis in the rabbit (110).

Some special indications for treatment of women during pregnancy should be mentioned. If a woman has been infected before pregnancy, it is unlikely that a toxoplasma infection will be passed to the fetus. If a primary infection begins during pregnancy, interruption of the pregnancy should be considered. In certain instances, it may be necessary to use drug therapy with pyrimethamine and sulfadiazine during pregnancy. For example, drug treatment may be indicated for a macula-threatening lesion in a mother's only functional eye. Since pyrimethamine carries a risk of teratogenesis, use of this drug could be considered an indication for therapeutic abortion. In the later stages of pregnancy, when an abortion would be inappropriate, the pregnancy should be allowed to go to term and the newborn should be evaluated clinically and serologically.

TOXOCARIASIS

Toxocara canis is the common intestinal ascarid found in dogs and *Toxocara cati* is the intestinal ascarid found in the cat. Both are true roundworms of the phylum Nematoda and measure 4–12 cm in length. *T. canis* is the most important etiologic agent in visceral larva migrans. The disease is caused by ingestion of infective ova, usually associated with the eating of dirt. The organism also produces ocular inflammatory disease which takes one of three forms: a posterior pole granuloma, a peripheral granuloma, and diffuse endophthalmitis.

Immunopathology

The dog is the definitive host for *T. canis* and the cat is the definitive host for *T. cati*. Man is an intermediate or accidental host in which the parasite cannot mature or reproduce. The life cycle of *Toxocara* is like that of other nematodes. Infective ova are ingested by the dog or cat and enter the gastrointestinal tract. Second-stage larvae gain access to the mesenteric vessels, enter the blood stream, and seed the liver, heart, brain, eyes, kidneys, and muscles. After a pulmonary phase, organisms are swallowed and descend to the gastrointestinal tract where they mature into adult larvae and reproduce. Infective ova are then deposited in the feces. Small children may be infected by ingesting soil contaminated with infective ova or by close contact with infected dogs. After ingestion of the ova, the larvae may enter the blood stream of the human through the mesenteric vessels, and migrate to various organs including the liver, lung, brain, and eye. The parasites do not mature into adult worms or complete their life cycle in man.

Certain laboratory abnormalities are found in patients with systemic visceral larva migrans; however, serologic abnormalities and systemic findings are minimal or nonexistent in patients with ocular toxocariasis. Because the diagnosis of the ocular disease in difficult, immunodiagnostic tests for the parasite have been eagerly sought.

Patients with visceral larva migrans generally have a leukocytosis in the range of 15,000–100,000. An eosinophilia of 30%–90% is often seen. Hyperglobulinemia, mostly of the γ fraction, is seen, as well as an elevated IgM and IgE. IgE may be 10–15 times the normal level. The heterophil antibody may be detected and anti-A and anti-B blood group antigens may be elevated (14). A skin test has been used in the past but this cross reacts with antigens of other nematodes.

Serologic tests including the indirect hemagglutination and bentonite flocculation tests are neither very sensitive nor very specific, and positive results correlate only with a very acute phase of the disease (23). A capillary tube precipitin test is fairly sensitive and specific (23). Cross reaction with *Ascaris* can be eliminated by absorption with *Ascaris* antigen. Recently, an enzyme-linked immunosorbent assay has been developed which shows promise for future serodiagnosis.

Clinical Features

General. For many years, clinicians observed a variety of disorders characterized by visceral lesions and eosinophilia. Frequently, parasites were considered to play an etiologic role. In 1950, Mercer *et al* (71) found nematode larvae in the liver of a 2-year-old patient with chronic eosinophilia. In 1952, Beaver *et al* identified a *Toxocara* larva in a liver biopsy from a child with a similar disorder and coined the term **visceral larva migrans** to describe this entity (6).

Patients may be asymptomatic, or they may present with fever, irritability, pallor, anorexia, and malaise. Hepatosplenomegaly is common and there may be transient migratory lung infiltrates. An erythematous, urticarial, or papular skin rash may be present over the abdomen or extremities, and generalized seizures or encephalomyelitis may occur. Stool examination will be negative since the parasite does not mature or reproduce in the human intestinal tract. Liver biopsy may demonstrate the larvae but many histologic sections may be required.

Ocular Findings. In 1950, Wilder reviewed 46 cases of pseudoglioma which showed larvae or their remnants (121). These were initially identified as third-stage hookworm larvae but were later correctly identified as *Toxocara*. Subsequently, three forms of ocular toxocariasis were identified: a posterior pole granuloma (4), a peripheral granuloma (51), and a diffuse endophthalmitis.

The average age of patients presenting with ocular toxocariasis is 7½ years. A history of dog or cat contact may be elicited but is not always obtained. Patients with ocular disease seldom have parasites in other tissues, and conversely patients with visceral disease seldom develop ocular disease. The patient may be asymptomatic, or may present with failing vision, a blind eye, strabismus, or leukocoria. Toxocariasis is a significant cause of uveitis, and in some series accounts for 10% of uveitis cases. In contrast to the systemic form of toxocariasis, laboratory tests are generally normal, patients are in an older age group, and there may be no history of ingesting dirt or of close contact with a pet.

Treatment

No therapy is currently available for the extraintestinal larvae of *Toxocara canis*. Thiabendazole destroys the tissue phase of some parasites and may be of some benefit in the treatment of visceral larva migrans. Corticosteroids are very effective in alleviating respiratory symptoms. The emphasis in managing a patient should be on the prevention of further ingestion of dirt. Children with this pica sometimes have an associated iron-deficiency anemia and this should be sought and treated appropriately. The ocular disease is frequently seen during an inactive stage. Often, only observation is necessary; however, malignancy must be ruled out. Thiabendazole has been used in only a few patients (13). Light coagulation and cryotherapy have also been employed but their effectiveness remains to be evaluated. It should be kept in mind that larval death in the eye may produce a severe inflammatory reaction which can be more damaging than the live larvae (18). For this reason, any therapy should be instituted with caution.

REFERENCES

1. Anderson HK, Spencer ES: Cytomegalovirus infection among renal allograft recipients. Acta Med Scand 186:7, 1969
2. Anderson SE Jr, Remington JS: Effect of normal and activated human macrophages on Toxoplasma gondii. J Exp Med 139:1154, 1974
3. Arjo JF, Remington JS: Effect of clindamycin on acute and chronic toxoplasmosis in mice. Antimicrob Agents Chemother 5:647, 1974
4. Ashton N: Larval granulomatosis of the retina due to Toxocara. Br J Ophthalmol 44:129, 1960
5. Axelrod AJ, Peyman GA, Apple DJ: Toxicity

of intravitreal injection of amphotericin B. Am J Ophthalmol 76:578, 1973

6. Beaver PC, Snyder CH, Carrera GM et al: Chronic eosinophilia due to visceral larva migrans. Report of three cases. Pediatrics 9:7, 1952

7. Beggs WH, Sarosi GA, Walker MI: Synergistic action of amphotericin B and rifampin against Candida species. J Infect Dis 133:206, 1976

8. Betts RF, George SD, Rundell BB et al: Comparative activity of immunofluorescent antibody and complement-fixing antibody in cytomegalovirus infection. J Clin Microbiol 4:151, 1976

9. Beverly JFA: A rational approach to the treatment of toxoplasmic uveitis. Trans Ophthalmol Soc UK 78:109, 1958

10. Bloomfield SE, Mondino B, Gray GF: Scleral tuberculosis. Arch Ophthalmol 94:954, 1976

11. Boniuk V, Boniuk M: The incidence of phthisis bulbi as a complication of cataract surgery in the congenital rubella syndrome. Int Ophthalmol Clin 12:77, 1972

12. Borges JS, Johnson WD Jr: Inhibition of multiplication of Toxoplasma gondii by human monocytes exposed to T lymphocyte products. J Exp Med 141:483, 1975

13. Brown DH: Ocular Toxocara. II. Clinical review. J Pediatr Ophthalmol 7:182, 1970

14. Brown DH: Ocular Toxocara. I. Experimental immunology. Ann Opthalmol 3:907, 1970

15. Brunell PA, Gershon AA, Uduman SA, Steinberg S: Varicella-Zoster immunoglobulins during varicella, latency and zoster. J Infect Dis 132:49, 1975

16. Bullock WE: Studies of immune mechanisms in leprosy. I. Depression of delayed allergic response to skin test antigens. N Engl J Med 278:298, 1968

17. Burns RP: Cytomegalic inclusion disease uveitis. Report of case with isolation from aqueous humor of virus in tissue culture. Arch Ophthalmol 61:376, 1959

18. Byers B, Kimura SJ: Uveitis after death of a larva in the vitreous cavity. Am J Ophthalmol 77:63, 1974

19. Char DH, Cogan DG, Sullivan WR Jr: Immunologic study of nonsyphilitic interstitial keratitis with vestibuloauditory symptoms. Am J Ophthalmol 80:491, 1975

20. Chien LT, Cannon NJ, Whitley RJ et al: Effect of adenine arabinoside on cytomegalovirus infections. J Infect Dis 130:32, 1974

21. Chumbley LC, Robertson DM, Smith TF, Campbell RJ: Adult cytomegalovirus inclusion retinouveitis. Am J Ophthalmol 80:807, 1975

22. Cogan DG: Syndrome of nonsyphilitic interstitial keratitis and vestibuloauditory symptoms. Arch Ophthalmol 33:144, 1945

23. Defalla AA: The serodiagnosis of human toxocariasis by the capillary-tube precipitin test. Trans R Soc Trop Med Hyg 69:146, 1975

24. Darrell RW: Acute tuberculous panophthalmitis. Arch Ophthalmol 78:51, 1967

25. Davidorf FH: The role of T lymphocytes in the reactivation of presumed ocular histoplasmosis scars. Int Ophthalmol Clin 15:111, 1975

26. Dent PB, Olsen GB, Good RA et al: Rubella virus—leukocyte interaction and its role in the pathogenesis of congenital rubella syndrome. Lancet 1:291, 1968

27. Donahue HC: Experience in a tuberculosis sanatorium. Am J Ophthalmol 64:742, 1967

28. Eales H: Primary retinal hemorrhage in young men. Ophthalmol Rev 1:41, 1882

29. Freemann CT, Knox DL: Variations in active toxoplasmic retinochoroiditis. Arch Ophthalmol 81:481, 1969

30. Frenkel JK: Pathogenesis of toxoplasmosis and of infections with organisms resembling Toxoplasma. Ann NY Acad Sci 64:215, 1956

31. Frenkel JK: Adoptive immunity to intracellular infection. J Immunol 98:1309, 1967

32. Ganley JP: Epidemiologic characteristics of presumed ocular histoplasmosis. Acta Ophthalmol [Suppl] (Kbh): 119, 1973

33. Ganley JP: The role of the cellular immune system in patients with macular disciform histoplasmosis. Int Ophthalmol Clin 15:83, 1975

34. Ganley JP, Smith RE, Thomas DB et al: Booster effect of histoplasmin skin testing in an elderly population. Am J Epidemiol 95:104, 1972

35. Gass JDM, Wilkinson CP: Follow-up study of presumed ocular histoplasmosis. Trans Am Acad Ophthalmol Otolaryngol 76:672, 1972

36. Gershon AA, Steinberg S, Smith M: Cell-mediated immunity to Varicella-Zoster virus demonstrated by viral inactivation with human leukocytes. Infect Immun 13:1549, 1936

37. Gradenigo PN: Tuberculosis of the iris. Boston M & Surg J 4:285, 1869

38. Green SH, Wirtschafter JD: Ophthalmoscopic findings in subacute sclerosing panencephalitis. Br J Ophthalmol 57:780, 1973

39. Gregg NM: Congenital cataract following German measles in the mother. Trans Ophthalmol Soc Aust 3:35, 1941

40. Guerrant RL, Humphries MK, Butler JE, Jackson RS: Tickborne oculo-glandular tularemia. Arch Intern Med 36:811, 1976

41. Gunderson T: Convalescent blood for treatment of herpes zoster ophthalmicus. Trans Am Ophthalmol Soc 38:124, 1940

42. Hedley-Whyte ET, Craighead JE: Generalized cytomegalic inclusion disease after renal homotransplantation. New Engl J Med 272:473, 1965

43. Hittner HM, Desmond MM, Montgomery JR: Optic nerve manifestations of human congen-

ital cytomegalovirus infection. Am J Ophthalmol 81:661, 1976

44. Hitzig WH, Grob PJ: Therapeutic uses of transfer factor. Prog Clin Immunol 2:69, 1974

45. Hoefnagels KLJ, Pijpers PM: Histoplasma capsulatum in a human eye. Am J Ophthalmol 63:715, 1967

46. Hoff GL, Bigler WJ, Prather EC: One-half century of tularemia in Florida. J Fla Med Assoc 62:35, 1975

47. Hope-Simpson RE: The nature of herpes zoster: a long-term study and a new hypothesis. Proc R Soc Med 58:9, 1965

48. Howard RJ, Miller J, Najarian JS: Cytomegalovirus-induced immune suppression. II. Cell-mediated immunity. Clin Exp Immunol 18:119, 1974

49. Howard RJ, Najarian JS: Cytomegalovirus-induced immune suppression. I. Humoral immunity. Clin Exp Immunol 18:109, 1974

50. Hyndiuk RA, Okumoto M, Damiano RA et al: Treatment of vaccinial keratitis with vidarabine. Arch Ophthalmol 94:1363, 1976

51. Irvine WC, Irvine AR Jr: Nematode endophthalmitis: Toxocara canis. Am J Ophthalmol 47:185, 1959

52. Jackson WB, O'Connor GR, Hall JM: Plate hemolysin test for the rapid screening of Toxoplasma antibodies. Appl Microbiol 27:896, 1974

53. Jaeger E: Veber choroidealtuberkel. Oesterr Z F Pract Heilk 1:9, 1855

54. Jones TC, Len L, Hirsch JG: Assessment in vitro of immunity against Toxoplasma gondii. J Exp Med 141:466, 1975

55. Kaariainen L, Klemola E, Paloheimo J: Rise of cytomegalovirus antibodies in infectious mononucleosis-like syndrome after transfusion. Br Med J 1:1270, 1966

56. Kantor GL, Goldberg LS, Johnson BM et al: Immunologic abnormalities induced by postperfusion cytomegalovirus infection. Ann Intern Med 73:553, 1970

57. Kaplan BS, Wigelsworth FW, Marks MI, Drummond KN: The glomerulopathy of congenital syphilis—an immune deposit disease. J Pediatr 81:1154, 1972

58. Kline LB, Jackson WB: Herpes zoster conjunctival ulceration. Can J Ophthalmol 12:66, 1977

59. Klintworth GK, Hollingsworth AS, Lutsman PA, Bradford WD: Granulomatous choroiditis in a case of disseminated histoplasmosis: histologic demonstration of Histoplasma capsulatum in choroidal lesions. Arch Ophthalmol 90:45, 1973

60. Knopf HLS, Blacklow NR, Glassman MI: Antibody in tears following intranasal vaccination with inactivated virus. III. Role of tear and serum antibody in experimental vaccinia conjunctivitis. Invest Ophthalmol 10:760, 1971

61. Knopf HLS, Blacklow NR, Glassman MI et al: Antibody in tears following intranasal vaccination with inactivated virus. II. Enhancement of tear antibody production by the use of polyinosinic: polycytidilic acid (poly I:C). Invest Ophthalmol 10:750, 1971

62. Krause AC, Hopkins WG: Ocular manifestations of histoplasmosis. Am J Ophthalmol 34:564, 1951

63. Lou P, Kazdan J, Bannatyne RM, Cheung R: Successful treatment of Candida endophthalmitis with a synergistic combination of amphotericin B and rifampin. Am J Ophthalmol 83:12, 1977

64. Maitre Jan A (Cited by Sorsby A): Systemic Ophthalmology. St Louis, Mosby, 1951, p 151

65. Makley TA, Long JW, Suie T, Stephan JD: Presumed histoplasmic chorioretinitis with special emphasis on present modes of therapy. Trans Am Acad Ophthalmol Otolaryngol 69:443, 1965

66. Manz L: Die Rinderpest, eine Sanitatspolizeiliche studie. Marburg Elwert, 1858, p 11

67. Marshall WC, Cope WA, Soothill JF, Dudgeon JA: In vitro lymphocyte response in some immunity deficiency diseases and in intrauterine virus infections. Proc R Soc Med 63:35, 1970

68. Matas BR, Spencer WH, Hayes TC et al: Morphology of experimental vaccinial superficial punctate keratitis. Invest Ophthalmol 10:348, 1971

69. McMaster PRB, Powers KG, Finerty JF, Lunde MN: The effect of two chlorinated lincomycin analogues against acute toxoplasmosis in mice. Am J Trop Med Hyg 22:14, 1973

70. Mendes NF, Kopersztych S, Mota NGS: T and B lymphocytes in patients with lepromatous leprosy. Clin Exp Immunol 16:23, 1974

71. Mercer RD, Lund HZ, Bloomfield RA et al: Larval ascariasis as a cause of chronic eosinophilia with visceral manifestations. Am J Dis Child 80:46, 1950

72. Miller DG: Immunologic Diseases. Boston, Little, Brown, 1965

73. Miller JM, Nelson JR, Reisner RM, Turner JA: Syphilis. Calif Med 115:47, 1971

74. Mizukawa T, Fujita N, Hara J: Autoradiographic and fluorescein antibody studies of susceptibility to virus of corneal stromal cells of the rabbit. Folia Ophthalmol Jpn 16:317, 1965

75. Morrison WL: Viral warts, herpes simplex and herpes zoster in patients with secondary immune deficiencies and neoplasms. Br J Dermatol 92:625, 1975

76. Mortada A: Orbital apex syndrome with contra-lateral hemiplegia due to tuberculoma of orbital apex. Mod Prob Ophthalmol 14:657, 1975

77. Newell FW, Krill AE: Treatment of uveitis

with azathioprine (Imuran). Trans Ophthalmol Soc UK 87:499, 1967

78. Nicholson DH, Wolchok EB: Ocular toxoplasmosis in an adult receiving long-term corticosteroid therapy. Arch Ophthalmol 94:248, 1976

79. Nozik RA, O'Connor GR: Studies on ocular toxoplasmosis in the rabbit. I. The effect of antigenic stimulation. Arch Ophthalmol 83:724, 1970

80. O'Connor GR: Ocular toxoplasmosis. Jpn J Ophthalmol 19:1, 1975

81. O'Connor GR: Uveitis of microbial origin: current and future trends. Trans Pac Coast Otoophthalmol Soc 57:223, 1976

82. O'Connor GR, Frenkel JK: Dangers of steroid treatment in toxoplasmosis. Arch Ophthalmol 94:213, 1976

83. Olsen GB, Dent PB, Rawls WE et al: Abnormalities of in vitro lymphocyte responses during rubella virus infection. J Exp Med 128:47, 1968

84. Pettit TH: The poxviruses: vaccinia and variola. Int Ophthalmol Clin 15:203, 1975

85. Poltkin SA: Editorial comment. J Pediatr 80:493, 1972

86. Quismorio FP, Rea TH, Levan NE et al: Immunoglobulin deposits in lepromatous leprosy skin. Arch Dermatol 111:331, 1975

87. Rawls WE: Congenital rubella: the significance of virus persistence. Prog Med Virol 10:238, 1968

88. Rawls WE: Virology and epidemiology of rubella virus. Int Ophthalmol Clin 12:21, 1972

89. Rea TH, Quismorio FP, Harding B et al: Immunologic responses in patients with lepromatous leprosy. Arch Dermatol 112:791, 1976

90. Rees RJW: Enhanced susceptibility of thymectomized and irradiated mice to infection with Mycobacterium leprae. Nature 211:657, 1966

91. Remington JA, Miller MJ, Brownless I: IgM antibodies in acute toxoplasmosis. Diagnostic significance in congenital cases and a method for their rapid detection. Pediatrics 41:1082, 1968

92. Rowe WP, Hartley JW, Waterman S et al: Cytopathogenic agent resembling human salivary gland virus recovered from tissue cultures of human adenoids. Proc Soc Exp Biol Med 92:418, 1956

93. Roy L, Alvarez L: Observation clinique du bacille de la tuberculose dans la cornée. Rev Clin Ocul Paris 5:185, 1885

94. Ruskin J, Remington JS: Toxoplasmosis in the compromised host. Ann Intern Med 84:193, 1976

95. Ryan SJ: Histopathological correlates of presumed ocular histoplasmosis. Int Ophthalmol Clin 15:125, 1975

96. Savir H, Kurz O: Fluorescein angiography in syphilitic retinal vasculitis. Ann Ophthalmol 8:713, 1976

97. Schlaegel TF: Essentials of Uveitis. Boston, Little, Brown, 1969

98. Schlaegel TF Jr: Histoplasmic choroiditis. Ann Ophthalmol 6:237, 1974

98a. Schlaegel TF, Weber JC, Helveston E, Kenney D: Presumed histoplasmic choroiditis. Am J Ophthalmol 63:919, 1967

99. Schlaegel TF, Weber JB: Follow-up study of presumed histoplasmic choroiditis. Am J Ophthalmol 71:1192, 1971

100. Shimada K, O'Connor GR: An immune adherence hemagglutination test for toxoplasmosis. Arch Ophthalmol 90:372, 1973

101. Shimada K, O'Connor GR, Yoneda C: Cyst formation by Toxoplasma gondii (RH strain) in vitro. Arch Ophthalmol 92:496, 1974

102. Smith JL, Israel CW: The presence of spirochetes in late seronegative syphilis. JAMA 199:126, 1967

103. Smith RE, Ganley JP, Knox DL: Presumed ocular histoplasmosis. II. Patterns of peripheral and peripapillary scarring in persons with nonmacular disease. Arch Ophthalmol 87:251, 1972

104. Smith RE, O'Connor GR, Halde CJ et al: Clinical course in rabbits after experimental induction of ocular histoplasmosis. Am J Ophthalmol 76:284, 1973

105. Solanes MP, Heatley J, Arenas F, Ibarra GG: Ocular complications in brucellosis. Am J Ophthalmol 36:675, 1953

106. Souri E, Green WR: Intravitreal amphotericin B toxicity. Am J Ophthalmol 78:77, 1974

107. Spaeth GC: Absence of so-called Histoplasma uveitis in 134 cases of proven histoplasmosis. Arch Ophthalmol 77:41, 1967

108. Spitler LE, Levin AS, Fudenburg HH: Transfer factor. Clin Immunobiol 2:153, 1974

109. Tabbara KF, Nozik RA, O'Connor GR: Clindamycin effects on experimental ocular toxoplasmosis in the rabbit. Arch Ophthalmol 92:244, 1974

110. Tabbara KF, O'Connor GR, Nozik RA: Effect of immunization with attenuated Mycobacterium bovis on experimental toxoplasmic retinochoroiditis. Am J Ophthalmol 79:641, 1975

111. Thygeson P: The changing characteristics of herpes zoster keratouveitis. Trans Pac Coast Otoophthalmol Soc 55:129, 1974

112. Tures JF, Townsend WF, Rose HD: Cephalosporin-associated pseudomembranous colitis. JAMA 236:948, 1976

113. Uduman SA, Gershon AA, Brunell PA: Should patients with zoster receive zoster immune globulin. JAMA 234:1049, 1975

114. Vail DT: A case of "squirrel plague" conjunctivitis in man. Ophthalmol Rec 23:487, 1914

115. Van Metre TE Jr, Maumenee AE: Specific

ocular uveal lesions in patients with evidence of histoplasmosis. Arch Ophthalmol 71:314, 1964

116. Venereal Disease Control Division, Bureau of State Services, Center for Disease Control. J Infect Dis 134:94, 1976

117. Von Pirquet CF: Klinische Studien Uber Vakzination and Vakzinale Allergie. Leipzig Deuticke, 1907

118. Waldorf DS, Sheagren JN, Trautman JR et al: Impaired delayed hypersensitivity in patients with lepromatous leprosy. Lancet 2:773, 1966

119. Weber JC, Schlaegel TF: Delayed skin test reactivity of uveitis patients: influence of age and diagnosis. Am J Ophthalmol 67:732, 1969

120. White LR, Leikin S, Villavicencio O et al: Immune competence in congenital rubella: lymphocyte transformation, delayed hypersensitivity, and response to vaccination. J Pediatr 73:229, 1968

121. Wilder HC: Nematode endophthalmitis. Trans Am Acad Ophthalmol Otolaryngol 55:99, 1950

122. Wong VG, Kwon-Chung KJ, Hill WB: Koch's postulates and experimental ocular histoplasmosis. Int Ophthalmol Clin 15:139, 1975

123. Woods AC: Influence of hypersensitivity on endogenous uveal disease. Trans Am Acad Ophthalmol Otolaryngol 51:75, 1946

124. Woods, AC: Experimental studies on the pathogenesis and treatment of ocular tuberculosis. Br J Ophthalmol 33:197, 1949

125. Woods AC, Whalen JE: The probable role of benign histoplasmosis in the etiology of granulomatous uveitis. Trans Am Ophthalmol Soc 57:318, 1959

126. Wuepper FD: "Red eye" as the presenting sign of syphilis d'Emblée. Calif Med 107:518, 1967

127. Yanoff M, Schaffer DB, Scheie HG: Rubella ocular syndrome: clinical significance of viral and pathologic studies. Trans Am Acad Ophthalmol Otolaryngol 72:896, 1968

SEVEN
SEVEN
SEVEN ocular diseases with immunologic features

There are a number of conditions which primarily affect the eye and seem to have an immunologic basis. In most cases, the immune pathogenesis of these diseases has not been established. However, certain clinical features or laboratory investigations have led us to categorize these entities as ocular conditions with immunologic features. While there is general agreement as to the importance of immune factors in certain conditions such as vernal conjunctivitis, sympathetic ophthalmia, and lens-induced uveitis, evidence for the immunologic nature of other diseases, such as retinitis pigmentosa and glaucoma, is tenuous at best. These diseases have been included in this chapter because they are being investigated by immunologic methods, and an immunologic abnormality may have been demonstrated even though its significance remains unknown.

VERNAL KERATOCONJUNCTIVITIS

Vernal keratoconjunctivitis ("vernal") is a bilateral and often severe disease, occurring mainly in children and associated with climatic factors. It is characterized by a stringy, mucinous discharge and giant papillae of the upper palpebral conjunctiva. Many features of vernal keratoconjunctivitis suggest an allergic etiology. A recently described entity with similar but milder manifestations has been described in individuals who wear hard or soft contact lenses.

Immunopathology

Patients with vernal keratoconjunctivitis frequently have a history of atopic disease such as hay fever, atopic eczema, or asthma (52). Sometimes, a history of atopy can be elicited only in a member of the patient's family. Increased levels of IgE can be detected in the tears of patients with vernal (1, 19), and even when the mean level of IgE in tears is not significantly greater than in control subjects, the serum IgE levels are significantly increased (1). In patients with vernal keratoconjunctivitis, it has been shown that IgA, IgD, and IgE are synthesized locally by conjunctival plasma cells in a ratio of approximately 4:1:2, respectively.

Histologically, the conjunctiva of patients with vernal keratoconjunctivitis contains many eosinophils, plasma cells, and fixed tissue mast cells (Figs. 7-1 and 7-2). Eosinophils and mast cells can also be demonstrated in scrapings of the conjunctiva. Additional histologic features have recently been described in this disease, including the presence of basophils, microvascular alterations of endothelial cells, and deposition of fibrin. These features have suggested the possibility of a delayed hypersensitivity component in vernal because they are similar to the typical histologic fea-

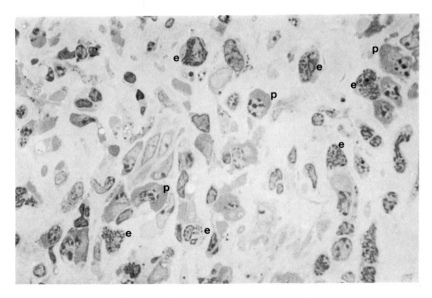

FIG. 7-1. Plasma cells (p) and eosinophils (e) in vernal keratoconjunctivitis.

tures of cutaneous basophil hypersensitivity reactions (33). Other histologic features of vernal include infiltration by lymphocytes and neutrophils, and epithelial invasion by mast cells and eosinophils.

Similar although milder histopathologic changes are present in the giant papillary conjunctivitis (Fig. 7-3) associated with wearing hard or soft contact lenses (2). In contrast to vernal conjunctivitis, this syndrome may not be more common in atopic patients, and itching is mild whereas in vernal it is severe. It has

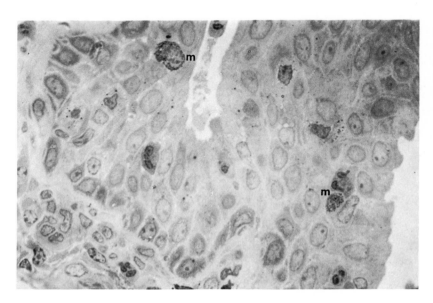

FIG. 7-2. Mast cells (m) in epithelium of giant papillae in vernal keratoconjunctivitis.

been suggested that the inciting antigen in this condition is the material which accumulates over a period of time on the surface of the contact lens. This material may incite a hypersensitivity reaction having both humoral and cellular immune components.

Clinical Features

Vernal keratoconjunctivitis begins in the prepubertal years and is more common in males than females. After the age of 20, the incidence in the two sexes is about the same. The peak incidence is between the ages of 11 and 13, and the disease is rare after age 30. Vernal is more common in warm climates than in temperate zones and is rarely seen in cold climates. Because of this geographic pattern, heat and other physical factors have been thought to contribute to the pathogenesis of the disease.

Patients complain of extreme itching and a ropy mucous discharge. The hallmark of vernal keratoconjunctivitis is the presence of giant papillae on the palpebral conjunctiva (Fig. 7-4). These papillae are polygonal and flat-topped, and contain tufts of capillaries. The conjunctiva has a milky appearance and many fine papillae may be present on the lower palpebral conjunctiva. A pseudomembrane may be present in severe cases (**Maxwell–Lyons sign**).

Corneal findings include superficial corneal ulcers and plaquelike deposits in the anterior cornea (Fig. 7-5). These contain mucus or many compacted layers of epithelial cells. The white dotlike deposits located at the limbus are known as **Trantas' dots** (Fig. 7-6). They contain large numbers of eosinophils and their presence parallels the activity of the disease. Other corneal complications include a diffuse epithelial keratitis, a micropannus, and a pseudogerontotoxon which is often adjacent to a limbal papilla. Conjunctival scarring does not occur in vernal unless the papillae have been treated with cryotherapy, irradiation, surgical removal, or other damaging procedures.

A limbal form of vernal keratoconjunctivitis with less involvement of the palpebral conjunctiva may also be seen. It is characterized

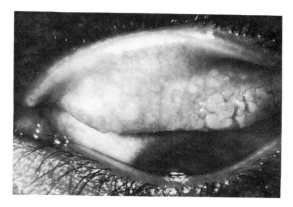

FIG. 7-3. Giant papillary conjunctivitis secondary to wearing contact lenses.

by gelatinous swellings at the limbus. This form of vernal is said to be more common in blacks.

Treatment

Vernal keratoconjunctivitis is a self-limited disease which runs a 5- to 10-year course. Treatment therefore should be conservative and aimed at relieving symptoms without producing serious iatrogenic side effects. Topical and systemic corticosteroids are frequently employed in treating this condition. While they decrease the symptoms, they do not significantly affect the corneal complications or shorten the duration of the disease, and they

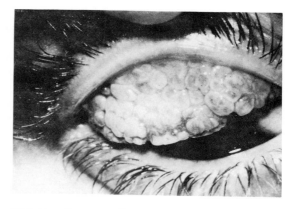

FIG. 7-4. Giant papillae on superior palpebral conjunctiva in vernal keratoconjunctivitis.

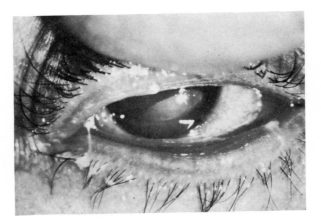

FIG. 7-5. Corneal plaque in patient with vernal keratoconjunctivitis. (Courtesy of Dr. K. Yamaguchi)

may be associated with serious side effects. A short course of topical steroids is useful in breaking the inflammatory cycle. Their use should be supplemented with vasoconstrictors, cold compresses, ice packs, and climatotherapy. Having the patient move to a cool, moist climate or sleep in a cool or air-conditioned room has been associated with marked relief of symptoms in many cases. Hyposensitization therapy with grass pollens and other antigens may be helpful in some instances but in general has not been rewarding.

Recently, cromolyn eye drops have been

used topically in a 1%–4% solution with good results (43, 143). This drug reduces itching, hyperemia, and mucous discharge. The giant papillae do not decrease in number with this therapy, but corneal complications seem to be lessened. This drug appears to hold great promise for the future treatment of vernal keratoconjunctivitis.

MOOREN'S ULCER

Mooren's ulcer is a chronic, progressive marginal corneal degeneration of unknown etiology. It is more common in older people and may be associated with marked pain and relentless melting of the peripheral cornea. Although some cases respond to surgical management, others are unresponsive to any form of therapy. Recently, autoimmune phenomena and collagenolytic enzymes have been implicated in the pathogenesis of Mooren's ulcer.

Immunopathology

Various etiologies have been proposed for Mooren's ulcer, including metabolic disorders (65), trophic disturbances secondary to local disease (57), neurotrophic disorders (144), he-

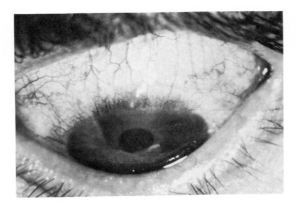

FIG. 7-6. Trantas' dots in vernal conjunctivitis. (Courtesy of Dr. H. B. Ostler).

reditary disease (110), and a variety of micro-organisms (40). Most recently, autoimmune phenomena have been proposed as contributing factors in the pathogenesis of Mooren's ulcer.

Circulating antibodies to human corneal epithelium have been demonstrated in patients with Mooren's ulcer (132), although antibodies could not be found deposited in the corneal epithelium. In a study of three patients with Mooren's ulcer (23), IgG, IgM, and the third component of complement (C3) were demonstrated by direct immunofluorescence in the intercellular spaces of the surface epithelium and within the epithelial cell cytoplasm in some portions of biopsy specimens. One of the patients had deposition of IgM along the conjunctival basement membrane and IgG and IgM within the conjunctival connective tissue. Another of the patients, with inactive disease, had IgG but no complement within epithelial cells. All three patients had circulating antibodies which bound to the epithelial cell cytoplasm of normal human corneas and conjunctivas. In two patients, the antibody titer was higher for conjunctival than for corneal antibody. Two patients also had a low titer of antibody to parietal cells. In all three patients the histocompatibility antigen HLA-A2 was present. Two patients had an elevated serum IgA (23).

In another patient with Mooren's ulcer, IgA and complement were deposited in the stroma and high concentrations of IgG, IgA, IgM, and C3 were found in the epithelium (108). This patient also had circulating antibodies to normal conjunctival and corneal epithelium, and the level of circulating antibodies correlated with the activity of the clinical disease. This patient also demonstrated antinuclear antibodies and antibodies to gastric parietal cells and to adrenal gland. An impaired response to phytohemagglutinin was present although the percentage of T cells was normal.

The authors (23, 108) concluded that Mooren's ulcer was unlikely to be a primary immunologic disturbance with production of autoantibodies against normal tissue antigens. Rather, they believe that antibodies develop secondary to persistent inflammation with re-

current epithelial defects in individuals already prone to develop autoimmune disease. Possibly the antigenic determinants of the conjunctiva and cornea become altered by tissue injury or by an infectious agent so that they are not recognized as "self."

Proteolytic enzymes have been demonstrated in the conjunctiva of patients with Mooren's ulcer (21). These enzymes may contribute to the corneal thinning which occurs in this disease. The conjunctiva also contains large numbers of plasma cells. Excision of the limbal conjunctiva adjacent to the ulcer is thought to remove the antibody-producing plasma cells and the cornea-destroying enzymes so that healing of the ulcer may take place (22).

Clinical Features

Mooren's ulcer is bilateral in at least 25% of cases and is more common in older people. It is usually painful and may be relentlessly progressive. The lesion may begin with one or two patches of gray infiltrate at the margin of the cornea which eventually coalesce. A shallow furrow forms and slowly spreads circumferentially and centrally. Scarring and vascularization follow and there may be central undermining of the ulcer with an overhanging superficial edge (Fig. 7-7).

Two types of Mooren's ulcer have been described (161). One responds to relatively conservative surgery and does not progress after one or two operative procedures. A second type, which is more common in young patients, is relentlessly progressive and involves the sclera as well as the peripheral cornea. Young Nigerians have a high incidence of this disease, with marked necrosis of the limbal sclera and episclera and a high percentage of perforations (81).

It should be noted that a furrowlike degeneration similar to Mooren's ulcer may develop in the paralimbal region as a complication of periarteritis nodosa, Wegener's granulomatosis, and Vogt–Koyanagi–Harada syndrome. The association of these diseases with autoimmune phenomena further suggests the im-

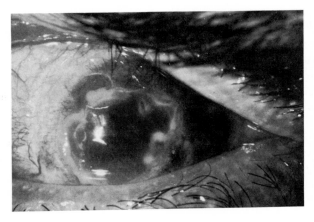

FIG. 7-7. Mooren's ulcer with marginal thinning and vascularization.

portance of immunologic factors in the pathogenesis of Mooren's ulcer.

Treatment

Medical treatment is frequently of no benefit in Mooren's ulcer (161). Peritomy and repeated freezing of the cornea have been advocated, and good results have also been obtained with excision of the limbal conjunctiva alone (22, 152). Lamellar keratoplasty and placement of a conjunctival flap have also been employed successfully. Hydrophilic contact lenses may give relief of severe ocular pain, but they do not appear to alter the progression of the corneal ulcers (79).

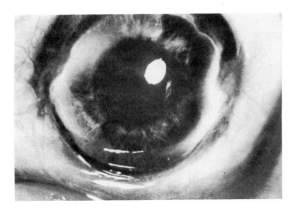

FIG. 7-8. Terrien's marginal degeneration with arcus-senilis–like deposits in the peripheral cornea.

TERRIEN'S MARGINAL DEGENERATION

This is another type of marginal corneal degeneration of unknown etiology. About 75% of cases occur in males and although any age group may be involved, it is most common below the age of 40. It is often bilateral and may progress to extreme thinning of the peripheral cornea. It usually begins in the superior cornea with a peripheral opacity closely resembling an arcus senilis (Fig. 7-8). A gutterlike furrow usually appears in the clear zone between the arcus and the limbus, but it may be more central. The gutter deepens and its floor may become vascularized. Eventually it may give way to the normal intraocular pressure and bulge forward, producing an ectasia. Rupture may occur with relatively mild trauma. The furrow spreads circumferentially, although the progression of the condition may be extremely slow. The disease may run a course lasting 10 to 20 years, with vision deteriorating gradually from an increasing amount of corneal astigmatism.

Two clinical types of the disease can often be distinguished (75). An inflammatory type is associated with marked corneal vascularization and congestion of the corneal and conjunctival vessels. A quiescent type is characterized by less vascular injection and vessel ingrowth. It has been suggested that the inflammatory type may be due to a hypersensitivity mechanism (75). Other proposed etiologies have included a lipid degeneration, an endocrine disturbance, or some type of infection. The relationship of marginal thinning to various connective tissue disorders, however, strongly suggests the interplay of immunologic mechanisms.

Treatment is disappointing in Terrien's marginal degeneration. A conjunctival or lamellar scleral flap may be used to reinforce the thin area (4). Application of trichloroacetic acid, cautery, and keratoplasty have also been advocated.

CHRONIC CYCLITIS

Chronic cyclitis, also known as **pars planitis** or **peripheral uveitis,** is a fairly common cause of bilateral uveitis in younger individuals. The etiology is unknown; however, immunologic mechanisms are thought to play a role.

Immunopathology

A hypersensitivity mechanism has been proposed as the basis for chronic cyclitis (83), but definitive immunologic studies have not been done in a large population of patients with this disorder. Clinical features such as "snowball"-type vitreous opacities can be produced in rabbits by injecting egg albumin into the vitreous (165). Some patients with chronic cyclitis are markedly sensitive to streptococcal antigens; however, they are not helped by desensitization therapy (151). Microscopic examination of the occasional eye with chronic cyclitis that is studied histologically demonstrates a low-grade inflammation of the uvea with infiltration of plasma cells and lymphocytes (83). In addition, fibroglial proliferation at the vitreous base and retinal phlebitis and periphlebitis can also be demonstrated (82). The ciliary body, which may in some ways be analogous to the kidney glomerulus in its filtration ability, could be a site of immune complex deposition which in turn might lead to inflammation in this region of the eye. Recently, elevated levels of circulating immune complexes have been detected in over 60% of a group of patients with chronic cyclitis and these levels could be correlated with increased disease activity (29a). An association has also been noted between peripheral uveitis and multiple sclerosis (58). Multiple sclerosis has many immunologic features. For example, elevated IgG is found in the cerebrospinal fluid, and a history of allergies or eczema can frequently be elicited in the patient or in his family. The inflammation of chronic cyclitis usually responds well to injections of steroids under Tenon's capsule or to other immunosuppressive agents (30, 59).

Clinical Features

Chronic cyclitis is most common in children and young adults and has an equal sex distribution. The disease has an insidious onset. Patients may be asymptomatic or they may complain of floaters and hazy vision. The external eye appears uninflamed but the anterior chamber usually reveals a mild reaction. Cells are usually present in the anterior vitreous and exudates may be found on the inferior pars plana, sometimes forming large "snowbanks." "Snowball" opacities are frequently present in the anterior vitreous. There may be sheathing of the retinal vessel both in the periphery and in the posterior pole. Diffuse edema of the posterior pole, including the disc and macula, may also occur.

Chronic cyclitis may run a benign course; however, complications occur in some patients which lead to visual loss. Many patients will develop cystoid macular edema, and this is the most frequent cause of visual loss in chronic cyclitis. If inflammation persists, the lens eventually becomes cataractous. Initially a posterior subcapsular cataract develops but subsequently the rest of the lens may become opaque. Permanent cystoid macular changes may develop if macular edema persists. Vitreous strands and inflammatory membranes may form along the vitreoretinal junction and lead to folding and shrinkage of the retina and sometimes to retinal detachment.

Treatment

Chronic cyclitis often runs a benign course and frequently does not require treatment. Usually synechiae do not form, and so the patient may not require dilation. Macular edema responds well to injections of steroids under Tenon's capsule. These can be given every 4 to 6 weeks with minimal side effects (59). Alternatively, 15–20 mg of prednisone can be given each day if subcapsular injections are not feasible. Treatment is continued until clinical or angiographic findings indicate that the macula is dry. In cases which are refractory to steroids, a course of cyproheptadine (Periactin) 4 mg orally three times a day may be tried. Cataracts can be removed when they are significantly impairing vision, and patients generally tolerate such procedures well.

FUCH'S HETEROCHROMIC IRIDOCYCLITIS

Fuchs' heterochromic iridocyclitis is an anterior uveitis characterized by a loss of iris pigment and heterochromia. The etiology is unknown, but most investigators feel that the disease is either an inflammatory or a degenerative process. Recently, immunologic and histologic studies have uncovered evidence that is consistent with an inflammatory etiology, possibly involving the deposition of immune complexes.

Immunopathology

Immune complexes have been detected in the aqueous humor, serum, or both in 9 of 11 patients with Fuchs' syndrome (37). These complexes were detected by their ability to inhibit exogenous rheumatoid factor or by inhibition of complement component C1q. These studies suggest a pathogenic role for immune complexes in Fuchs' syndrome, possibly the same mechanism as is responsible for endogenous uveitis produced experimentally in rabbits (70).

Cellular immune mechanisms may also play a role in Fuchs' syndrome (63). Hypersensitivity to the alpha crystallin component of lens protein has been demonstrated using both the lymphocyte transformation and leukocyte migration inhibition tests. No hypersensitivity to uveal pigment could be demonstrated using the same methods (63).

Other immunologic studies suggesting a hypersensitivity mechanism in this disorder have demonstrated positive skin tests to tuberculin, *Streptococcus,* or *Toxoplasma* antigens in 30% of patients studied (139). Hyposensitization therapy using these allergens has been advocated but not widely accepted.

Histopathologic studies (60) have demonstrated a mononuclear inflammatory infiltrate involving the anterior surface and the superficial stroma of the iris. This infiltrate consists chiefly of plasma cells, lymphocytes, and histiocytes. The prominence of plasma cells in this disease further suggests a possible immunologic component involving antibody.

Clinical Features

Fuchs' syndrome accounts for at least 2%–3% of uveitis cases in various clinics. The time of onset ranges from puberty to age 35 and both sexes are affected equally. Patients complain of blurred vision, which is usually associated with cataract formation or vitreous veils. Usually the disease is unilateral, although a few bilateral cases have been reported. The onset is insidious since the eye usually appears to be uninflamed. Often the first sign is a discoloration of the iris. Usually, the involved iris is lighter in color (Fig. 7-9) and transilluminates in a patchy distribution. If the anterior stroma of the iris atrophies before the pigment epithelium does, the affected eye may be darker.

A mild to moderate anterior chamber reaction is usually observed, but synechia formation is rare. Widespread keratic precipitates are typically small and white. Koeppe nodules are occasionally present. Fine, rubeotic vessels can be seen in the filtration angle and may be related to the increased intraocular pressure which frequently accompanies this syndrome. These vessels tend to bleed and produce a filiform hemorrhage upon paracentesis (**Amsler's sign**). A few inflammatory cells may be found in the anterior vitreous, and occasionally a moderate reaction is observed. The remainder of the fundus examination, however, is usually normal. Glaucoma is a major complication which is seen in about 20% of cases and may occur at any time during the course of the dis-

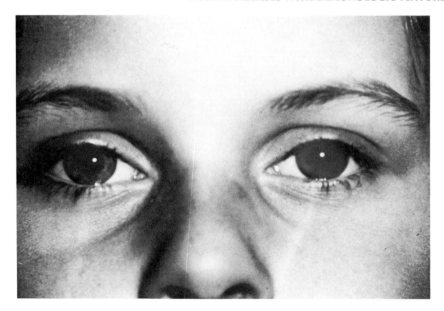

FIG. 7-9. Depigmentation of the right iris in Fuchs' heterochromic iridocyclitis. (Courtesy of Dr. G. Mintsioulis)

ease (64). Cataracts develop in up to 70% of patients, and may be due to inflammation or to steroid therapy.

Treatment

Corticosteroids do not seem to alter the course of the disease. They may, however, decrease the amount of anterior chamber inflammation as well as the number of keratic precipitates. The major disadvantages of steroids are that they may enhance the progression of cataract formation and may induce glaucoma or worsen this problem. A brief course of topical steroids can be tried, but if patients fail to respond dramatically the drops should be discontinued.

Management of these patients includes a lifetime of follow-up examinations for glaucoma and cataract formation. Glaucoma can be treated medically in the same way as other types of open-angle glaucoma. Some cases prove intractable and may require filtering surgery. Cataract extraction may be undertaken when necessary, since cataract surgery in Fuchs' syndrome appears to be only slightly more complicated then routine cataract surgery (141).

LENS-INDUCED UVEITIS

Lens-induced uveitis is a general term for inflammatory reactions in the eye related to sensitization or toxicity to lens material. The toxic properties of lens material were first pointed out in 1899 by Schirmer (129), who stressed the delayed and severe irritant properties of lens protein following extracapsular cataract extraction. Others confirmed his findings and expanded the concept of lens-induced uveitis to include inflammation occurring after dislocation and breakdown of the lens.

Immunopathology

The possibility that immune factors may play a role in lens-induced uveitis was first suggested by Verhoeff and Lemoine (148) in 1922. They applied the term **endophthalmitis phacoanaphylactica** to this type of lens-induced uveitis. They found that each of their 12 patients gave a positive skin reaction to lens protein, unlike 28 patients with rupture of the lens capsule without uveitis, who had negative skin tests.

A second type of lens-induced uveitis, known as **phacotoxic** or **phacogenic uveitis,**

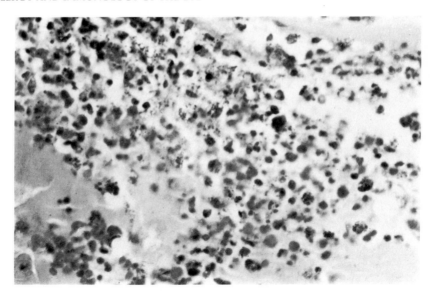

FIG. 7-10. Neutrophils invading and phagocytosing lens material in lens-induced uveitis.

should be distinguished from endophthalmitis phacoanaphylactica. This entity may be due to simple toxicity of lens protein or it may involve some degree of hypersensitivity. It is a somewhat poorly defined condition; however, it does have certain characteristic histologic features (90). Another related entity, is **phacolytic glaucoma.** This is not a true uveitis, but involves the phagocytosis of hypermature lens material by macrophages, and leads to glaucoma from mechanical obstruction of the filtration angle.

The Irvines have distinguished three types of lens-induced uveitis reactions (74). 1) In endophthalmitis phacoanaphylactica, the pathologic changes involve the anterior segment and neutrophils invade the lens (Fig. 7-10), while giant cells are seen in the iris and surrounding lens fragments. 2) The phacotoxic type of reaction occurs in the presence of a mature or hypermature lens. Protein content in the aqueous is high and keratic precipitates are frequently present. The iris is infiltrated by plasma cells, and lens material in the aqueous and vitreous is phagocytosed by large eosinophilic macrophages. 3) In phacolytic glaucoma, elevated intraocular pressure occurs in the presence of a hypermature cataract. The filtration angle is

blocked by macrophages engorged with lens material. There is considerable overlap between the first two entities and the relative importance of hypersensitivity and toxic factors is not entirely known.

In 1903, Uhlenhuth (145) demonstrated that lens protein has organ specificity. He immunized rabbits intravenously with saline homogenates of bovine lens. Antiserum produced in this way precipitated homogenates of bovine lens but not other antigenic preparations of bovine origin. Surprisingly, the lens antiserum also reacted with lens protein from other vertebrate species such as man, horse, pig, deer, guinea pig, mouse, and rat. Even more surprising was that the lens antiserum also precipitated lens preparations originating from the rabbit, the species which had produced the antiserum. Thus, antibodies produced by the rabbit acted as autoantibodies. Uhlenhuth found this result to be somewhat annoying at first. Three years previously, Ehrlich and Morganroth (44) had proposed their theory of *horror autotoxicus*, or fear of self-poisoning. This concept has been updated by Burnet and Fenner (27), who postulated that immunologic mechanisms are capable of distinguishing between "self" and "nonself." It was expected that an organism would not make antibodies against its own tissues and the idea than an animal had produced antibodies against its own lens tissue seemed quite strange. Uhlenhuth's studies, however, were soon confirmed by other investigators and the concept of organ-specific antigens became incontestable.

We now know that very strong organ-specific antigens and hardly any species-specific antigens are found in the lens. We now know also that organ-specific antigens are not confined to the lens. They have also been demonstrated in the brain, thyroid, adrenal, pituitary, submaxillary gland, kidney, liver, and testes. Organ-specific antigens frequently stimulate the formation of autoantibodies. Most organ-specific antigens are localized within the protoplasm of cells (53). Presumably these antigens are "sequestered" and under normal circumstances do not evoke an antibody response. Organ-specific antigens may act as haptens in their own species. They are capable of combining with antibodies that were previously formed but they do not ordinarily stimulate antibody formation in their host. The organ-specific antibodies may, however, elicit an immune response if their structure is altered in a particular way or if they are administered with adjuvants. Apparently, antigenic sites which were previously masked can become uncovered by this method.

Organ-specific antigens do not usually produce any pathologic changes in their host. Three experimental diseases, however, may be related to autoimmune responses to organ-specific antigens. Allergic encephalomyelitis can be produced by immunization with brain or spinal cord (109), thyroiditis (155) by immunization with thyroid tissue, and aspermatogenesis by immunization with testicular tissue or seminal fluid (53). Similarly, experimental lens-induced uveitis appears to be an autoimmune response induced by an organ-specific antigen.

Early attempts to produce lens autoantibodies in the rabbit, using whole lens extracts, were unsuccessful (96). Autoantibodies could, however, be produced with relative ease using heterologous lens tissue. In 1924, Hektoen (66) was able to induce autoantibody formation by immunization with crudely fractionated alpha and beta lens crystallin. He concluded that fractionation had denatured the alpha crystallin, exposing new antigenic sites. Halbert et al (61) demonstrated that rabbit lens could be made antigenic by combining it with Freund's adjuvant. It is not entirely clear why immunization without adjuvant fails to stimulate an autoantibody response, but it has been suggested that the adjuvant or fractionation alters the normal protein of lens tissue which the host recognizes as self (96).

Recently, it has been shown that homologous lens protein can induce a detectable immune response in rabbits without the addition of adjuvant (106). The intensity of the response is low and specific antibodies can be detected only by sensitive techniques such as the hemagglutination test. In contrast, heterologous lens protein will induce an antibody response which is detectable by less sensitive methods. Homologous lens antibodies are of the IgG class and cross react with extraocular tissues, in which the antigens are related to cell mitochondria, microsomes, and proteins associated with contractile elements. Autologous lens protein injected in complete Freund's adjuvant may also be antigenic when sensitive antibody detection methods are employed (123). Intravitreal injection of autologous lens protein in preimmunized animals leads to an Arthus type of acute endophthalmitis. The response to lens antigens varies in both magnitude and duration in different rabbits, which suggests a central control mechanism involving immune-response genes or possibly an antigenic competition between various antigens.

The major lens antigen is alpha crystallin. This substance has a molecular weight of $7.5 \cdot 10^5$, and in young, normal lenses it consists of three polypeptide chains: two A chains and one B chain. In cataractous lenses and in the periphery of old, normal lenses, eleven polypeptide chains have been identified (126).

An artifactual protein complex known as albuminoid is composed of all lens protein antigens. This macrocomplex can be dissociated by acidification or isoelectric precipitation. Albuminoid may act as an adjuvant for autologous lens protein. However, it is alpha crystallin which is felt to be the important antigen in the immunopathology of lens-induced uveitis.

The evidence that lens-induced uveitis is an immunologic disease is derived mainly from animal studies. Most have involved sensitization of various laboratory animals with homologous lens protein either with or without adjuvants. Following sensitization, the lens is frequently traumatized (96). This leads to a severe inflammation of both the lens and the uveal tract. Antilens antibodies, especially to alpha crystallin, are produced by these procedures. It has been suggested that inflammation produced by crystallins involves a humoral immune mechanism while that produced by other albuminoid components is mediated by cellular components (96).

The histopathologic findings in experimental models of lens-induced uveitis are often at variance with the findings in human disease. Recently, Marak (98) has created an experimental lens-induced granulomatous endophthalmitis (ELGE) in the rat which is virtually identical histologically to endophthalmitis phacoanaphylactica in man. Rats are immunized with six subcutaneous injections of whole lens protein in incomplete Freund's adjuvant at 2-week intervals. Lens capsules are ruptured 1 week after the last injection and the eyes are removed and examined 1 week later. A granulomatous inflammation with a typical zonal pattern is produced. Neutrophils infiltrate the lens fibers, histiocytes phagocytose lens material, and eosinophils and plasma cells are prominent features. Moreover, ELGE can be passively transferred with serum to virgin animals whose lenses are injured 24 h after injection of antilens serum. Fluorescent antibody studies in ELGE demonstrate IgG and the third component of complement (C3) in the injured lenses. In addition, cobra venom factor, which depletes C3, prevents the development of ELGE in most animals. These findings suggest that an immune-complex mechanism may be involved in the immunopathogenesis of ELGE and possibly even in endophthalmitis phacoanaphylactica.

The immune etiology of the human disease has in the past been difficult to establish. Verhoeff and Lemoine (148) originally suggested an immune etiology and demonstrated de-layed skin reactions to bovine or swine lens protein. Skin test responses have not been consistently positive in lens-induced uveitis, and positive tests may in fact be demonstrated in patients with other types of lens pathology as well as in normal subjects. Circulating antilens antibodies have been demonstrated by Luntz and Wright (94) and by Kinces and Szabo (84). However, these antibodies are not specific for lens-induced uveitis and may be found after lens injury, in patients with uveitis, or in normal subjects with cataracts. Witmer has found high aqueous titers of antilens antibodies using a hemagglutination technique (156) and has demonstrated local antibody formation in the iris by a fluorescent antibody technique (157). Still, the significance of antilens antibody in human disease remains unclear.

The role of cellular immunity in the development of lens-induced uveitis has also been investigated. Luntz and Wright (94) were able to produce passively transferred hypersensitivity to lens protein in guinea pigs, using a patient's leukocytes. Other investigators have reported a cellular immune response, using the leukocyte migration inhibition test following lens trauma, in addition to antibody formation (84, 91).

It is clear from experimental studies that lens protein has potent immunogenic properties and can produce an autoimmune disease. The observations of human lens-induced disease are not as clear-cut; however, circumstantial evidence suggests that endophthalmitis phacoanaphylactica may represent an autoimmune response to lens protein.

Clinical Features

Endophthalmitis phacoanaphylactica (Fig. 7-11) presents as a severe, generalized uveitis which may be chronic or relapsing. It can follow extracapsular cataract extraction, discission, trauma, or, rarely, spontaneous capsular rupture. The severity of the reaction varies with the amount of lens material remaining in the eye. The Irvines (74) reported that in 50% of cases in which lens material was left in the eye a uveitis did not develop. In 25%, it was uncertain whether inflammation was caused by lens material or by some other underlying disease. In 25%, lens material appeared to be responsible for the inflammation. It was in these patients that either allergic or toxic factors appeared to be responsible for lens-induced uveitis. Usually a latent period of 24 h to 14 days preceded the onset of inflammation. This variable time period may have been related to the presence or absence of previous sensitization to lens protein. "Mutton-fat" keratic precipitates and extensive posterior synechiae may be present. Secondary glaucoma may develop as a consequence of severe anterior segment inflammation or iris bombé. Lid edema, chemosis, and corneal clouding may also be present. Late in the disease, an affected eye may become phthisical.

It has been reported that endophthalmitis phacoanaphylactica may occur more commonly than expected in association with sympathetic ophthalmia (16). Of 170 eyes excised for sympathetic ophthalmia, 23% had histologic evidence of endophthalmitis phacoanaphylactica. Easom and Zimmerman (42) studied eleven sympathizing eyes enucleated for sympathetic ophthalmia. Six showed histologic evidence of both sympathetic ophthalmia and endophthalmitis phacoanaphylactica, while another four had findings compatible with the latter entity only. The two diseases can be differentiated clinically even when they are both bilateral. In endophthalmitis phacoanaphylactica, the first eye involved is usually inactive when the inflammation begins in the second. In addition, the lens of the first eye is opaque at the onset of the disease but may be clear in sympathetic ophthalmia.

Phacogenic or **phacotoxic uveitis** represents a far more heterogeneous group. It may follow an injury or extracapsular cataract extraction and develops after a latent period of 24 h to 2 weeks. Presumably, the toxicity of lens protein is responsible for the inflammatory process. A phacotoxic response may be produced by a dislocated lens or a degenerating cataractous lens. Whether normal lens protein is toxic or whether an aging change confers toxic properties upon it is unclear. Conceivably, phacotoxic reactions are mediated by an immune response to various degrees of sensitization.

Phacotoxic uveitis may present as a mild iri-

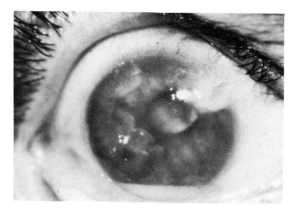

FIG. 7-11. Lens-induced uveitis with hypopyon and degenerative lens changes.

docyclitis or a violent endophthalmitis. The histologic picture is not granulomatous; however, mutton-fat keratic precipitates may be observed. Intraocular pressure may be elevated as well.

Phacolytic glaucoma is not a true uveitis. However, it is generally discussed in connection with other types of lens-induced reactions. It occurs in association with hypermature cataracts. The lens capsule may be thin, ruptured, or intact. Presumably, the lens substance in a morgagnian cataract becomes completely liquefied and can escape even through an unbroken lens capsule. The patient does not become sensitized, either because the lens protein has lost its antigenicity or because of the patient's inability to mount an immune response. The inflammatory response primarily involves macrophages, which engulf the lens material and accumulate in the filtration angle. This leads to a mechanical obstruction of the trabecular meshwork and an elevated intraocular pressure. Typically, keratic precipitates and fibrin deposition are absent.

Diagnosis and Treatment

The diagnosis of lens-induced uveitis can frequently be made from the history and physical examination. A history of ocular inflammation following an extracapsular cataract extraction or lens injury should lead one to consider the diagnosis. An anterior chamber paracentesis may be helpful in situations where the diagnosis is being considered. In endophthalmitis phacoanaphylactica, eosinophils may be numerous, sometimes accounting for more than 30% of total inflammatory cells. Macrophages containing lens material are characteristically found in phacolytic glaucoma and can be found by passing aspirated fluid through a millipore filter, staining the filter, and viewing it under the light microscope.

Definitive treatment for lens-induced uveitis involves surgical removal of the lens or its remnants as early as possible after the diagnosis has been made (124). Irrigation of the anterior chamber may temporarily relieve the mechanical obstruction of the filtration angle and lower intraocular pressure. Topical steroids may have some effect on reducing inflammation of the anterior segment, but they are not curative and do not substitute for surgical treatment.

SYMPATHETIC OPHTHALMIA

The immunologic aspects of sympathetic ophthalmia have been more widely studied than those of almost any other ocular disease. The concept that an injury to uveal tissue could lead to immunization and an attack on the uninjured eye makes this disease an attractive model for investigation of autoimmune phenomena. It has not in fact been easy to establish the immunopathogenesis of sympathetic ophthalmia and it remains unclear which antigen and which effector mechanisms are important in this disease.

Immunopathology

Infectious Theory. Various infectious agents have been implicated in sympathetic ophthalmia. The association with trauma and the exposure of uveal tissue, as well as the characteristic granulomatous appearance of the inflammation, is suggestive of an infection. The tubercle bacillus, *Bacillus subtilis,* and later rickettsias (131) and viruses (72, 73, 140) were at one time thought to play a role. Although sporadic reports of infectious agents in sympa-

thetic ophthalmia still appear, no studies thus far have fulfilled Koch's postulates, and therefore the possibility of an infectious etiology must remain in doubt.

Immunologic Theory. The first suggestion that sympathetic ophthalmia might be a hypersensitivity disease was made in 1903 by Pusey (119). Elschnig (46) proposed that uveal pigment was the offending antigen. Evidence in favor of a hypersensitivity mechanism was obtained by injecting an emulsion of eye tissue from a patient with sympathetic ophthalmia into guinea pigs passively sensitized with the patient's serum, and thereby producing anaphylaxis.

The presence of circulating antibody in patients with sympathetic ophthalmia has been considered by some to be a nonspecific finding which results from tissue injury (99). Indeed, the histopathology of the ocular reaction in animals sensitized to uveal antigen is a nongranulomatous inflammation of the iris and ciliary body that does not resemble the human disease (142). Although uveal tissue is a weak antigen, its antigenicity can be increased by using adjuvants such as staphylococcal toxin (26, 92) or complete Freund's adjuvant (34, 35). While this type of immunization produces a severe uveitis in guinea pigs and monkeys, it is also nongranulomatous and does not resemble the classic description of sympathetic ophthalmia. Implanting whole rabbit eyes in rabbits is said to cause a reaction that more closely simulates the histologic changes of sympathetic ophthalmia (147). However, some authors have found no abnormal clinical or morphologic findings using this procedure (71).

Woods was unable to demonstrate complement-fixing antibodies against bovine uveal pigment antigen in the serum of six patients with sympathetic ophthalmia (162). Antiuveal antibodies may, however, develop during the normal healing process of a penetrating uveal injury. Woods hypothesized that these antibodies exert a protective influence after uveal injury and prevent the development of sympathetic ophthalmia. Mills and Shedden were also unable to demonstrate circulating antibodies to uveal tissue in the serum of five patients with sympathetic ophthalmia, using several methods of antibody detection (105). Marak *et al* were unable to demonstrate agglutinating or precipitating antibodies against uveal tissue in one patient with sympathetic ophthalmia (101). Luntz (93) was unable to demonstrate either antiuveal or antilens antibodies in three patients with sympathetic ophthalmia, although a high incidence of these antibodies was found in patients with other types of nontraumatic uveitis.

Uveal autoantibodies have been found in a high percentage of sympathetic ophthalmia patients by Aronson (5). However, antibody determinations were performed on serum which had been concentrated threefold and a pathologic diagnosis of sympathetic ophthalmia was only made in a small number of cases.

Recent studies have concentrated on the possible role of cellular immunity in the pathogenesis of sympathetic ophthalmia. Marak *et al* demonstrated blastogenic activity when lymphocytes from two patients with sympathetic ophthalmia were cultured in the presence of retinal pigment epithelium antigens, retinal antigens, and lens antigens (99).

Wong *et al* also demonstrated enhanced lymphocyte transformation in eight histologically proven cases of sympathetic ophthalmia when peripheral leukocytes were exposed to homologous uveal–retinal antigen (160). Patients with the highest degree of transformation often had the least clinical evidence of active disease. Hammer (62) demonstrated increased blast transformation in three patients with sympathetic ophthalmia and in two patients with Vogt–Koyanagi–Harada syndrome (see in Ch. 9) using bovine uveal pigment as an antigen. Increased lymphocyte transformation with homologous retina but not with choroid was also reported in two cases from Germany (87). It would appear from several of these studies that the retina is far more immunogenic than the choroid and that melanin is an unlikely antigen to elicit a hypersensitivity response (97).

A recent study has analyzed the subpopulations of lymphocytes in the blood of nine patients with sympathetic ophthalmia (17). While a normal distribution was present in most patients, one had low numbers of T cells and two had increased numbers of "null" cells. The function of this latter population of lymphocytes is presently unclear.

An intradermal skin test was used at one time to aid in the diagnosis of sympathetic ophthalmia (103). Although hypersensitivity to uveal pigment could be demonstrated in this fashion, the skin test was sometimes positive in other types of uveitis as well. Examination of skin test sites 2 weeks after intradermal challenge revealed a histologic picture similar to that found in the uveal tract in sympathetic ophthalmia (54). The uveal skin test antigen is no longer used because of the difficulty in obtaining a stable preparation and because of the possible danger of stimulating a uveal hypersensitivity response.

Histopathology

Similar histopathologic changes are found in both the exciting and the sympathizing eye. A diffuse, granulomatous uveitis occurs, with massive lymphocytic infiltration and nests of epithelioid cells (Fig. 7-12). The latter may be larger and more numerous in black patients. Epithelioid and giant cells (Fig. 7-13) contain pigment granules, and this is a key feature in making a diagnosis. Dalen–Fuchs nodules (Fig. 7-14) are present but are not considered pathognomomic of sympathetic ophthalmia. Eosinophils may be found in substantial numbers in many cases of sympathetic ophthalmia (100). The choriocapillaris and retina are relatively spared from the inflammatory process. The posterior layers of the iris are generally more involved than the anterior layers. Focal infiltration by lymphocytes occurs in and around the large veins of the choroid. A perivasculitis may involve the vessels of the retina and optic nerve (104). Posterior synechiae, cataracts, and necrosis of the iris and ciliary body may also be seen. Evidence of a preceding injury or surgical procedure can often be demonstrated on pathologic examination of the exciting eye.

Sympathetic ophthalmia is associated with phacoanaphylactic uveitis in 23% of cases (16). This association is much greater than could occur by chance alone and adds strength to the evidence that these two diseases are immunologic in nature.

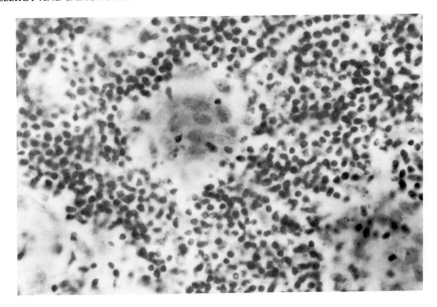

FIG. 7-12. Granuloma of uveal tract in sympathetic ophthalmia. Epithelioid cells are seen centrally.

Numerous authors have attempted to produce the histologic picture of sympathetic ophthalmia in laboratory animals (34, 35, 147). None of these models has yet demonstrated the typical histopathologic features of sympathetic ophthalmia.

Clinical Features

Sympathetic ophthalmia is a bilateral granulomatous uveitis which occurs as a rare event after unilateral ocular trauma or surgery. The incidence has declined dramatically in the last

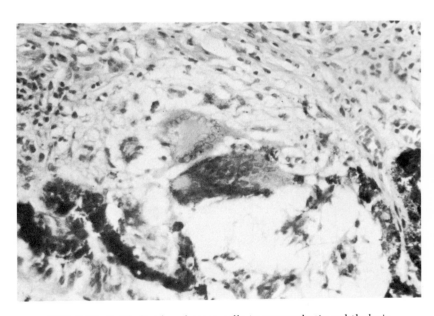

FIG. 7-13. Epithelioid and giant cells in sympathetic ophthalmia.

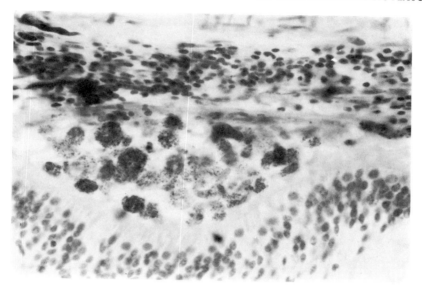

FIG. 7-14. Dalen–Fuchs nodule in sympathetic ophthalmia.

few decades and the condition is presently seen in about 0.1% of eye injuries (6). Most cases follow perforating injuries of the globe in which uveal tissue, especially the ciliary body, is traumatized. Accidental wounds account for about 65% of cases in the literature while surgical wounds account for another 25%. Surgical procedures in which the iris or lens capsule is incarcerated in the wound are particularly prone to produce sympathetic ophthalmia. It has been stated that the condition of an eye undergoing a glaucoma procedure is a more important factor than the actual type of operation (133). Glaucoma surgery is felt to be particularly hazardous in this respect for blind eyes with absolute glaucoma (133).

Occasionally, sympathetic ophthalmia has been reported after perforation of corneal ulcers, subconjunctival rupture of the sclera (80, 163), or contusions without rupture of the globe (125), and with intraocular malignant melanomas (125). However, some doubt has been cast on the association of melanomas with sympathetic ophthalmia (41), since most of the reported cases have had associated penetrating wounds. Sympathetic ophthalmia rarely occurs with endophthalmitis; however, about 22 such cases have been reported in the literature (120). I have seen one case of sympa-

thetic ophthalmia that developed in a man who had a nonperforating injury in which the exciting eye was severely burned with molten lead (Figs. 7-15 and 7-16).

Inflammation of the second, or sympathizing, eye usually occurs 1 to 3 months after injury to the exciting eye. The disease has been reported as early as 9 days after injury (80) and as late as 50 years (130). Sympathetic ophthalmia usually begins as a low-grade, persistent uveitis. It may be associated with mutton-fat or small white keratic precipitates, and nodules may be present on the surface of the iris or at the pupillary margin. A similar clinical picture may be seen in the sympathizing eye with early involvement of the anterior segment.

The choroid may contain multiple yellowish white spots resembling drusen in the peripheral fundus. These are thought to correspond histologically to Dalen–Fuchs nodules. Other findings include vitreous clouding, subretinal edema, and an optic papillitis. Lens opacities, posterior synechiae, and secondary glaucoma are common complications of anterior segment involvement. Sympathetic ophthalmia runs a chronic course and has a marked tendency to relapse. The disease may end in phthisis bulbi and eventual blindness.

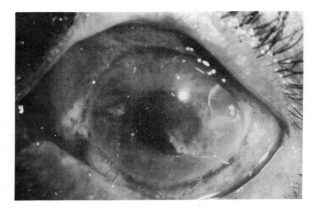

FIG. 7-15. Exciting eye in sympathetic ophthalmia secondary to molten lead injury.

Occasionally, vitiligo and poliosis of the eyelashes and brows may develop (18, 24). Meningeal involvement and auditory defects have also been reported (153). These striking similarities to the findings in the Vogt–Koyanagi–Harada syndrome (see in Ch. 9) suggest a possible relationship between these two diseases.

Treatment

It is generally agreed that if the injured eye is enucleated within the first 10 days to 2 weeks after injury, the possibility of developing sympathetic ophthalmia is minute. If an eye is hopelessly injured, enucleation should be car-

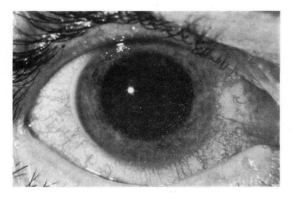

FIG. 7-16. Sympathizing eye in sympathetic ophthalmia.

ried out promptly (95). If the injured eye has a possibility of recovering significant vision, every effort should be made to save it. It is widely held that a 2-week safe period exists during which a decision can be made about enucleation. After this period, enucleation of the injured eye is less likely to prevent the development of sympathetic ophthalmia (95). Many authors feel that the injured eye should not be removed once the disease becomes established in the sympathizing eye since the exciting eye may eventually be the better of the two.

Clinical management of sympathetic ophthalmia is directed toward reduction of the inflammatory response and prompt dilation of the pupil to prevent synechia formation. Corticosteroids are the mainstay of treatment in the disease, and these may be given topically, subconjunctivally, or, in very severe inflammation, systemically. High doses of prednisone may be given initially (68). The dosage should be reduced to the lowest level which controls inflammation, and this should be continued for as long as the inflammation persists. As in other chronic disorders, complications of corticosteroid therapy should be kept in mind. Prophylactic steroid therapy has been recommended for potential cases of sympathetic ophthalmia (164). However, there is presently no evidence to support the efficacy of this type of therapy following perforating injuries, and some authorities believe that steroids should definitely not be used in these circumstances (32, 102). Besides measures to control inflammation and prevent synechiae, antibiotics and glaucoma therapy should be employed as needed.

Antimetabolite drugs have been used recently in the treatment of sympathetic ophthalmia. They are especially useful when corticosteroids have been ineffective in suppressing inflammation. Agents used in the past have included chlorambucil (68), methotrexate (89, 158), cyclophosphamide (158, 159), azathioprine (107, 112), and mercaptopurine (113, 118). A trial of immunosuppressive treatment should last several weeks, and one should not consider these agents ineffective until they have been given for some time (6). These drugs must be used with great caution because of their life-threatening toxic side effects, which involve the bone marrow and various organ systems. Usually an internist should monitor a patient when these drugs are being administered. Antilymphocyte serum has also been used to treat sympathetic ophthalmia (45, 118); however, the side effects of this agent are so numerous that its use should probably be considered only under the most extreme circumstances.

OPEN-ANGLE GLAUCOMA

While there is no direct evidence that open-angle glaucoma is mediated by immunologic mechanisms, several studies of immune aspects have been carried out in patients with this disease.

Immunopathology

In 1962, Becker and his associates (9) performed immunofluorescent studies on the trabecular meshwork of eyes obtained at autopsy from patients with glaucoma. Almost two-thirds showed positive staining of the trabecular meshwork for γ-globulin, compared with only 15% of nonglaucomatous eyes. In a later study, 75% demonstrated fluorescent staining of the trabecular meshwork, as did 79% of surgically excised or autopsied eyes from patients with primary open-angle glaucoma (13).

Plasma cells could be demonstrated in 82% of autopsied glaucomatous eyes and in 61% of surgically-treated glaucomatous eyes. Only 20% of eyes obtained from routine autopsy procedures had plasma cells in the trabecular meshwork. These findings might suggest an antibody-mediated reaction in the trabecular meshwork of glaucoma patients. Over 10 years later, however, Shields and coworkers were unable to demonstrate specific immunoglobulins or complement components in the trabecular meshwork (134). The complement component C3 could occasionally be demonstrated in small amounts in both glaucomatous eyes and controls. Although most ocular structures contain immunoglobulins, the trabecular meshwork of normal eyes usually does not (3).

Serologic studies have been carried out to determine whether systemic evidence of sensitization exists in patients with glaucoma. Waltman and Yarian (150) demonstrated antinuclear antibodies (ANA) in the serum of 44% of patients with open-angle glaucoma. More recently, however, Felberg and his colleagues (48) found no significant increase in ANA among glaucoma patients. They theorized that positive ANA reactions may be found at low serum dilutions but are actually a nonspecific finding. No significant difference in antibodies to DNA could be demonstrated in glaucoma patients and control subjects (48). Abnormalities in humoral and cellular immunity have occasionally been shown in glaucoma patients (121). However, Henley and associates (67) did not find a consistent abnormality when measuring cellular immunity by the leukocyte migration inhibition test.

As in many other diseases, HLA antigens have been studied in patients with open-angle glaucoma. HLA-B7 and B12 were significantly increased in patients with primary open-angle glaucoma as compared to a nonglaucomatous population (137). B12 was found in 50% of the glaucoma population while B7 was present in 49%, and either one antigen or the other could be detected in 88% of glaucoma patients. Furthermore, HLA-B7 and B12 were of value for predicting the development of glaucomatous visual field loss in patients with ocular hypertension. The presence of these antigens, however, did not relate to the level of intraocular pressure (135).

Henley *et al* (66a) described an association between HLA-A9, B8, and Bw35 in patients with open-angle glaucoma. Black patients with primary open-angle glaucoma had an increased prevalence of HLA-B7 and B12 and a decreased prevalence of HLA-A1 and A11 (11). Although white patients demonstrated an increase of A3 and a decrease of Bw35, these associations were not found among blacks. A recent study (133a) found no statistically significant alteration in HLA antigen frequencies among black patients with open-angle glaucoma. Patients with HLA-B7 or B12 were thought to be at higher risk of developing glaucomatous visual field loss, while the presence of HLA-A11 and Bw35 was thought to be associated with protection from glaucomatous damage (136). The significance of the association between HLA antigens and glaucoma is at present unclear. A recent study (124a) showed no significant HLA differences between glaucoma patients and a normal population. Another report (80a) concluded that the association of HLA antigens with open-angle glaucoma was not impressive as previously reported.

Several studies recently have examined the sensitivity to corticosteroids of lymphocytes taken from glaucoma patients. The transformation of lymphocytes by phytohemagglutinin and their uptake of tritiated thymidine can be inhibited by corticosteroids (28, 47, 115). Phytohemagglutinin-induced transformation is inhibited by lower concentrations of steroid in glaucoma patients than in controls. Individuals who possess HLA-B12 also respond to significantly lower concentrations of steroid whether or not they have glaucoma (10, 12). This association does not hold true for those who possess HLA-B7. Increased cellular sensitivity to steroids was found both in patients with open-angle glaucoma and in individuals who respond to topical steroids with increased pressures of greater than 31 mm Hg (15). Lymphocytes from patients with primary open-angle glaucoma are also more responsive to epinephrine than are lymphocytes from a control population (117), possibly owing to an increase in intracellular cyclic AMP.

Foon and associates also found an increased cellular sensitivity to corticosteroids among glaucoma patients (51). In contrast, Benezra and associates (14) found no specific response pattern in patients with steroid-induced glaucoma or with increased intraocular pressures. No clear-cut difference could be found in the behavior of lymphocytes from glaucoma patients and in those from controls. The mechanism by which glucocorticoids inhibit lymphocyte function is currently thought to involve several steps. The steroid molecule is first taken up by the cell and binds to a cytoplasmic receptor. The receptor–steroid complex is then taken up by the nucleus and a nuclear complex is formed (154). The binding of this complex affects the DNA template and synthesis of RNA, and this in turn initiates the synthesis of a protein which inhibits glucose transport and cellular activity (111). Obviously the question of lymphocyte sensitivity to glucocorticoids requires further study. This subject is of immense importance because of the possibility of developing a blood test which would be useful in the early detection of open-angle glaucoma.

ACUTE POSTERIOR MULTIFOCAL PLACOID PIGMENT EPITHELIOPATHY (APMPPE)

APMPPE is a recently described inflammatory disease in which the pigment epithelium, choriocapillaris, or both are affected (56). Ocular manifestations of APMPPE has also been associated with optic neuritis, uveitis, keratitis, episcleritis, and retinal vasculitis (76). With increased recognition of this clinical entity, there have been numerous reports of inflammatory signs in this disease as well as associations with systemic inflammatory conditions. Recent evidence suggests that APMPPE may be the result of an immunologic response to a systemic viral infection (8, 25).

APMPPE may be preceded by an acute viral infection in some cases (50, 127, 128). Previous mycobacterial infection (20) and an increased incidence of positive tuberculin skin tests (84a, 88) have also been associated with APMPPE. Erythema nodosum, a condition which complicates many infectious diseases and which is probably due to immune-complex deposition, has been reported in association with APMPPE (39, 146). A type 5 adenovirus has been cultured from the throat and tonsils of a 19-year-old black patient with APMPPE and the same patient demonstrated a rise in complement-fixing antibodies to this virus (8). There have also been reports of APMPPE associated with multifocal cerebral vasculitis (69) and with acute thyroiditis (76). A cerebrospinal fluid pleocytosis and increased CSF protein have been noted in some patients (25, 69). At present, it seems likely that APMPPE is part of a systemic vasculitis which occurs following acute viral infections.

Recent fluorescein angiography studies show that a vascular ischemic process occurs in APMPPE which is due to a precapillary choroidal arteriolitis and results in nonprofusion of lobules of choriocapillaris (38). This acute occlusion may be part of a generalized vasculitis.

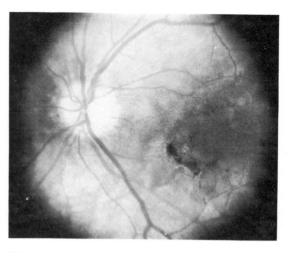

FIG. 7-17. Acute posterior multifocal placoid pigment epitheliopathy.

Clinical Features

The disease is characterized clinically by a rapid loss of central vision and multifocal yellow-white placoid lesions at the level of retinal pigment epithelium and choroid (Fig. 7-17). These lesions resolve rapidly, leaving permanent alterations in the affected layers, with depigmentation of the retinal pigment epithelium and irregular clumping of pigment. Gradually, inactive pigmented scars form. Improvement is usually seen within 6 weeks of the onset of the disease.

RETINAL VASCULITIS

Retinal vasculitis is a poorly defined clinical entity which is usually regarded as inflammatory and treated empirically. Although retinal vasculitis may accompany a variety of systemic disorders, the entity we are concerned with here does not have any obvious extraocular manifestations. A vasoobliterative vasculitis known as **Eales' disease** occurs mainly in young males and involves the peripheral venules or the central retinal vein. Other types of retinal vasculitis involve arterioles and venules or sometimes just arterioles.

The etiology of retinal vasculitis is still obscure. Eales' disease was at one time attributed to a tuberculous infection or an allergy to tuberculoprotein (7). Serum IgG and IgA may be elevated in Eales' disease (78), and IgM has been reported to be reduced (85). Some studies of retinal vasculitis have shown an elevated serum IgM and a slight increase in autoantibodies, mainly to smooth muscle (31). Some studies have demonstrated neither autoantibodies nor an abnormality in the complement system (77). The absence of complement abnormalities, however, does not rule out the possibility that retinal vasculitis may be secondary to immune-complex deposition within the walls of the retinal vessels. This mechanism, *i.e.*, intravascular immune-complex deposition, is responsible for many types of vasculitis (36). A vasculoocclusive retinopathy may be seen as a part of experimental allergic encephalomyelitis (EAE), in which monkeys are immunized with injections of guinea pig spinal cord antigen in complete Freund's adjuvant (149). EAE (see under Multiple Sclerosis, Ch. 10) is an autoimmune process in which cellular immune mechanisms have been implicated, since it can be transferred with lymphocytes but not with serum, and *in vitro* tests for cellular immunity are positive. While

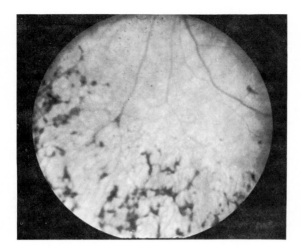

FIG. 7-18. Retinitis pigmentosa. (Courtesy of Dr. R. Dennis)

colloid and microsomal antibodies, and adrenocortical antibodies, were demonstrated in a patient with retinitis pigmentosa and Graves' disease (116). This patient's sibling had retinitis pigmentosa and an adrenal abnormality. Possibly, retinitis pigmentosa in this instance was part of a disease spectrum associated with an inherited abnormal immune response.

Cellular immune mechanisms have been investigated in retinitis pigmentosa. Cellular hypersensitivity can be demonstrated by the leukocyte migration inhibition test and by activity against a retinoblastoma cell line using a cytotoxicity test (29). As in other situations, it is difficult to tell whether sensitization to retinal elements is involved in the pathogenesis of the disease or whether immunologic findings are secondary to tissue damage inflicted by nonimmunologic means.

antibodies can be demonstrated, they do not correlate positively with production of the disease.

Retinal vasculitis is characterized clinically by sheathing of vessels and sometimes by narrowing, segmentation, and obliteration of vessels. Neovascularization and hemorrhage are sometimes seen (77). Other ocular findings include swelling of the optic nerve, macular edema and exudates, vitreous haze, and anterior uveitis (114).

Treatment depends on the severity and progression of the disease. The vasculitis may remit spontaneously without treatment (77), or corticosteroids (114) or other immunosuppressive agents may be required.

RETINITIS PIGMENTOSA

Pigmentary degenerations of the retina (Fig. 7-18) are usually considered to be hereditary conditions. However, the possibility of immune factors in their pathogenesis cannot be ruled out (138). Rheumatoid factor is found in 40% of patients with primary retinitis pigmentosa (49). Increased levels of serum IgM have also been reported by others (55, 86, 122). The significance of these immunoglobulin alterations is unclear at present. Recently, thyroid

REFERENCES

1. Allansmith MR, Hahn GS, Simon MA: Tissue, tear and serum IgE concentrations in vernal conjunctivitis. Am J Ophthalmol 81:506, 1976
2. Allansmith MR, Korb DR, Greiner JV et al: Giant papillary conjunctivitis in contact lens wearers. Am J Ophthalmol 83:697, 1977
3. Allansmith MR, Whitney CR, McClellan BH et al: Immunoglobulin in the human eye. Arch Ophthalmol 89:36, 1973
4. Anderson FG: Repair of marginal furrow perforation. Ophthalmic Surg 8:25, 1977
5. Aronson SB: The role of non-specific tests in uveitis. In Aronson SB et al: Clinical Methods in Uveitis. St Louis, Mosby, 1968, p 191
6. Aronson SB, Elliott JH: Ocular Inflammation. St Louis, Mosby, 1972
7. Ashton N: Pathogenesis and etiology of Eales' disease. In Pandit YK (ed): XIX Concilium Ophthalmologicum, Vol 2. Bombay, The Times of India Press, 1962, p 828
8. Azar P Jr, Gohd RS, Waltman D, Gitter KA: Acute posterior multifocal placoid pigment epitheliopathy associated with an adenovirus type 5 infection. Am J Ophthalmol 80:1003, 1975
9. Becker B, Keates EU, Coleman SL: Gamma-globulin in the trabecular meshwork of glaucomatous eyes. Arch Ophthalmol 68:643, 1962
10. Becker B, Palmberg PF, Shin DH: Glucocorticoid responsiveness associated with HLA-B12. Invest Ophthalmol Vis Sci 16:61, 1977

11. Becker B, Shin DH: HLA antigens and primary open-angle glaucoma in black Americans. Invest Ophthalmol Vis Sci 16:175, 1977

12. Becker B, Shin DH, Palmberg PF, Waltman SR: HLA antigens and corticosteroid response. Science 194:1427, 1976

13. Becker B, Unger H-H, Coleman SL, Keates EU: Plasma cells and gamma-globulin in trabecular meshwork of eyes with primary open-angle glaucoma. Arch Ophthalmol 70:38, 1963

14. Benezra D, Tichio U, Sachs U: Lymphocyte sensitivity to glucocorticoids. Am J Ophthalmol 82:866, 1976

15. Bigger JF, Palmberg PF, Becker B: Increased cellular sensitivity to glucocorticoids in primary open-angle glaucoma. Invest Ophthalmol 11:832, 1972

16. Blodi FC: Sympathetic uveitis as an allergic phenomenon. Trans Am Acad Ophthalmol Otolaryngol 63:642, 1959

17. Boone WB, Gupta S, Hansen J, Good RA: Lymphocyte subpopulations in patients with sympathetic ophthalmitis and nongranulomatous uveitis. Invest Ophthalmol 15:957, 1976

18. Bor S, Feiwel M, Chanarin I: Vitiligo and its etiological relationship to organ-specific autoimmune disease. Br J Dermatol 81:83, 1969

19. Brauninger GE, Centifanto YM: Immunoglobulin E in human tears. Am J Ophthalmol 72:558, 1971

20. Brown M, Eberdt A, Lodos G: Pigment epitheliopathy in a patient with mycobacterial infection. J Pediatr Ophthalmol 10:278, 1973

21. Brown SI: Mooren's ulcer: histopathology and proteolytic enzymes of adjacent conjunctiva. Br J Ophthalmol 59:670, 1975

22. Brown SI: Mooren's ulcer. Treatment by conjunctival excision. Br J Ophthalmol 59:675, 1975

23. Brown SI, Mondino BJ, Rabin BS: Autoimmune phenomenon in Mooren's ulcer. Am J Ophthalmol 82:835, 1976

24. Bruno MG, McPherson SD Jr: Harada's disease. Am J Ophthalmol 32:513, 1949

25. Bullock JD, Fletcher RL: Cerebrospinal fluid abnormalities in acute posterior multifocal placoid pigment epitheliopathy. Am J Ophthalmol 84:45, 1977

26. Burky EL: Experimental endophthalmitis phaco-anaphylactica in rabbits. Arch Ophthalmol 12:536, 1934

27. Burnet FM, Fenner F: The production of antibodies. New York, Macmillan, 1949

28. Caron GA: Prednisolone inhibition of DNA synthesis by human lymphocytes induced in vitro by phytohemagglutinin. Int Arch Allergy 32:191, 1967

29. Char DH, Bergsma DR, Rabson AS et al: Cell-mediated immunity to retinal antigens in patients with pigmentary retinal degenerations. Invest Ophthalmol 13:198, 1974

29a. Char DH: Immune complexes in uveitis. Ocular Microbiology and Immunology Group, Annual meeting, Kansas City, Mo., Oct 21, 1978

30. Charamis I, Skouras I: Die Behandlung der chronischen Zyklitis nebst Zystenodem der Makula mit Azathioprin. Klin Monatsbl Augenheilkd 170:362, 1977

31. Chilman T: Specific and non-specific antibody activity in retinal vasculitis. Trans Ophthalmol Soc UK 93:193, 1973

32. Coles RS: Uveitis—a review. Surv Ophthalmol 5:355, 1960

33. Collin HB, Allansmith MR: Basophils in vernal conjunctivitis in humans: an electron microscopic study. Invest Ophthalmol 16:858, 1977

34. Collins RC: Experimental studies on sympathetic ophthalmia. Am J Ophthalmol 32:1687, 1949

35. Collins RC: Further experimental studies on sympathetic ophthalmia. Am J Ophthalmol 36 Part 2:150, 1955

36. Conn DL, McDuffie FC, Holley KE, Schroeter AL: Immunologic mechanisms in sytemic vasculitis. Mayo Clin Proc 51:511, 1976

37. Dernouchamps JP, Vaerman JP, Michiels J, Masson PL: Immune complexes in the aqueous humor and serum. Am J Ophthalmol 84:24, 1977

38. Deutman AF, Lion F: Choriocapillaris nonperfusion in acute multifocal placoid pigment epitheliopathy. Am J Ophthalmol 84:652, 1977

39. Deutman AF, Oosterhuis JA, Boen-Tan TN, Aan deKerk AL: Acute posterior multifocal placoid pigment epitheliopathy. Br J Ophthalmol 56:863, 1972

40. Duke-Elder S, Leight AG: Diseases of the outer eye. In System of Ophthalmology, Vol 8, Pt 2. St Louis, Mosby, 1965, p 916

41. Easom HA: Sympathetic ophthalmia associated with malignant melanoma. Arch Ophthalmol 70:786, 1963

42. Easom HA, Zimmerman LE: Sympathetic ophthalmia and bilateral phacoanaphylaxis. A clinicopathologic correlation of the sympathogenic and sympathizing eyes. Arch Ophthalmol 72:9, 1964

43. Easty D, Rice NSC, Jones BR: Disodium cromoglycate (Intal) in the treatment of vernal kerato-conjunctivitis. Trans Ophthalmol Soc UK 91:491, 1971

44. Ehrlich P, Morgenroth J: Ueber Haemolysine Dritte Mittheilung. Ber Klin Wocehnschr 21:453, 1900

45. Ellis P: Noncorticosteroid anti-inflammatory drugs. In Symposium on Ocular Pharmacol-

ogy and Therapeutics (Transactions of the New Orleans Academy of Ophthalmology). St Louis, Mosby, 1970, pp 62–63

46. Elschnig A: Zur Frage der sympatischen Ophthalmie. Klin Monatsbl Augenheildk 80:289, 1928

47. Elves MW, Gough J, Israels MCG: The place of the lymphocyte in the reticuloendothelial system. A study of the in vitro effect of prednisolone on lymphocytes. Acta Heamatol (Basel) 32:100, 1964

48. Felberg NT, Leon SA, Gasparini J, Spaeth GL: A comparison of antinuclear antibodies and DNA-binding antibodies in chronic open-angle glaucoma. Invest Ophthalmol Visual Sci 16:757, 1977

49. Fessel WJ: Serum protein disturbance in retinitis pigmentosa. Am J Ophthalmol 53:640, 1962

50. Fitzpatrick PJ, Robertson DM: Acute posterior multifocal placoid pigment epitheliopathy. Arch Ophthalmol 89:373, 1973

51. Foon KA, Yuen K, Ballantine EJ, Rosenstreich DL: Analysis of the systemic corticosteroid sensitivity of patients with primary open-angle glaucoma. Am J Ophthalmol 83:167, 1977

52. Frankland AW, Easty D: Vernal keratoconjunctivitis: an atopic disease. Trans Ophthalmol Soc UK 91:479, 1971

53. Freund J, Lipton MM, Thompson GE: Aspermatogenesis in guinea pig induced by testicular tissue and adjuvants. J Exp Med 97:711, 1953

54. Friedenwald JS: Notes on the allergy theory of sympathetic ophthalmia. Am J Ophthalmol 17:1008, 1934

55. Fugiwara H: Biochemical studies on retinitis pigmentosa by Cyanogum gel electrophoresis. Folia Ophthalmol Jpn 16:667, 1965

56. Gass JDM: Acute posterior multifocal placoid pigment epitheliopathy. Arch Ophthalmol 80:177, 1968

57. Gasteiger H: Uber das Ulcas rodens corneae nebst Bemerkungen uber Hornhautveranderungen bei Sklero-Perikeratitis. Klin Monatsbl Augenheilkd 114:112, 1949

58. Giles CL: Peripheral uveitis in patients with multiple sclerosis. Am J Ophthalmol 70:17, 1970

59. Godfrey WA, Smith RE, Kimura SJ: Chronic cyclitis: corticosteroid therapy. Trans Am Ophthalmol Soc 74:178, 1976

60. Goldberg MF, Croxan Y, Duke JR, Frost JK: Cytopathologic and histopathologic aspects of Fuchs' heterochromic iridocyclitis. Arch Ophthalmol 74:604, 1965

61. Halbert SP, Locatcher-Khorazo D, Swick L, Witmer R, Seegal B, Fitzgerald P: Homologous immunological studies of ocular lens. I. In vitro observation. J Exp Med 105:439, 1957

62. Hammer H: Lymphocyte transformation test in sympathetic ophthalmitis and Vogt-Koyan-agi-Harada syndrome. Br J Ophthalmol 55:850, 1971

63. Hammer H, Olah M: Hypersensitivity towards alpha-crystalline in the heterochromia syndrome. Albrecht von Graefes Arch Klin Ophthalmol 197:61, 1975

64. Hart CT, Ward DM: Intraocular pressure in Fuchs' heterochromic uveitis. Br J Ophthalmol 51:739, 1967

65. Heintz G: Uber Ulcas rodens. Z Augenheilk 77:289, 1932

66. Hektoen L: Further observations on lens precipitins. Antigenic properties of alpha and beta crystallins. J Infect Dis 34:433, 1924

66a. Henley WL, Leopold IH, Aviner Z: Glaucoma and HLA antigens. Lancet 2:1273, 1974

67. Henley WL, Okas S, Leopold IH: Cellular immunity in chronic ophthalmic disorders. 4. Leukocyte migration inhibition in diseases associated with glaucoma. Am J Ophthalmol 76:60, 1973

68. Hogan MJ: Treatment of endogenous uveitis. In Ophthalmology—Proceedings of the XXI International Congress, Mexico. Amsterdam, Excerpta Medica Foundation, 1971, p 531

69. Holt W, Regan C, Trempe C: Acute posterior multifocal placoid epitheliopathy. Am J Ophthalmol 81:403, 1976

70. Howes EL Jr, McKay DG: Circulating immune complexes. Effects on ocular vascular permeability in the rabbit. Arch Ophthalmol 93:365, 1975

71. Hussman H, Hübner H, Böke W: Zur Frage nach der Immunogenese der sympathischen Ophthalmie. Albrecht von Graefes Arch Klin Ophthalmol 185:22 1972

72. Ikui H, Kimura K, Kwaki S: Electron microscopic study of ultrathin sections of sympathetic ophthalmia (preliminary report). Jpn J Ophthalmol 2:13, 1958

73. Ikui H, Kimura K, Nishio T, Furuyoshi Y: Etiology of sympathetic ophthalmia. 18th Int Congr Ophthalmol 2:1285, 1959

74. Irvine SR, Irvine AR Jr: Lens-induced uveitis and glaucoma. Part II. The phacotoxic reaction. Am J Ophthalmol 35:370, 1952

75. Iwamoto T, DeVoe AG, Farris RL: Electron microscopy in cases of marginal degeneration of the cornea. Invest Ophthalmol 11:241, 1972

76. Jacklin HN: Acute posterior multifocal placoid pigment epitheliopathy and thyroiditis. Arch Ophthalmol 95:995, 1977

77. Jampol LM, Isenberg SJ, Goldberg MF: Occlusive retinal arteriolitis with neovascularization. Am J Ophthalmol 81:583, 1976

78. Johnson GJ, Bloch KJ: Immunoglobulin levels in retinal vascular abnormalities and pseudoxanthoma elasticum. Arch Ophthalmol 81:322, 1969

79. Joondeph HC, McCarthy WL, Rabb M, Constantaras AA: Mooren's ulcer: two cases occurring after cataract extraction and treated with hydrophilic lens. Ann Ophthalmol 8:187, 1976

80. Joy HH: A survey of cases of sympathetic ophthalmia occurring in New York State. Arch Ophthalmol 14:733, 1935

80a. Kass MA, Palmberg P, Becker B, Miller JP: Histocompatibility antigens and primary open-angle glaucoma: A reassessment. Arch Ophthalmol 96:2207, 1978

81. Keitzman B: Mooren's ulcer in Nigeria. Am J Ophthalmol 65:679, 1968

82. Kenyon KR, Pederson JE, Green WR, Maumenee AE: Fibroglial proliferation in pars planitis. Trans Ophthalmol Soc UK 95:391, 1975

83. Kimura SJ, Hogan MJ: Chronic cyclitis. Trans Am Ophthalmol Soc 61:397, 1963

84. Kinces E, Szabo G: Cell-mediated and humoral immune response after lens injury. Mod Prob Ophthalmol 16:95, 1976

84a. Kirkham TH, Ffytche TJ, Sanders MD: Placoid pigment-epitheliopathy with retinal vasculitis and papillitis. Br J Ophthalmol 56:875, 1972

85. Koliopoulos JX, Perkins ES, Seitanides BE: Serum immunoglobulins in retinal vasculitis. Br J Ophthalmol 54:233, 1970

86. Krachmer JH, Smith JL, Tocci PM: Laboratory studies in retinitis pigmentosa. Arch Ophthalmol 75:661, 1966

87. Kraus-Mackiw E, Schopf E, Muller-Ruchholtz W: Comparison of cell-mediated immune reactions in sympathetic and phacogenic ophthalmia with reactions in uveitis of other origin. Mod Prob Ophthalmol 16:106, 1976

88. Laatikainen L, Erkkila H: Clinical and fluorescein angiographic findings of acute multifocal central subretinal inflammation. Acta Ophthalmol (Kbh) 5:645, 1973

89. Lazar M, Weiner MJ, Leopold IH: Treatment of uveitis with methotrexate. Am J Ophthalmol 67:383, 1969

90. Leigh AG: Lens induced uveitis. Trans Ophthalmol Soc UK 75:51, 1955

91. Leopold IH: The role of lymphocyte (cell-mediated) immunity to ocular disease. Am J Ophthalmol 76:619, 1973

92. Lucie H: Sensitization of rabbits to uveal tissue by the synergic action of staphylotoxin. Arch Ophthalmol 22:359, 1939

93. Luntz MH: Anti-uveal and anti-lens antibodies in uveitis and their significance. Exp Eye Res 7:561, 1968

94. Luntz MH, Wright R: Lens-induced uveitis. Exp Eye Res 1:317, 1962

95. Makley TA, Leibold JE: Modern therapy of sympathetic ophthalmia. Arch Ophthalmol 64:809, 1960

96. Manski W: Immunological studies on normal and pathological lenses. In The Human Lens in Relation to Cataract Formation. CIBA Foundation Symposium. New York, Association of Scientific Publishers, 1973

97. Marak GE Jr: Immunopathology of sympathetic ophthalmia. Mod Prob Ophthalmol 16:102, 1976

98. Marak GE Jr, Font RL, Alepa FP: Experimental lens induced granulomatous endophthalmitis: passive transfer with serum. Ophthalmol Res 8:117, 1976

99. Marak GE Jr, Font RL, Johnson MC, Alepa FP: Lymphocyte-stimulating activity of ocular tissues in sympathetic ophthalmia. Invest Ophthalmol 10:770, 1971

100. Marak GE Jr, Font RL, Zimmerman LE: Histologic variations related to race in sympathetic ophthalmia. 78:935, 1974

101. Marak GE, Tischler SM, Evans PY, Alepa FP: Pathogenesis of sympathetic ophthalmia. Invest Ophthalmol 10:162, 1971

102. McLean JM: Steroid prophylaxis in sympathetic ophthalmia. Am J Ophthalmol 45 (Pt 2):162, 1958

103. McPherson SD Jr, Wood AC: The significance of the intracutaneous test for hypersensitivity to uveal pigment. Am J Ophthalmol 31:35, 1948

104. Meller J: Chronische Iridocyclitis und Neuritis retrobulbaris. Abrecht von Graefes Arch Klin Ophthalmol 105:299, 1921

105. Mills PV, Shedden WIH: Serological studies in sympathetic ophthalmia. Br J Ophthalmol 49:29, 1975

106. Misra RN, Rahi AHS, Morgan G: Immunopathology of the lens. II. Humoral and cellular immune responses to homologous lens antigens and their roles in ocular inflammation. Br J Ophthalmol 61:285, 1977

107. Moore CE: Sympathetic ophthalmitis treated with azathioprine. Br J Ophthalmol 52:688, 1968

108. Mondino B, Brown SI, Rabin BS, Lemp MA: Autoimmune phenomena of the conjunctiva and cornea. Arch Ophthalmol 95:468, 1977

109. Morgan IM: Allergic encephalomyelitis in monkeys in response to injection of normal monkey cord. J Bacteriol 51:614, 1946

110. Muller HK, Sollner F: Ulcus roden de la cornée familial. J Genet Hum 5:81, 1956

111. Munck A: Glucocorticosteroid inhibition of glucose uptake by peripheral tissues. Old and new evidence, molecular mechanisms, and physiological significance. Perspect Biol Med 114:265, 1971

112. Newell FW, Krill AE: Treatment of uveitis with azathioprine (Imuran). Trans Ophthalmol Soc UK 87:499, 1967

113. Newell FW, Krill AE, Thompson A: The

treatment of uveitis with six-mercaptopurine. Am J Ophthalmol 81:628, 1969

114. Nolan J, Cullen JF: Retinal vasculitis associated with anterior uveitis. Br J Ophthalmol 51:361, 1967

115. Nowell PC: Inhibition of human leucocyte mitosis by prednisolone in vitro. Cancer Res 21:1518, 1961

116. Nye FJ, Howel Evans W: Retinitis pigmentosa and autoimmune endocrine abnormalities in identical twins. Br Med J 1:616, 1977

117. Palmberg PF, Hajek S, Cooper D, Becker B: Increased cellular responsiveness to epinephrine in primary open-angle glaucoma. Arch Ophthalmol 95:855, 1977

118. Polack FM: Heterologous antilymphocyte serum. In Kaufman HE (ed): Ocular Anti-Inflammatory Therapy. Springfield, IL. Thomas, 1970, p 131

119. Pusey B: Cytotoxins and sympathetic ophthalmia. Arch Ophthalmol 32:334, 1903

120. Pusin SM, Green WR, Tasman W et al: Simultaneous bacterial endophthalmitis and sympathetic uveitis after retinal detachment. 81:57, 1976

121. Putintseva LS, Doronina TF: Autoallergic reactions in glaucomatous patients. Vestn Oftalmol 1:3, 1975

122. Rahi AHS: Autoimmunity and the retina. II. Raised IgM in retinitis pigmentosa. Br J Ophthalmol 57:904, 1973

123. Rahi AHS, Misra RN, Morgan G: Immunopathology of the lens. III. Humoral and cellular immune responses to autologous lens antigens and their roles in ocular inflammation. Br J Ophthalmol 61:371, 1977

124. Riise P: Endophthalmitis phacoanaphylactica. Am J Ophthalmol 60:911, 1965

124a. Ritch R, Podos SM, Henley W et al: Lack of association of histocompatibility antigens with primary open-angle glaucoma. Arch Ophthalmol 96:2204, 1978

125. Riwchun MH, DeCoursey E: Sympathetic ophthalmia caused by non-perforating intraocular sarcoma. Arch Ophthalmol 25:848, 1941

126. Roy D, Spector A: Human alpha-crystallin-III isolation and characterization of protein from normal infant lenses and old lens peripheries. Invest Ophthalmol 15:394, 1976

127. Ryan SJ, Maumenee AE: Acute posterior multifocal placoid pigment epitheliopathy. Am J Ophthalmol 74:1066, 1972

128. Savino PJ, Weinberg RJ, Yassin JG, Pilkerton AR: Diverse manifestations of acute posterior multifocal placoid pigment epitheliopathy. Am J Ophthalmol 77:659, 1974

129. Schirmer O: IX Int Congr Ophthalmol Utrecht 402, 1899

130. Schlaegel TF Jr: Essentials of Uveitis. Boston, Little, Brown, 1969, pp 123–124

131. Schreck E: Uber den Erreger der sympatischen Ophthalmie. Albrecht von Graefes Arch Klin Ophthalmol 151:46, 1951

132. Shaap OL, Feltkamp TEW, Breebaart AC: Circulating antibodies to corneal tissue in a patient suffering from Mooren's ulcer (ulcus rodens corneae). Clin Exp Immunol 5:365, 1969

133. Shammas HF, Zubyk NA, Stanfield TF: Sympathetic uveitis following glaucoma surgery. Arch Ophthalmol 95:638, 1977

133a. Shaw JF, Levene RZ, Sowell JG: The incidence of HLA antigens in black primary open-angle glaucoma patients. Am J Ophthalmol 86:501, 1978

134. Shields MB, McCoy RC, Shelburne JD: Immunofluorescent studies on the trabecular meshwork in open-angle glaucoma. Invest Ophthalmol 15:1014, 1976

135. Shin DH, Becker B: The prognostic value of HLA-B12 and HLA-B7 antigens in patients with increased intraocular pressure. Am J Ophthalmol 82:871, 1976

136. Shin DH, Becker B: HLA-A11 and HLA-Bw35 and resistance to glaucoma in white patients with ocular hypertension. Arch Ophthalmol 95:423, 1977

137. Shin DH, Becker B, Waltman SR et al: The prevalence of HLA-B12 and HLA-B7 antigens in primary open-angle glaucoma. Arch Ophthalmol 95:224, 1977

138. Shore B, Leopold IH, Henley WL: Cellular immunity in chronic ophthalmic disorders. II. Leukocyte migration inhibition in diseases of the cornea. Am J Ophthalmol 73:62, 1972

139. Shpak NI, Gladkova NR: The role of infectious allergy in etiopathogenesis of Fuchs' syndrome. Oftalmol Zh 39:89, 1975

140. Sie-Boen-Lian: Cultivation of virus in a case of sympathetic ophthalmia. Ophthalmologica 146:43, 1963

141. Smith RE, O'Connor GR: Cataract extraction in Fuchs' syndrome. Arch Ophthalmol 91:39, 1974

142. Suie T, Dodd MC: An immunologic study in rabbits sensitized with homologous uveal tissue. Am J Ophthalmol 39:377, 1955

143. Tabbara KF, Arafat NT: Cromolyn effects on vernal keratoconjunctivitis in children. Arch Ophthalmol 95:2184, 1977

144. Triebenstein O: On the question of Ulcus rodens corneae. Klin Monatsbl Augenheilkd 82:212, 1929

145. Uhlenhuth P: Zur Lehre von der Unter-scheidung verschiedener eiweissarten mit Hilfe spezifischer Sera. In Festschrift zum Sechzigsten Geburtstage von Robert Koch. Gustav Fischer, Jena, 1903, p 49

146. Van Buskirk EM, Lesell S, Friedman E: Pigmentary epitheliopathy and erythema nodosum. Arch Ophthalmol 85:369, 1971

147. Vannas S, Nordman E, Teir H: Uveitis resembling sympathetic ophthalmia induced by

sensitization of intraperitoneally implanted eye. Acta Ophthalmol (Kbh) 38:618, 1960

148. Verhoeff F, Lemoine AN: Hypersensitiveness to lens protein. Am J Ophthalmol 5:700, 1922

149. von Sallman L, Meyers RE, Lerner EM, Stone SH: Vasculo-occlusive retinopathy in experimental allergic encephalomyelitis. Arch Ophthalmol 78:112, 1967

150. Waltman SR, Yarian D: Antinuclear antibodies in open-angle glaucoma. 13:695, 1974

151. Welch RB, Maumenee AE, Whalen HE: Peripheral posterior segment inflammation, vitreous opacities, and edema of the posterior pole. Arch Ophthalmol 64:540, 1960

152. Wilson FM II, Grayson M, Ellis FD: Treatment of peripheral corneal ulcers by limbal conjunctivectomy. Br J Ophthalmol 60:713, 1976

153. Wilson P: Sympathetic ophthalmitis simulating Harada's disease. Br J Ophthalmol 46:626, 1962

154. Wira CR, Munck A: Glucocorticoid receptor complexes in rat thymus cells. J Biol Chem 249:5328, 1974

155. Witebsky E, Rose NR, Terplan KL, Paine JR, Egan RW: Chronic thyroiditis and autoimmunization. JAMA 164:1439, 1957

156. Witmer R: Phacogenic uveitis. Ophthalmologica 133:326, 1953

157. Witmer R: Phaco-antigenic uveitis. Doc Ophthalmol 16:271, 1962

158. Wong VG: Immunosuppressive therapy of ocular inflammatory disease. Arch Ophthalmol 81:628, 1969

159. Wong VG: Immunosuppressive agents in ophthalmology. Surv Ophthalmol 13:290, 1969

160. Wong VG, Anderson R, O'Brien PJ: Sympathetic ophthalmia and lymphocyte transformation. Am J Ophthalmol 72:960, 1971

161. Wood TO, Kaufman HE: Mooren's ulcer. Am J Ophthalmol 71:417, 1971

162. Woods AC: Immune reactions following injuries to the uveal tract. JAMA 77:1317, 1921

163. Woods AC: Sympathetic ophthalmia. Am J Ophthalmol 19:9, 1936

164. Woods AC: Personal communication, quoted by McLean JM: Steroid prophylaxis in sympathetic ophthalmia. Am J Ophthalmol 45 (pt 2):162, 1958

165. Zimmerman LE, Silverstein AM: Experimental ocular hypersensitivity. Am J Ophthalmol 48:447, 1959

EIGHT
EIGHT
EIGHT arthritic and connective tissue disorders

Ocular involvement is a characteristic feature of many rheumatologic and connective tissue disorders. Autoimmune mechanisms are thought to play a significant role in a number of these conditions and a wide variety of immunologic abnormalities have already been demonstrated. Immunologic elements are generally measured in a sample of the patient's blood, or in tissues which can be conveniently biopsied, such as the skin or blood vessels. Since the eye is only one of many organs affected by the rheumatic disorders and related conditions, it is likely that a study of immunologic abnormalities in these tissues may lead us to an understanding of the pathogenesis of the ocular lesions as well.

ANKYLOSING SPONDYLITIS

Ankylosing spondylitis is a chronic, progressive, inflammatory arthritis primarily involving the sacroiliac joints and spine. Approximately 25% of cases are associated with iridocyclitis. Males are affected much more frequently than females, accounting for 80%–90% of all patients. The highest incidence of the disease occurs between ages 20 and 40. Over 90% of patients with ankylosing spondylitis possess the histocompatibility antigen HLA-B27. This represents one of the highest known correlations between an HLA type and a disease entity.

Immunopathology

The basic pathogenesis of ankylosing spondylitis is unknown. For many years it was considered a variant of rheumatoid arthritis but it is now known to differ in several respects from rheumatoid disease. There is no strong evidence for an autoimmune mechanism, and rheumatoid factor is absent except in about 5% of cases.

It has been known for many years that genetic factors play a role in the development of ankylosing spondylitis. The disease is 40 times more common among first-degree relatives of spondylitis patients than in the general population (33), and the concordance rate in identical twins is 70% (60). Family pedigrees suggest that ankylosing spondylitis is inherited as a mendelian dominant trait with 70% penetrance in males and 10% penetrance in females (33). It is also known that the frequency of ankylosing spondylitis is high among certain American Indian groups, such as the Haida, the Bella Coola, and the Pima (44). In contrast, the disease is relatively rare among African black populations (45).

In April 1973, Schlosstein and his colleagues (106) in Los Angeles, and Brewerton and his colleagues (10) in England reported a strikingly high incidence of HLA-B27 in patients with ankylosing spondylitis. This histocompatibility antigen, which has a frequency of 4%–9% in control populations (the antigen is found in 8% of Caucasians), was found in 95%

of patients with ankylosing spondylitis. Other investigators have confirmed a high incidence of HLA-B27 in patients with spondylitis. American blacks in general have an incidence of HLA-B27 of 4%, while 89% of black patients with ankylosing spondylitis are positive for the antigen (106).

Histocompatibility antigens are cell surface determinants that are present on the vast majority of human cell membranes (see Histocompatibility Antigens, Ch. 1, and Transplantation Immunology, Ch. 11). The frequency of an antigen is determined by genetic and racial factors. Frequency of an HLA type can be computed by using panels of donor lymphocytes of known antigenicity together with specific antiserums.

Although HLA typing has been used primarily to match donors and recipients for organ transplantation, much interest recently has been generated in the association of HLA genotypes with specific disease entities. Perhaps the highest association of any HLA type with a specific disease is that of B27 with ankylosing spondylitis and Reiter's syndrome. Although B27 is detected in only 4%–9% of the general population it is found in over 90% of patients with these diseases. The vast majority of patients who develop postinfectious arthropathies resembling Reiter's syndrome are also positive for B27.

Ankylosing spondylitis is common in families which carry the HLA-B27 antigen. It has been estimated that if the risk of spondylitis in an antigen-negative female is 1, then the risk in a B27-positive female is 276 times greater. For a B27-positive male, the risk is 1,937 times greater (73).

The significance of this high frequency of HLA-B27 in ankylosing spondylitis patients is uncertain. The antigen is also found in 90% of patients with a spondylitis that occurs following infection with *Yersinia enterocolitica*, a gram-negative bacterium. This organism causes a transient inflammatory bowel disorder which may be followed by a polyarthritis and a sacroiliitis. In patients who recover uneventfully from the infection, the incidence of HLA-B27 is the same as for the general population. Of those patients who develop arthritis,

however, B27 is found in about 90%. This pattern of events suggests that a disease caused by an infectious agent can produce a spondylitis in a genetically susceptible individual. The disease might develop in those who have a defective immune response to *Yersinia* or other infectious agents. This reasoning has also been used to support an infectious etiology for Reiter's syndrome and even for ankylosing spondylitis.

Clinical Features

General. Approximately 50% of patients with ankylosing spondylitis are entirely asymptomatic. Others complain of low back pain, stiffness, and pain and tenderness of the sacroiliac joints. There may also be spasm of the paravertebral muscles. Although the sacroiliac joints and spine are primarily involved, peripheral joint involvement is found in onefifth of affected patients. If the disease progresses, advanced changes may be found. These include complete fusion of the sacroiliac joints and vertebrae, loss of the normal lumbar lordosis, dorsocervical kyphosis, and decreased chest expansion.

Radiographic changes are often helpful in making a proper diagnosis (Fig. 8-1). These include demineralization of bone adjacent to the sacroiliac joints, and subchondral sclerosis. The involvement of the sacroiliac joints is usually visible in advanced disease. Squaring of the vertebral bodies on lateral x-ray and sclerosis and fusion of the vertebrae produce a characteristic "bamboo" appearance of the spine. Calcification and ossification of the paraspinal ligaments may also be seen.

The extraarticular manifestations of ankylosing spondylitis include iritis in 25% of patients, carditis in 10% and aortitis with aortic insufficiency in 1%–4%. Rare complications include a pericarditis and pulmonary fibrosis.

Ocular Findings. The uveitis associated with ankylosing spondylitis is generally an acute, recurrent, bilateral iridocyclitis (Fig. 8-2). The patient usually complains of pain, redness, and photophobia during the acute attacks. Examination reveals an injected conjunctiva,

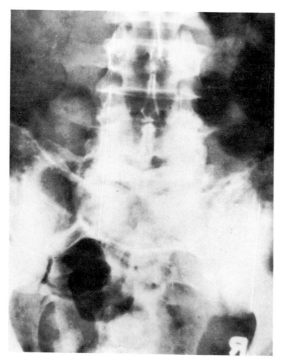

FIG. 8-1. Ankylosing spondylitis with fusion of sacroiliac joints.

with cells and flare in the anterior chamber. Fibrin is sometimes seen in the anterior chamber, and formation of synechia is common. These may be irregular and extend virtually 360° (Fig. 8-3). Glaucoma may occur either secondary to complete synechia and iris bombé or may accompany the anterior segment inflammation. Vitreous reaction may be seen to a variable extent, but is not generally a prominent feature of the disease. Keratic precipitates are frequently present.

Ankylosing spondylitis is one of the most common systemic diseases found among uveitis patients. Laitinen and his colleagues (68) found ankylosing spondylitis in 23% of young patients with acute, recurrent iridocyclitis and symptoms suggesting ankylosing spondylitis in another 10%. Kimura and associates (65) showed that in 191 patients with joint disease and iridocyclitis, 41, or 21.5% had definite ankylosing spondylitis. Another 27 cases had probable ankylosing spondylitis and

if these are counted, 35.6% of the patients with uveitis and joint disease had ankylosing spondylitis.

Diagnosis

Ankylosing spondylitis should be suspected in any patient complaining of low back pain, particularly if there is an associated iritis. One of the most helpful laboratory tests is the sedimentation rate, which is elevated in 80% of cases (65). A mild anemia may also be present. Rheumatoid factor, hypergammaglobulinemia, and antinuclear antibodies are not usually found in ankylosing spondylitis. Electrocardiographic abnormalities, such as atrioventricular block, left or right bundle branch block, and left ventricular hypertrophy, may reflect cardiac involvement.

While x-ray findings are most helpful in the diagnosis of ankylosing spondylitis, newer radiographic techniques appear to be even more sensitive. A bone scan using technetium-99m stannous pyrophosphate can detect early osteoblastic activity at the sacroiliac joints. By scanning the sacrum and sacroiliac joints, a sacroiliac-to-sacrum radioactivity ratio can be calculated. If this ratio is greater than 1.20, it is considered abnormal. This sensitive technique of scintigraphy involves 450 millirads of radiation, approximately half that received from a conventional x-ray of the lumbosacral spine. It appears to be a sensitive method for detecting sacroiliitis before radiologic evidence of this condition appears (98). When patients with acute anterior uveitis are studied by this technique, abnormal bone scans can be found in several who do not have radiographic changes of ankylosing spondylitis. While many of these patients are HLA-B27–positive, a number do not have this antigen. Scintigraphy, while not specific for ankylosing spondylitis, may prove useful in associating acute anterior uveitis with various spondylitic conditions (99).

Treatment

The treatment of ankylosing spondylitis involves the use of antiinflammatory agents to

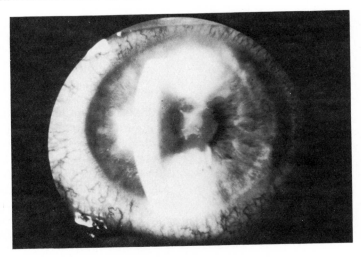

FIG. 8-2. Acute iridocyclitis in patient with ankylosing spondylitis. (Courtesy Dr. G. Mintsioulis)

decrease inflammation and pain, and the use of physical therapy to maintain muscle strength and functional joints. Phenylbutazone or indomethacin can be given but both of these agents are associated with significant toxic side effects, and hematologic function should be monitored in patients receiving them. Postural exercises such as lying flat for several periods during the day, breathing exercises and sleeping without a pillow are also useful. Collars and braces for back and neck support are sometimes used. Local heat treatment is also a part of the usual physical therapy.

The ocular disease is generally treated with frequent topical corticosteroid drops and cycloplegic–mydriatic drops. These should be instituted at the onset of acute inflammation

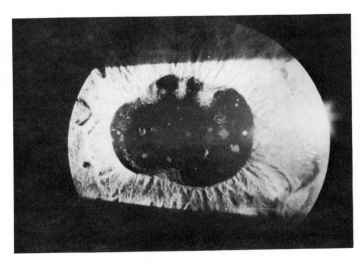

FIG. 8-3. Extensive posterior synechia formation in ankylosing spondylitis. (Courtesy Dr. G. Mintsioulis)

since synechia formation can develop rapidly. Patients who are prone to develop this type of iritis may find it beneficial to have these drops on hand so that they may be started as soon as a flare-up occurs. Because of the possibility of lens changes and glaucoma associated with steroid drops, their use should be limited to the acute phase of the iritis. Salicylates may be taken for long periods of time by patients who are able to tolerate this type of medication. Aspirin not only may help to control joint inflammation, but may reduce the frequency of uveitis flare-ups.

REITER'S SYNDROME

Reiter's syndrome consists of the triad of acute conjunctivitis, nonspecific urethritis, and arthritis. It usually occurs in sexually active males but may be seen following dysenteric infections with *Shigella*, *Yersinia*, or *Salmonella*. Of particular interest is the high incidence of HLA-B27 among patients developing Reiter's syndrome.

Immunopathology

Over 90% of patients with Reiter's syndrome have the histocompatibility antigen HLA-B27. The cause of Reiter's syndrome and the reason for its association with HLA-B27 are not actually known. There are, however, a number of theories. The B27 antigen may act as a favorable receptor site for certain pathogenic infectious agents. Various infectious agents, including *Chlamydia*, *Mycoplasma*, and *Shigella*, have been irregularly associated with Reiter's syndrome. A second possibility is that infectious agents which cause Reiter's syndrome and other rheumatoid variants share common antigens with the patient's own connective tissues. This could result in an inability to recognize and defend against the invading microbe or, alternatively, it could result in an immune response directed against the patient's tissues as well as against the infectious agent. A third possibility and the most widely accepted is that HLA-B27 is linked on the genetic material to an immune response gene, and that it is this

immune response gene which is responsible for the clinical syndrome. The immune response may be appropriately directed against an infectious agent or inappropriately directed against the patient's own tissues.

The immunologic abnormalities in patients with Reiter's syndrome are few. Cellular immunity is intact. Lymphocyte transformation has been demonstrated with *Chlamydia* and prostatic antigens (2). Cell-mediated immunity to autologous IgG has also been found in some patients with Reiter's syndrome (125).

Infectious agents have frequently been implicated in Reiter's syndrome. Schachter and associates were able to isolate and propagate a *Bedsonia* (*Chlamydia*) agent from synovial fluid, synovial membranes, urethras, and conjunctivas of patients with Reiter's syndrome (101). When the organism is recovered from the synovial membrane of a patient with Reiter's syndrome and inoculated into the anterior chamber of rabbits, ocular disease can be produced, consisting of papillary conjunctivitis, corneal edema, corneal opacities and neovascularization, and iritis (88). Several cases of Reiter's syndrome have also been reported in association with dysentery due to *Shigella* and other enteric pathogens (47). Thus it may be that certain infectious agents are capable of producing this syndrome in genetically susceptible individuals.

Clinical Features

The first manifestation of Reiter's syndrome is usually urethritis. This may be mucoid or mucopurulent and may be associated with dysuria. At other times, the patient may be entirely asymptomatic. Prostatitis is often associated with the urethritis. Several days after the urethritis begins, conjunctivitis develops. It is generally bilateral and mucopurulent. Papillary hypertrophy, lid edema, chemosis, and conjunctival hemorrhage are frequently present. A preauricular node is occasionally found. The conjunctivitis lasts for 2–4 weeks and then subsides spontaneously. Corneal involvement in Reiter's syndrome usually consists of a superficial punctate keratitis with underlying subepithelial opacities. Occasionally, pleomorphic anterior stromal infiltrates, marginal subepithelial opacities, epithelial bullae, and erosions may be seen.

Iritis has been reported in 8%–40% of patients with Reiter's syndrome. A hypopyon may be seen occasionally. Other ocular manifestations of Reiter's syndrome include episcleritis, recurrent retinal edema, and optic neuritis.

The arthritis is polyarticular and usually involves the large weight-bearing joints. A tendinitis particularly involving the Achilles tendon is fairly common. The sacroiliac joints and vertebral column may also become involved. While the skin and mucous membrane lesions are not part of the original triad, they are quite characteristic. One may see stomatitis, circinate balanitis, and a skin rash involving the palms and soles known as keratoderma blennorrhagicum. Other constitutional symptoms, including fever, minor weight loss, diarrhea, pericarditis, and myocarditis, have been reported. A leukocytosis of 10,000–20,000 with eosinophilia and anemia may occur.

Treatment

Reiter's syndrome is a self-limited disease and no specific therapy is available or usually necessary. Systemic tetracycline 1–1.5 g/day for 3 weeks has been recommended, since this drug is active against chlamydia, although its value is considered limited (88). A number of antiinflammatory agents, including aspirin, indomethacin, and phenlybutazone, may be effective in suppressing inflammation; however, salicylate hepatotoxicity has been associated with Reiter's syndrome (47). Iritis may be treated with topical steroids and cycloplegic–mydriatic drops to prevent synechia formation.

RHEUMATOID ARTHRITIS

Rheumatoid arthritis is a chronic, recurrent systemic inflammation which involves mainly the peripheral joints. It affects 2%–3% of the population and is three times more frequent in females than in males. The onset usually occurs between ages 30 and 50. The peripheral joints are involved first, in a symmetric fashion, and the arthritis usually progresses centripetally. There is no consistent pattern of inheritance and no known prevalence of any HLA antigen.

Immunopathology

The stimulus which initiates joint inflammation in rheumatoid arthritis is unknown. Certain microorganisms have been implicated in the pathogenesis of the disease; however, an infectious etiology is currently unproven. Viruses, particularly the slow viruses, may play a role, although no virus particles have definitely been identified. Attempts at isolation of *Mycoplasma* organisms and rubella virus from the joints of rheumatoid arthritis patients have been inconclusive (32). Hepatitis B virus, like many other infectious agents, can give rise to rheumatoid factor in serum. Hepatitis B virus, moreover, can form immune complexes and can produce a serum-sicknesslike syndrome with polyarthralgias and vasculitis during the prodromal phase of hepatitis. This virus seems to be the first known virus to produce a chronic rheumatic disorder in man. The clinical syndrome, however, does not resemble rheumatoid arthritis or systemic lupus erythematosus.

Other infectious etiologies in rheumatoid arthritis have been investigated. Rheumatoid synovial cells show a decreased sensitivity to infection with Newcastle disease virus and rubella virus. *Mycoplasma* antibodies have been isolated from rheumatoid arthritis patients, especially those with long-standing disease (58). Recently a very slow-growing infectious agent has been isolated from the synovial fluid of patients with rheumatoid arthritis. This agent has some properties of a *Mycoplasma*. However, other investigators have not found evidence of previous *Mycoplasma* infection in rheumatoid arthritis patients (21).

A variety of immunologic abnormalities have been noted in rheumatoid arthritis patients. Much evidence has been accumulated to support placing rheumatoid disease in the category of autoimmune diseases. Antibodies against IgG are formed in the blood and synovial fluid. Recently, it has been shown that IgG molecules in the serum of patients with rheumatoid arthritis have a conformational anomaly in the hinge region (59). This altered IgG may be recognized as abnormal by B lymphocyte receptors, and this in turn may lead to a humoral autoimmune response directed against IgG. Immune complexes are formed and are deposited in the joints (130) and other tissues. Immune complexes may even be found within plasma cells of the synovial membrane, a finding unparalleled in any other immunopathological disorder (83, 84). The immune complexes activate the complement system through the classic and alternate pathways, and it is felt that the interaction between immune complexes and the complement system contributes to the inflammation (84). Activation of the complement system results in a number of inflammatory phenomena, including chemotaxis of leukocytes, histamine release, and membrane damage with cell lysis. Enzymes released by the synovial leukocytes produce inflammatory changes in the joints and destruction of normal structures. The inflammatory response is amplified by the various humoral amplification systems.

The humoral immune system appears to be highly active and important in the pathogenesis of rheumatoid arthritis (Fig. 8-4). An increase in synovial B lymphocytes, which are precursors of antibody-producing plasma cells, is frequently found. Over 50% of the synovial plasma cells produce IgG rheumatoid factor, an antibody directed against other IgG molecules (82). While peripheral B cells are generally found in increased numbers, estimation of their numbers is hampered by the presence of antilymphocyte antibodies (127). When these antibodies are removed, peripheral B cells may in fact be found to be decreased. A variety of other antibodies have been identified in the serum of rheumatoid arthritis patients. These include antibodies to double-stranded DNA (7), antibodies to human native and denatured collagen (5), and antinuclear antibodies.

A number of defects in cellular immunity have also been associated with rheumatoid arthritis. Some 20% of rheumatoid arthritis patients are anergic when tested with multiple skin test antigens (4). T lymphocytes in the pe-

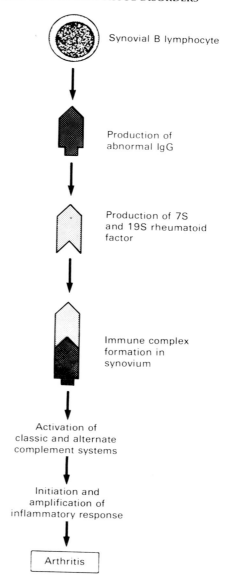

Synovial B lymphocyte

Production of abnormal IgG

Production of 7S and 19S rheumatoid factor

Immune complex formation in synovium

Activation of classic and alternate complement systems

Initiation and amplification of inflammatory response

Arthritis

FIG. 8-4. Hypothetical immunopathogenesis in rheumatoid arthritis. (Reproduced with permission from Fye K et al: Rheumatoid Diseases in Fudenberg H H et al: Basic and Clinical Immunology, Los Altos, Lange, 1976, p 366)

ripheral blood may be slightly increased, although some investigators have reported abnormally low percentages of T lymphocytes in the blood during active disease (126). An increased number of T cells are found, however, in synovial fluid obtained from actively inflamed joints (39). It has also been shown that heat-aggregated IgG, and to a lesser extent native IgG, causes inhibition of the migration of leukocytes from rheumatoid arthritis patients. This T cell mediated response to IgG antigens suggests a cellular immune component in rheumatoid arthritis. The soluble mediators of lymphocytes may also contribute to the inflammatory changes that exist in the rheumatoid joint.

A third population of lymphocytes, which are lacking in conventional B and T cell markers, may be important in the pathogenesis of rheumatoid disease. This population, known as "null cells," includes the so-called "killer" lymphocytes (K cells), which are cytotoxic to IgG-coated target cells (39). These K cells may be responsible for the formation of "rheumatoid rosettes," which are formed by lymphocytes interacting with IgG-coated erythrocytes. It should also be noted that peripheral blood leukocytes obtained from patients with rheumatoid arthritis may be cytotoxic for synovial cells (89).

Preparations of uvea–retina antigen, synovial membrane antigen, and articular cartilage antigen inhibit the migration of leukocytes taken from patients with rheumatoid arthritis (119). In ankylosing spondylitis, inhibition is induced only by synovial membrane antigens. Moreover, lymphocytes from the blood and synovial fluid of patients with rheumatoid arthritis demonstrate a markedly diminished blastogenic response to phytohemagglutinin and pokeweed mitogen (52).

The reason for depressed cellular immunity in rheumatoid arthritis is unknown. It may result from a preoccupation of the patient's immune mechanisms with cell-mediated immune reactions related to the pathogenesis of the disease. The depression of cellular immunity may also be related to a systemic viral infection. Immune-complex formation may suppress cellular immunity. In some instances, cellular immunity may be depressed by therapy for rheumatoid arthritis.

Clinical Features

General. Rheumatoid arthritis is a chronic, recurring inflammation which affects multiple joints in a symmetric pattern. It may be associated with constitutional symptoms such as malaise, fever, and weight loss. The arthritis begins in the distal joints, especially the proximal interphalangeal and the metacarpophalangeal joints, and progresses centripetally. Rheumatoid arthritis is characterized by early morning stiffness which improves with movement of the joints and is better later in the day. In the early stages there is fusiform swelling of the soft tissues around the involved joints. Later in the disease typical deformities occur, such as the boutonniere deformity (flexed proximal interphalangeal joints forced through the extensor hood) and the swan-neck deformity (hyperextension of the proximal interphalangeal joints and flexion of the distal interphalangeal joints). Subcutaneous nodules may be seen, especially over the bony eminences. Rheumatoid factor may be detected by immunologic means in most rheumatoid arthritis patients.

Extraarticular manifestations occur in a large number of patients. These include prominent atrophy of the skin and muscles of the extremities. Lymphadenopathy, splenomegaly, and leukocytopenia may be present. A diffuse vasculitis may occur, as well as interstitial lymphocytic pneumonitis or fibrosis. Rheumatoid cardiac disease may include a myocarditis, valvular insufficiency, and conduction disturbances. Pericarditis is found in 40% of autopsied rheumatoid patients. Peripheral neuropathy may occur secondary to an obliterative vasculitis. Sjögren's syndrome (to be discussed subsequently) may occur in up to 30% of rheumatoid arthritis patients.

Ocular Findings. Iridocyclitis often occurs in juvenile rheumatoid arthritis. In adults, by contrast, the association between iridocyclitis and rheumatoid arthritis is unusual and probably coincidental (65). Scleritis (Fig. 8-5) and sclerouveitis, however, occur frequently in rheumatoid arthritis patients and are important ocular complications of this disease. Frequently scleritis may be accompanied by inflammatory cells in the anterior chamber; however, this is considered a "spillover" reaction from the inflamed sclera and not a true iridocyclitis.

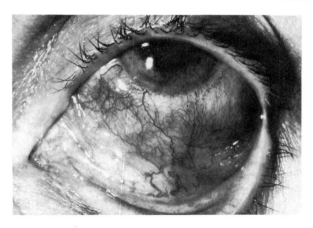

FIG. 8-5. Scleritis in patient with rheumatoid arthritis.

Scleritis and episcleritis have been classified by Watson and Hayreh (124). Scleritis may be broadly divided into anterior scleritis and a much less frequent posterior scleritis. Anterior scleritis in turn may be divided into diffuse anterior scleritis, nodular scleritis, and necrotizing scleritis. Necrotizing scleritis may occur with or without inflammation; the latter condition is often termed **scleromalacia perforans** (Fig. 8-6). Episcleritis may be classified as simple or nodular in type.

Both scleritis and episcleritis present with similar symptoms. The patient complains of redness of the eyes, lacrimation, and photophobia. Pain is a prominent feature of both conditions but is generally worse in scleritis. It may be a boring pain and may radiate to the orbital margin, the temple, or the jaw. Pain is rarely complained of in scleromalacia perforans, in which there is no surrounding inflammation. Severe pain is not a feature of episcleritis, but patients do complain of discomfort which is not sharp and aching. Frank discharge does not occur in either condition, and if it is found the diagnosis of scleritis or episcleritis should be questioned.

In addition to a good history, careful examination is required for differentiating between scleritis and episcleritis. This involves an examination in daylight and a slit-lamp examination, which may include the use of red-free light. A thorough eye examination, including funduscopy, and a systemic medical examination should be included in the workup of all scleritis patients.

The slit-lamp examination is directed toward the detection of scleral edema. This can be diagnosed when both the superficial and deep episcleral blood vessels are elevated. If only the superficial plexus is elevated, episcleritis rather than scleritis is probably present (Fig. 8-7). Injection of the deep episcleral vessels produces a bluish discoloration in scleritis. There may be tenderness over the involved sclera. Ischemic patches can be detected in 27% of patients with scleritis. Funduscopic changes such as serous detachment of the retina and proptosis are infrequent

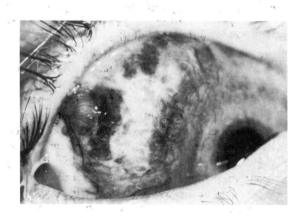

FIG. 8-6. Scleromalacia perforans.

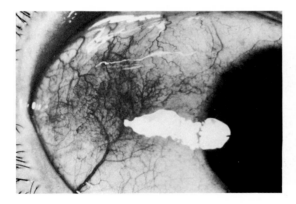

FIG. 8-7. Episcleritis with injection of the conjunctival vessels and superficial episcleral plexus.

findings and generally indicate a posterior scleritis. Nodule formation can occur in either scleritis or episcleritis. As the scleral inflammation progresses, marked thinning may occur. In severe scleritis, scleral thinning may lead to prolapse of uveal tissue, and scleral grafting may be required.

Episcleritis is characterized by injection of the superficial episcleral plexus and the overlying conjunctival vessels. There may be intense redness which is often sectoral. Episcleral edema and deposits may sometimes be observed. Tenderness is also a feature of episcleritis. Episcleritis most frequently occurs in the interpalpebral region; however, scleritis has a fairly even distribution over all four quadrants of the anterior sclera.

It is helpful, in differentiating scleritis and episcleritis, to put a drop of 10% phenylephrine (Neo-Synephrine) or epinephrine 1:1000 in the conjunctival sac. These adrenergic agents will constrict the conjunctival and superficial episcleral vessels more than the deep episcleral vessels. Frequently this allows one to observe scleral injection and edema.

Scleritis and episcleritis may be associated with decreased vision if there is an accompanying keratitis. This may take the form of a sclerosing keratitis or peripheral gutter formation (Fig. 8-8). Corneal changes in scleritis may occur in up to 29% of patients. Lipid deposition and vascularization may follow a severe keratitis. The most severe corneal complica-

tion is keratolysis. This rare complication may be seen in patients who have a very severe necrotizing scleritis and is accompanied by rapid disappearance of the corneal stroma. Although cataract formation may occur after long-term use of topical or systemic steroids, keratitis may be considered the major cause for decreased vision associated with scleritis. Keratitis is less common in episcleritis but is sometimes seen in the superficial and midstromal layers.

Scleritis is accompanied by a systemic illness in 46% of patients (124). In 15%, a connective tissue disorder can be diagnosed, and in 10% a diagnosis of rheumatoid arthritis can be made. Other commonly associated systemic diseases include gout and chronic granulomatous disease. In episcleritis, it is rare to find an associated systemic disease. However, allergy, gout, and herpes zoster may sometimes be diagnosed. In most studies the frequency of scleritis in the rheumatoid arthritis population is less than 1% (76). The incidence of rheumatoid arthritis in a scleritis population, however, may be as high as 33%.

Diagnosis

A variety of laboratory abnormalities may accompany rheumatoid arthritis. The mainstay of laboratory diagnosis is the detection of rheumatoid factor. This antibody directed against IgG is found in over 75% of rheuma-

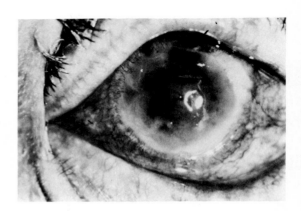

FIG. 8-8. Corneal furrow formation in rheumatoid arthritis. (Courtesy Dr. G. Mintsioulis)

toid arthritis patients. Rheumatoid factor may be an IgM molecule or it may be of the IgG or IgA class. It can be detected by several methods. The most commonly used screening methods involve inert particles such as latex and bentonite (Fig. 8-9). These inert particles are coated with denatured IgG. When serum containing rheumatoid factor is added to the slide, flocculation occurs and indicates a positive test. While a slide test is generally used, the semiquantitative tube test is somewhat more accurate. The best test for rheumatoid factor is the Rose–Waaler test. It depends on specific antibody binding and is the most reliable test in common use. Tanned sheep red blood cells are coated with rabbit antibody against the red cells. These sensitized sheep cells will agglutinate in the presence of rheumatoid factor. More complicated tests include a radioimmunoassay for IgM rheumatoid factor and an immunodiffusion assay. It should be kept in mind that a negative rheumatoid factor test does not rule out a diagnosis of rheumatoid arthritis. Seronegative patients may have IgG or IgM rheumatoid factor or circulating IgG–anti-IgG complexes. Conversely, a positive rheumatoid factor does not necessarily indicate rheumatoid arthritis. False-positive tests are found in a large number of diseaes, including systemic lupus erythematosus, Sjögren's syndrome, scleroderma, and polymyositis. In addition, positive latex or bentonite tests may occur in individuals with hypergammaglobulinemia, liver disease, kala azar, sarcoidosis, and syphilis. In these conditions, the sheep red cell test is generally negative. In some chronic conditions, including leprosy and tuberculosis, both latex and sheep red cell tests may be positive.

Besides rheumatoid factor, certain other laboratory abnormalities are found in rheumatoid arthritis. α_2-Globulin may be increased or there may be a polyclonal hypergammaglobulinemia. Albumin may be decreased. Cryoprecipitins may be present, and serologic tests for syphilis are positive in 5%–10% of cases. LE cell preparation are positive in 8%–10% and antinuclear antibodies are found in 20%–70% of rheumatoid arthritis patients. Serum complement levels are generally nor-

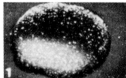

Positive result   Negative result

FIG. 8-9. Rheumatoid factor (RF) test: Agglutination of IgG-coated latex particles by serum from rheumatoid arthritis patient.

mal; however, complement levels in synovial fluid are generally decreased due to immune-complex deposition. The sedimentation rate is generally elevated in active rheumatoid disease and in 37% of patients with scleritis and 14% of patients with episcleritis (124). Other laboratory abnormalities are unusual in scleritis and episcleritis but may include a positive latex fixation test, positive serologic tests for syphilis, and an elevated serum uric acid.

Treatment

The treatment of rheumatoid arthritis frequently involves the use of salicylates. Most patients can tolerate 3.6–6 g/day. High-dosage aspirin therapy is associated with numerous side effects, including tinnitus, gastric upset, and gastrointestinal blood loss. Since aspirin also causes decreased platelet adhesiveness, it should be used only with great caution in patients with bleeding tendencies and in those taking anticoagulants. Other nonsteroidal agents which have been used include indomethacin, phenylbutazone, ibuprofen, and naproxen. These drugs may also be accompanied by serious side effects, particularly hematologic ones; however, they may be useful in patients who cannot tolerate aspirin.

Antimalarial drugs are frequently used in the treatment of rheumatoid arthritis. These agents also have side effects, including nausea and vomiting, skin rashes, and corneal and retinal changes. A doughnut-shaped or bull's-eye–shaped macular lesion is characteristic of chloroquine toxicity. Ocular toxicity in general is related to excessively high drug dosages. In patients whose dosage has been moderate, ocular toxicity rarely occurs and may represent an idiosyncratic reaction (105). The corneal deposits which are typical of chloroquine keratopathy are observed in about 10% of treated patients and are generally reversible. Ocular examination should probably be repeated every 3–6 months in patients receiving long-term chloroquine therapy.

Other forms of systemic therapy have been advocated. Gold salts are thought to act by stabilizing lysosomal membranes; however, their exact mode of action is unclear. Corticosteroids and antimetabolites are frequently used in the treatment of rheumatoid disease for their antiinflammatory properties. Penicillamine has proved to be a useful drug although its mechanism of action is currently unknown.

Besides drug therapy, a treatment program in rheumatoid arthritis should include physiotherapy. Surgical procedures are sometimes carried out to correct or compensate for joint damage. Some authorities suggest synovectomy to prevent joint damage and deformity.

Treatment of episcleritis usually involves the use of topical steroids for a short period of time; often no treatment at all is necessary.

Topical steroids alone are not generally effective in scleritis. Systemic medication is often necessary. This may be in the form of systemic steroids or nonsteroidal antiinflammatory agents such as oxyphenbutazone or indomethacin. Treatment is continued until the condition has been lessened for 7 days. Periocular steroid injections have also been recommended in the treatment of scleritis, but there is some feeling that they may contribute to scleral thinning in some patients. If the sclera becomes unusually thin and perforation is imminent, scleral grafting may be required. Surgery, however, is rarely necessary. Corneal grafting may occasionally be required in patients with marked corneal gutter formation.

JUVENILE RHEUMATOID ARTHRITIS

Juvenile rheumatoid arthritis (JRA) is a major chronic and progressive crippling disease of childhood. It has a peak incidence between the ages of 2 and 4, and a smaller peak between the ages of 10 and 12. It occurs twice as often in females as in males and has an average duration of about 6½ years. A major complication of juvenile rheumatoid arthritis is chronic iridocyclitis. This may be associated with significant visual disability, and is one of the leading causes of uveitis in childhood. Juvenile rheumatoid arthritis is conveniently divided into three forms: 1) an acute, toxic form, or **Still's disease;** 2) a polyarticular form; and 3) a monoarticular or a pauci- or oligoarticular form. It is this last group which has the highest incidence of iridocyclitis.

Immunopathology

Unlike the case in adult rheumatoid arthritis, rheumatoid factor is not commonly found in patients with juvenile rheumatoid arthritis. In JRA, the incidence of positive tests is between 10% and 20%, whereas in the adult disease it is between 50% and 85%. On the other hand, antinuclear antibodies (ANA) are found in 20%–40% of children with JRA (103). Antinuclear antibodies are found mainly in children with pauciarticular and polyarticular JRA, and rarely in the systemic form (Still's disease). Of considerable interest is the fact that ANA are found in 88% of JRA patients who have chronic iridocyclitis (102). Antinuclear antibodies are predominantly of the IgG immunoglobulin class and titers are 1:50 or higher in most patients. The consistent homogeneity of the nuclear fluorescence pattern is typical of reactivty against deoxyribonucleoprotein (38). Antibodies to DNA and RNA have generally not been demonstrated, although there have been recent reports of antibodies against double-stranded RNA in children with JRA and iridocyclitis (34). A positive finding of ANA usually precedes the onset of iridocyclitis and this may provide a useful test for identifying patients with JRA who are at risk of developing chronic iridocyclitis. The reason for a positive ANA finding in this disease is not known. Both infectious processes and immune defects have been associated with the formation of ANA and other autoantibodies.

Smooth-muscle antibodies, usually of the IgM class, are found in 15%–23% of patients with JRA and iridocyclitis; however, this incidence is no greater than that found among control groups. HLA antigens have been examined in patients with JRA. Some investigators report an increased incidence of HLA-B27 (13, 90). Other investigators have not found an increased incidence of B27 among JRA patients (80, 87), and suggest that earlier studies included patients with ankylosing spondylitis, which may mimic JRA in the early stages.

The clinical picture of Still's disease suggests the possibility of a disseminated infection. The evidence for an infectious etiology is scanty, however. A rise in antibody titer to coxsackie B3 and A9 virus and the isolation of adenovirus 7 have been reported (61). An increased titer of rubella virus antibody as well as isolation of rubella virus antigen from synovial fluid has also been reported. Perhaps a viral infection combined with defective immune responses allows the infection to persist, and this may account for the clinical findings in JRA.

Clinical Features

General. The acute toxic form (Still's disease) accounts for 20%–25% of all patients with JRA. The mean age at onset is 4½ years. Patients present with arthralgias and fever as high as 106˚. Other findings include lymphadenopathy, splenomegaly, myocarditis, pericarditis, and pneumonitis. The polyarticular form accounts for 50% of patients with JRA. Systemic findings are less common; however, 20% have a tachycardia that is out of proportion to the fever. The most common joints involved are the knees, followed by the wrists, ankles, and cervical spine. In older children, the joints of the hands and feet are typically involved.

The monoarticular or oligoarticular variety accounts for 25%–30% of JRA patients. They present with pain, stiffness, and swelling of the affected joints. The pain is mild unless the hip is involved, in which case pain may be severe. The knees are the most frequent joints involved, followed by the hips, ankles, elbows, and heels. Systemic symptoms are occasionally present, but in general the patient appears to be in good health. Iridocyclitis is most common in this group of patients, occurring in about 20%. The ocular involvement usually

follows the arthritis but may occasionally precede it.

Other clinical findings in JRA include a salmon-pink rash in 30%–40% of patients, subcutaneous nodules in less than 10%, and myocarditis, pericarditis, and splenomegaly in 10%–25%. The prognosis for the joint disease is most favorable in the monoarticular or oligoarticular form; however, as mentioned, it is this group that is most likely to develop ocular disease. The ultimate course of the arthritis is more severe when polyarthritis develops.

Ocular Findings. The mean age at onset of ocular disease if 5½ years, with a range of 3–12 years. Girls are affected four times more frequently than boys (112). The disease is bilateral in two-thirds of the cases, and the second eye becomes involved within a few months of the first or not at all. Often there are no symptoms and in over half of the cases the ocular disease is entirely silent. The earliest signs may be a minimal transient redness of the eye, an irregular pupil, or leukocoria.

The classic ocular triad of JRA includes chronic iridocyclitis, band keratopathy, and complicated cataract. The iridocyclitis is usually low-grade, smoldering, chronic, and nongranulomatous. The eyes are minimally injected. Inflammatory cells are seen in the anterior chamber, and posterior and anterior synechiae may be present. Posterior uveitis rarely occurs. Secondary glaucoma is not uncommon and calcific band keratopathy is quite common (Fig. 8-10). A complicated cataract frequently occurs, especially in patients who are taking long-term steroid therapy. The duration of the uveitis ranges from 1 to 21 years, with a median of 5–6 years (62). The activity of the uveitis appears to be independent of the activity of the joint disease.

The ultimate prognosis for visual acuity is variable. In one study, 30% of patients had vision reduced to 20/200 or less (62). Cataract surgery in this disease also meets with varying degrees of success. Some have found that vision improved in most cases following cataract surgery (62), while others have found the results of surgery disappointing (113).

An acute iridocyclitis has been described in association with JRA. Many such cases even-

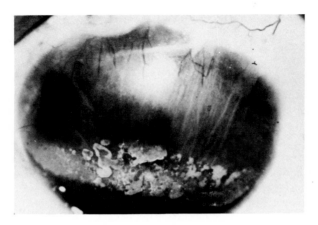

FIG. 8-10. Band keratopathy in juvenile rheumatoid arthritis. (Courtesy Dr. I Wong)

tually develop a spondylitis with radiographic changes and may represent a variant of ankylosing spondylitis rather than juvenile rheumatoid arthritis.

Treatment

In general, treatment of the uveitis associated with JRA should include cycloplegics and mydriatics to prevent posterior synechiae. Topical steroids should be given when necessary to treat acute exacerbations. Long-term use of topical steroids, however, should be avoided. Steroid injections beneath Tenon's capsule or oral steroids may be given if persistent macular edema develops. Again, these agents should be used with caution. Band keratopathy responds well to chelation with edetate (EDTA).

Treatment of the joint disease must be individualized. Exercise in association with drug therapy is generally used. Salicylates are usually the first choice because of their analgesic and antiinflammatory effects. They inhibit the production of kallikrein enzymes and the release of prostaglandins from platelets and the spleen. They also decrease joint inflammation. Gold salt therapy and antimalarials have been used in conjunction with aspirin, but the latter are not recommended in children because they can cause arterial hypotension and central nervous system depression. Indomethacin and phenylbutazone are less useful in JRA than in certain other diseases. Repeated

routine eye examinations are essential in children with juvenile rheumatoid arthritis.

SYSTEMIC LUPUS ERYTHEMATOSUS

Systemic lupus erythematosus (SLE) is a multisystem collagen vascular disease. The etiology is unknown; however, hereditary, immunologic, and microbiologic factors seem to be involved. SLE is characterized by a tendency to form autoantibodies, especially to constituents of the cell nucleus. The main organ systems affected are the joints, skin, kidneys, lungs, and heart. The eye and central nervous system may also be involved. SLE occurs most commonly in women of the child-bearing age and has a greater incidence in nonwhites than in whites.

Immunopathology

Recent investigations have shown that genetic susceptibility, possible viral infection, and abnormal control of the immune system interact in the pathogenesis of SLE. Antibody formation to double-stranded DNA (ds-DNA) occurs frequently and is associated with disease activity. Depressed T cell activity, enhanced B cell activity, and decreased serum complement are also prominent features of SLE.

Much of our current understanding about SLE is derived from animal studies using the

New Zealand black (NZB) mouse, an animal model for SLE. NZB mice have a deficiency of suppressor T cells and a related decrease in the concentration of a circulating thymic hormone known as thymosin. NZB mice are immunologically impaired and are susceptible to various infections, including those caused by oncogenic viruses. NZB mice and hybrids between NZB and New Zealand white mice have been studied extensively. NZB and hybrid mice as well as humans with SLE produce antinuclear antibodies in their blood. Both the mice and humans with SLE have deposits of immune complexes, as well as components of the complement system, in their kidneys. These complexes contain DNA and antibodies against DNA. The source of the DNA is not known. It could be released from damaged cells, possibly as the result of viral infection. Alternatively, the DNA could itself be of viral origin. Viruses have been implicated in the development of human SLE and in the mouse disease. A virus has been identified in NZB mice and it is transmitted genetically from parent to progeny in the egg and sperm. Thus, copies of the viral genome can be incorporated into the cellular genome. It has been suggested that a genetic defect in NZB mice permits genetic expression of the virus and that this in turn results in an autoimmune disease. The pathologic changes might be due to the development of antibodies against viral components which could form immune complexes with viral antigen and be deposited in the kidneys and other organs. A second possibility is that viral antigens on cell surfaces provoke an immunologic attack on these infected cells, which are not recognized by the host as "self." Antigens related to those of type C virus have been identified on the lymphocytes and in the kidneys of some individuals with SLE.

Currently the most popular hypothesis for the pathogenesis of SLE is as follows: The infectious agent is a type C RNA virus which is known to be transmitted genetically in animals. Owing to a genetic predisposition of the host, the virus is allowed to avoid the immune surveillance system and home in on, replicate, or express itself in the thymus. The thymic alteration may eventually destroy T cell function either directly or through an autoimmune mechanism. Further viral replication and dissemination is allowed because of the resulting defect in cellular immunity. This leads to an enhanced humoral immune response, so that immune complexes are formed, circulated, and deposited in various organs. Inflammatory reactions against these complexes result with activation of the complement system. Inflammation and clinical disease then develop.

Studies of lymphocytes from patients with SLE indicate that T cells are markedly reduced in active SLE. The population of null cells, however, is increased. The number of B cells is usually found to be normal. The T cell lymphopenia may be due to an increase in the number of null cells, which may simply be immature T cells. Exposure to thymus tissue may allow these null cells to mature and increase the population of T cells.

The function of monocyte/macrophages has also been shown to be depressed early in the course of SLE. Since these cells are involved in the processing of antigen and in lymphokine activity, this defect could result in a depression of cellular immunity (69). A lupus like syndrome has also been associated with a deficiency of the second component of complement (C2) (31). Perhaps an inherited deficiency of this component could predispose individuals to lupus or to faulty handling of viral infections.

Histocompatibility antigens have been investigated in SLE and also in discoid lupus erythematosus (DLE), a cutaneous variant of SLE. In female patients, SLE shows a significant association with HLA-B8, while patients with DLE show an increased incidence of HLA-B7 and HLA-B8 (77, 78).

Clinical Features

General. Virtually any organ system can be affected in SLE. At least 90% of patients have constitutional symptoms, with fever being the most common. A polyarthritis may involve any peripheral joint, with those of the hands, wrists, and knees being most commonly affected. Skin lesions are seen in at least 75% of patients with SLE; however, the characteristic butterfly rash occurs in a relatively small number of patients. Vasculitic lesions, purpura, bullae, urticaria, and alopecia have all been reported. Raynaud's phenomenon occurs in about 50% of patients with SLE.

Two-thirds of patients will develop serositis, with pleurisy and pericarditis being common. Cardiopulmonary lesions, including myocarditis and endocarditis, may also be seen. Pneumonitis is relatively rare.

Renal involvement occurs in 75% of patients with SLE. Four fairly distinct histologic types of lupus nephritis may be seen. 1) Focal proliferative disease shows electron-dense deposits in mesangial areas. These lesions are associated with mild to moderate proteinuria and respond to corticosteroid therapy. 2) Diffuse proliferative glomerlonephritis occurs, with extensive proliferation of endothelial and mesangial cells. Inflammation extends to the tubules and the interstitium. Deposits of DNA–anti-DNA complexes can be demonstrated by immunofluorescence. This kidney lesion is associated with hematuria, proteinuria, and cylindruria and if untreated will progress to renal failure within 1–3 years. 3) Membranous lupus nephritis is associated with electron-dense deposits at subepithelial and intramembranous sites, with thickening and deformity of glomerular capillary walls. There is diffuse thickening of the basement membrane, and immunofluorescence reveals a characteristic "lumpy bumpy" staining pattern. This form of nephritis presents with the nephrotic syndrome and progresses to renal failure. 4) Interstitial disease is marked by substantial or complete sparing of the glomeruli. Immunofluorescence shows bright, granular deposits along the tubular basement membranes and the interstitium.

Another area of involvement is the central nervous system. Convulsions, cranial nerve palsies, lethargy, and cerebral vascular accidents may be seen. Peripheral neuritis is uncommon. The gastorintestinal system may be involved by a vasculitis. Pancreatitis, hepatomegaly, and splenomegaly may be seen. Sjögren's syndrome occurs in 5%–10% of patients with SLE.

A drug-induced lupuslike syndrome is seen with certain common medications, including hydralazine and procainamide. Other agents which have been implicated are phenytoin, trimethadione, mephenytoin, isoniazid, penicillamine, penicillin, tetracycline, sulfonamides, streptomycin, griseofulvin, phenylbutazone, oral contraceptives, methyldopa, and levodopa.

Ocular Findings. SLE may affect most areas of the eye. The skin of the lids may be involved in the typical butterfly eruption. Telangiectasias and purpura may be seen. The so-called "Boston lids" are characterized by multiple telangiectatic vessels lying just above the cilia line of the upper lids. This finding is most obvious when the disease is active. The conjunctiva may be involved and may demonstrate simple hyperemia (Fig 8-11) or isolated, sharply marginated, phlyctenulelike necrotic patches. Keratoconjunctivitis sicca with filamentous keratopathy may occur and tears may show an absence of lysozyme. Conjunctivitis and conjunctival scarring have also been reported with SLE (122).

Corneal lesions include a punctate epithelial keratitis with hyperkeratosis and recurrent erosions. Vascularized peripheral infiltrations have also been reported. A bilateral, band-shaped accumulation of grayish white granular material has been described in the deep stroma of some patients with SLE (93). This deep or disciform keratitis is avascular and may be complicated by large ulcerations with sharp margins. The keratitis may lead to corneal opacities or even perforation. Corneal staining is a frequent sign of SLE. It occurs just inside the limbus where the upper lid touches the cornea. It is seen in almost 90% of patients with SLE (114).

Rarely, the anterior uvea may be involved in association with corneal infiltrates. The posterior uvea occasionally contains grayish white or yellowish foci of miliary infiltrates (107). A nodular necrotizing scleritis may rarely be seen.

The retina is the ocular tissue most frequently involved in SLE. Cotton-wool spots are observed in about 20% of cases. This is particularly characteristic of the later stages of the disease, and is associated with an occlusive vasculitis of the ganglion cell layer. The cot-

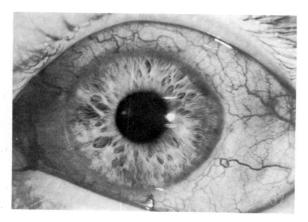

FIG. 8-11. Conjunctival hyperemia in systemic lupus erythematosus.

ton-wool spots are white and not sharply outlined, and are located in the posterior pole, where two or three are often seen. They are usually about one-quarter disc diameter in size. They may disappear after a few weeks, sometimes leaving atrophic patches. Scattered hemorrhages and exudates may also be seen in the retina. Sometimes these are associated with hypertensive retinopathy. Basically, two types of retinopathy are seen. In classic retinopathy, cotton-wool spots are usually present. These are probably related to narrowing or occlusion of miniscule arterioles. The second type of retinopathy is associated with disease of larger vessels and is manifested by thrombotic and vasospastic occlusions of larger arterioles (23). It has been suggested that the slow flow of blood in the retinal vessels prolongs the contact between antigen–antibody complexes and the vessel wall, a process which leads to sheathing and necrosis (23).

Fluorescein angiography in SLE frequently shows microaneurysms, capillary dilation, leakage of dye, and drusen (100). Retinal microangiopathy may be demonstrated by fluorescein angiography even when no ophthalmoscopic abnormalities are seen (100).

Other ocular manifestations of SLE include papilledema due to intracranial hypertension, ischemic papillitis, perivasculitis, detachment of the retina, and central retinal artery occlu-

sions. Numerous complications occur as a result of therapy with steroids or antimalarial drugs. These include posterior subcapsular cataracts due to steroids, and the characteristic corneal and retinal changes associated with chloroquine (Fig. 8-12).

Diagnosis

The hallmark of SLE is the demonstration of antinuclear antibodies in the serum. Immunoglobulins of all classes may form antinuclear antibodies. Several patterns of staining have been reported that are characteristic of certain types of antibodies or antigens (Table 8-1). 1) A homogeneous staining pattern is typical with antideoxyribonucleoprotein antibodies and is strongly associated with active SLE. 2) The peripheral rim, or "shaggy," pattern is associated with anti–double stranded DNA antibodies and antibodies to soluble nucleoprotein. It is also characteristic of active SLE. 3) The speckled pattern results from fluorescence scattered throughout the nucleus. It is associated with two antigens: one, the Sm antigen, is a macromolecule resistant to ribonuclease and slowly destroyed by trypsin; the other is an antigen associated with ribonucleoprotein which is sensitive to both ribonuclease and trypsin. The speckled pattern is seen less frequently in SLE but is seen commonly with scleroderma. 4) The nucleolar pattern is asso-

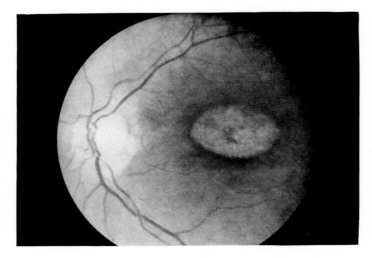

FIG. 8-12. Chloroquine retinopathy. (Courtesy Dr. R. Dennis)

ciated with ribosomal antigen and is also seen commonly in scleroderma and less frequently in SLE. All patterns of immunofluorescence staining should be interpreted with caution. The sensitivity may vary with different techniques, and a homogeneous pattern may obscure other underlying patterns.

Anti-DNA antibodies, including those to single-stranded and double-stranded DNA, are usually of the IgG or IgM type. Antibodies to double-stranded RNA, antierythrocyte anti-bodies, circulating anticoagulants, and anti-platelet antibodies may also be demonstrated. False-positive serologic tests for syphilis, including both the VDRL and, less often, the FTA-ABS tests, may be present in SLE (111). Other autoantibodies may be detectable in SLE, including rheumatoid factor and organ-specific antibodies to muscle, liver, kidney, and joint tissue, as well as anticytoplasmic antibodies (antimitochondrial, antiribosomal, and antilysosomal).

TABLE 8-1. RELATIONSHIP OF ANTINUCLEAR ANTIBODIES TO IMMUNOFLUORESCENT PATTERN AND TO DISEASE

Disease	Pattern of nuclear staining (immunofluorescence)	Specificity of antibody
Systemic lupus erythematosus	Rim	DNA or nucleoprotein
	Diffuse	Nucleoprotein
	Speckled	Sm antigen or ribonucleoprotein
Drug-induced lupus (procainamide, hydralazine)	Diffuse	Nucleoprotein
Mixed connective tissue disease (MCTD)	Speckled	Ribonucleoprotein
Scleroderma (Progressive systemic sclerosis; PSS)	Speckled	Ribonucleoprotein (low incidence); others unknown
	Nucleolar	4–6S RNA; others unknown
Sjögren's syndrome	Speckled	Unknown
	Nucleolar	4–6S RNA; others unknown
	Diffuse	Unknown
Rheumatoid arthritis	Diffuse	Unknown

(Adapted from Tan EM, Northway JD, Pinnas JL: Postgrad Med 54:148, 1973. In Freedman SO, Gold P (eds): Clinical Immunology, 2nd ed. Hagerstown, Harper & Row, 1976, p 264)

Another immunologic laboratory finding in SLE is the LE cell phenomenon. The LE cell is a neutrophil which has ingested a large homogeneous mass of deoxyribonucleoprotein. The formation of the LE cell is dependent upon an IgG antibody which reacts with nuclear protein of damaged leukocytes in the presence of complement and leads to destruction of the normal chromatin pattern. The positive LE cell test is observed in 75%–80% of patients with SLE.

Treatment

Corticosteroids are the mainstay of treatment for the systemic disease. When arthritis is the predominant symptom and activity of the disease is low, aspirin and antimalarials may be of great benefit. Treatment for the ocular disease is symptomatic. It usually involves tear replacement, dilation of the pupils to prevent posterior synechiae when iritis is severe, and sometimes topical corticosteroids. Cytotoxic and immunosuppressive agents have been used for the treatment of systemic disease.

SJÖGREN'S SYNDROME

Sjögren's syndrome is a chronic inflammatory disease of unknown origin which primarily affects the lacrimal and salivary glands. Clinically, the hallmark of this disease is dryness of the oral mucosa, conjunctiva, and other mucous membranes. Half of the patients with Sjögren's syndrome have rheumatoid arthritis and a smaller group have other connective tissue diseases.

Immunopathology

Patients with Sjögren's syndrome develop lymphocytic infiltrates and tissue destruction in the salivary and lacrimal glands as well as in other tissues. Both T and B lymphocytes have been detected in the salivary gland infiltrates (92). Examination of the peripheral blood of patients with Sjögren's syndrome generally shows a modest increase in peripheral B lymphocytes. T lymphocytes are reduced in about one-third of the patients. The lymphocytes infiltrating the salivary glands synthesize IgM and IgG locally, as well as rheumatoid factor and other autoantibodies.

Hypergammaglobulinemia is the most frequent finding in Sjögren's syndrome and is usually of the polyclonal type. Rheumatoid factor is found in at least three-fourths of the patients, and the titers are especially high in those with keratoconjunctivitis sicca and xerostomia alone. Antinuclear antibody is found in about 90% of patients with Sjögren's syndrome; staining is usually of the homogeneous or speckled pattern (8). Anti–double-stranded DNA antibodies and LE cells are found in a smaller percentage of patients. Autoantibodies against salivary duct antigens may be detected in about 50% of Sjögren's syndrome patients.

While antibody formation in Sjögren's syndrome is exuberant, cellular immunity appears to be somewhat depressed. Patients may not develop delayed hypersensitivity to contact allergens (109), and peripheral blood lymphocytes do not respond normally to mitogens. Cellular hypersensitivity to salivary gland extracts has been demonstrated in patients with Sjögren's syndrome using peripheral blood lymphocytes. Perhaps T lymphocyte sensitization to salivary gland antigens with production of lymphokines occurs and is responsible for the pathologic changes. It is felt that in Sjögren's syndrome, as in other autoimmune disorders, a defect in T suppressor cells exists. A deficiency of T suppressor cells may allow B cells to proliferate in an uncontrolled fashion and to make overactive immune responses, including the formation of autoantibodies.

Patients with Sjögren's syndrome have a predisposition to develop lymphoproliferative disorders (26). These include lymphomas, leukemias, and Waldenstrom's macroglobulinemias. An intermediate stage of lymphoproliferation, known as "pseudolymphoma," may occur. Whether Sjögren's syndrome is the result of a slow or latent viral disease or is a disorder of immunologic regulation remains to be determined.

Clinical Features

General. Sjögren's syndrome has an insidious onset and usually occurs in middle age. Over

90% of patients are female. Most often the course is benign and chronic. However, when the sicca complex occurs, the onset is frequently rapid and is associated with episodic keratitis. Clinically, a dry mouth due to salivary gland hyposecretion is present. Patients complain of difficulty in chewing or swallowing foods, and of dry lips and mouth. Parotid gland enlargement occurs in about 50% of patients with Sjögren's syndrome. The nasal mucosa may become dry and crusted, with recurrent epistaxis. The larynx and respiratory tract may also be dry leading to hoarseness and a dry throat. The vaginal mucosa may be dry, causing a burning sensation or dyspareunia. Splenomegaly occurs in 25%, and hepatomegaly in about 20% of patients. Raynaud's phenomenon is seen in 20% of cases and chronic thyroiditis of Hashimoto's type is occasionally seen. Gastrointestinal involvement is sometimes seen and is manifested by dysphagia. A high incidence of adverse drug reactions is also known to occur. Penicillin, gold salts, antibiotics, aspirin, and barbiturates are most frequently implicated. Sjögren's syndrome has a benign course; however, the ultimate fate of the patient is determined by the severity of the associated connective tissue disorder.

Ocular Findings. The ocular symtoms in Sjögren's syndrome are due to deficient secretion of the lacrimal glands. Patients with Sjögren's syndrome have a dry eye syndrome and keratoconjunctivitis sicca. They complain of ocular irritation, redness, a foreign body sensation, itching, burning, and photophobia. They may report a lack of tears in response to emotional stimuli.

Clinically, one may observe a bilateral condition with injected conjunctivas, chemosis, and sometimes redness of the lid margins. Corneal filaments which are true epithelial filaments may be present. The tear film is thin and more viscous than usual, with epithelial and mucous debris. The corneal epithelium contains opacities which are small, gray, and poorly defined. The corneal surface may have an irregular or pitted appearance. Punctate staining may be observed on the cornea and bulbar conjunctiva, especially in the interpalpebral region. Tear breakup time may be rapid and the extent of moisture in the Schirmer test is usually less than 5mm. Tear lysozyme can be measured by use of the Schirmer test strips and the *Micrococcus,* a microorganism which is very sensitive to it. Tear lysozyme will be deficient or absent in Sjögren's syndrome. Keratinized epithelial cells can usually be demonstrated by a Giemsa stain of conjunctival scrapings (Fig. 8-13).

Complications that occur in Sjögren's syndrome are often due to the deficiency of tears. These include ulceration and vascularization of the cornea, and sometimes scarring and perforation (67). Perforation is a particular hazard when topical corticosteroids are used in treating patients with keratoconjunctivitis sicca.

A probable diagnosis of Sjögren's syndrome can be made if two of the following three features are present: 1) recurrent or chronic idiopathic swelling of the salivary glands, 2) unexplained xerostomia, and 3) a connective tissue disease. A definite diagnosis of Sjögren's syndrome can be made if objective evidence of keratoconjunctivitis sicca is present or if typical histopathologic changes are present in the lacrimal or salivary glands.

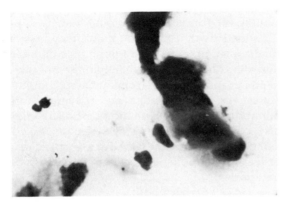

FIG. 8-13. Keratinized epithelial cells and filament from conjunctival scraping in keratoconjunctivitis sicca. (Courtesy Mr. M. Okumoto)

Treatment

Treatment of Sjögren's syndrome is often based on the symptoms of the associated connective tissue disease. For the oral manifestations, it is important for the patient to maintain good oral hygiene, with regular dental examinations and use of mouth washes. Frequent sips of water and use of gum or candy will stimulate the salivary secretions and may be helpful in relieving the xerostomia.

Since Sjögren's syndrome is usually not in itself life-threatening, systemic immunosuppressive or corticosteroid therapy is generally not used. Some improvement in the sicca symptoms has, however, been noted during treatment with cyclophosphamide for serious complications of other associated diseases (3).

Management of keratoconjunctivitis sicca is directed toward maintaining hydration and lubrication of the corneal and conjunctival epithelium. Frequent use of artificial tears such as methylcellulose or polyvinyl alcohol may provide some help. A humidifier in the patient's room may be of considerable benefit. Those who are more frequently exposed to air conditioning may have increased difficulties. Moisture shields may be placed over the eyes at night. Occlusion of the lacrimal puncta may be tried if tear replacement is insufficient.

POLYARTERITIS NODOSA

Polyarteritis nodosa is a connective tissue disorder, and one of a number of arteritis-vasculitis syndromes. The hallmark of polyarteritis nodosa (also known as periarteritis nodosa) is a widespread inflammation of medium- and small-sized arteries. Nearly any organ system may be involved, and ocular manifestations occur in 10%–20% of patients. A number of factors suggest that the disease is immunologic in nature and probably mediated by immune-complex deposition within vessels. Several other clinical entities may be included under the heading of arteritis–vasculitis syndromes. These include hypersensitivity angiitis, temporal arteritis, vasculitis associated with rheumatic fever, and allergic granulomatous angiitis. These syndromes have been classified by Zeek (129) and an expanded classification has been proposed by Hawkins (49) (Table 8–

TABLE 8–2. THE ARTERITIS–VASCULITIS SYNDROMES

I. Polyarteritis nodosa
II. Hypersensitivity angiitis
    Drug-induced
    Serum sickness arteritis
    Anaphylactoid purpura (Henoch–Schönlein syndrome)
III. Vasculitis associated with connective tissue diseases
    Rheumatoid arthritis
    Systemic lupus erythematosus
    Progressive systemic sclerosis (scleroderma)
    Polymyositis, dermatomyositis
    Sjögren's syndrome
IV. Vasculitis associated with rheumatic fever
V. Vasculitis with a granulomatous component
    Allergic granulomatous angiitis (Churg and Strauss)
    Wegener's granulomatosis
    Lethal midline granuloma
    Limited Wegener's granulomatosis
    Lymphomatoid granulomatosis
    Giant cell or temporal arteritis
    Aortic arch syndrome (Takayasu's disease)
VI. Other vasculitides and disorders associated with vasculitis
    Mixed cyroglobulinemia
    Drug abuse (methamphetamines)
    Hepatitis-associated antigenemia with vasculitis (Australia antigenemia)
    Nonsuppurative inflammatory bowel disease
    Postcoarctation resection
    Pulmonary hypertension
    Systemic hypertension
    Reticuloendothelial malignancies
    Goodpasture's syndrome
    Syphilis
    Erythema nodosum
    Nodular vasculitis
    Weber-Christian disease
    Cogan's syndrome

(Adapted from Zeek PM: Am J Clin Pathol 22:777, 1952. In Freedman SO, Gold P (eds): Clinical Immunology, 2nd ed. Hagerstown, Harper & Row, 1976, p 270)

2). Many of these entities are thought to have a similar etiology and pathogenesis.

Immunopathology

Although most cases of polyarteritis nodosa appear to be related to hypersensitivity, the nature of the antigen has rarely been identified. The vascular inflammation may, however, be the result of hypersensitivity to a number of antigens. Humoral factors may play a role in the development of polyarteritis nodosa. Repeated intravenous injections of heterologous protein antigens in rabbits produce an arteritis similar to polyarteritis nodosa. Bovine γ-globulin administration will not only induce a polyarteritis but can also lead to immune-complex deposition in the kidneys. Injection of immune complexes intravenously in rats will also lead to a vasculitis.

In human cases of polyarteritis nodosa, immune-complex deposition has been demonstrated in vessel walls during active disease. The work of Gocke *et al* has shown the presence of circulating immune complexes composed of Australia antigen and immunoglobulin in the serum of patients with biopsy-proven polyarteritis nodosa (42). Some of these patients also show deposition of Australia antigen, IgM, and complement in blood

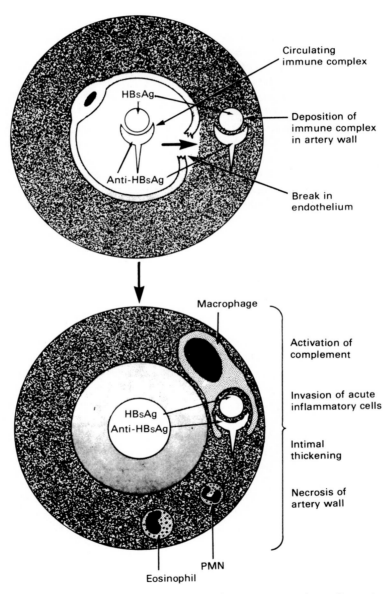

FIG. 8-14. Hypothetical immunopathogenesis in Australia-antigen–associated polyarteritis nodosa. (Reproduced with permission from Fye K, et al: Rheumatoid Diseases. In Fudenberg H H et al: Basic and Clinical Immunology, Los Altos, Lange, 1976, p 380)

vessel walls (Fig. 8-14). Although this intriguing finding suggests a relationship between polyarteritis nodosa and exposure to a microorganism, most cases of polyarteritis nodosa do not show circulating immune complexes containing Australia antigen. Renal biopsies from patients with polyarteritis nodosa have shown deposition of immune reactants such as immunoglobulins, complement, and fibrin. The findings, however, are not consistent and may in fact be nonspecific.

Microbial antigens, drugs, and autoantigens may all play a role in widespread vascular inflammation. Streptococcal antigens have been associated with polyarteritis, hypersensitivity angiitis, and Henoch–Schönlein purpura. Drugs, including sulfonamides, penicillin, phenytoin, arsenicals, thiouracil, iodides, and thiazides, have also been implicated. There is also a strong association between the abuse of methamphetamine and polyarteritis nodosa. Since many such drug abusers eventually develop hepatitis, an association between polyarteritis nodosa and Australia antigen seems even more valid.

Histologically, the typical lesion of polyarteritis nodosa is an infiltration of neutrophils and eosinophils around medium and small arteries in a necrotizing inflammatory process. Bifurcation sites of vessels are the most common locations for such lesions. Round-cell infiltration develops in the chronic phase of inflammation, and fibrinoid necrosis is eventually seen.

Clinical Features

General. Polyarteritis nodosa is a widespread disease with variable features that depend upon the organ system involved. The disorder is unusual for a connective tissue disease in that it is three times more common in men than women, especially in those over the age of forty. It may present as an abrupt febrile systemic illness with musculoskeletal pain, anorexia, and weight loss. Polyarthralgias and myalgias are common. Skin lesions include petechiae, purpura, urticaria, hemorrhagic nodules, bullae, and periungual infarcts. Tender subcutaneous nodules are sometimes

seen in the skin along vessels and these may lead to superficial necrosis and ulceration.

Renal disease occurs in 70%–80% of patients with polyarteritis nodosa. Glomerulonephritis and hypertension are the most frequent manifestations. Renal infarction and perirenal hematomas may follow renal artery inflammation, and hemorrhagic cystitis may also develop. Pulmonary involvement occurs in 25% of patients and usually presents with cough and hemoptysis following an upper respiratory infection, with generalized arteritis and eosinophilia. Pericarditis, coronary insufficiency, or myocardial infarction in a younger person should lead the clinician to suspect the possibility of polyarteritis nodosa. Abdominal complaints may develop owing to ischemia or infarction secondary to arteritis of abdominal vessels. Testicular pain secondary to testicular arteritis is sometimes seen. Peripheral vascular phenomena may develop, including Raynaud's phenomenon or ischemic peripheral angiopathy. Neurologic lesions may be seen owing to a nutrient vessel arteritis. The radial and peroneal nerves are most frequently involved and present with wrist drop or foot drop respectively. Neuropsychiatric syndromes with vertebral, cerebral, and meningeal arteritis may develop when the central nervous system is affected.

Ocular Findings. Between 10% and 20% of patients with polyarteritis nodosa have ocular signs of the disease. Conjunctival hyperemia and edema may be seen, occasionally with subconjunctival hemorrhage (Fig. 8-15). Sjögren's syndrome may occur in association with polyarteritis nodosa, as with other connective tissue disorders.

Scleritis or episcleritis is sometimes seen in association with polyarteritis nodosa. A nodular or necrotizing nodular picture may develop. A sclerokeratitis with marginal furrow formation may develop and circumferential spread may take place. This can be associated with severe pain and involvement of both eyes. Scarring, vascularization, and perforation may ensue. The appearance of these ring ulcers may be similar to Mooren's ulcer. However, an adjacent area of scleritis may help to differentiate these two entities. Histologically,

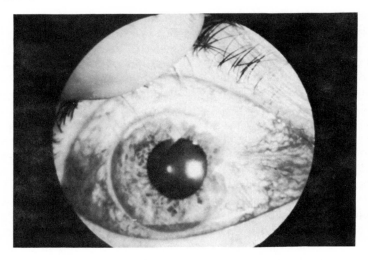

FIG. 8-15. Conjunctival hypermia and peripheral corneal opacities in polyarteritis nodosa. (Courtesy Dr. G. Mintsioulis)

an occlusive vasculitis has been demonstrated, involving the ciliary body and sclera (17), and episcleral nodules have been shown to contain granulomas and areas of scleral necrosis (55).

Polyarteritis nodosa has been associated with Cogan's syndrome (41). In this entity, an interstitial keratitis with patchy deep infiltration and vascularization of the corneal stroma is seen. The audiovestibular disease associated with Cogan's syndrome may also be caused by a widespread vascular disturbance.

The uveal tract may be involved in polyarteritis nodosa. An iridocyclitis or yellow to white subretinal patches may be seen. These focal areas of choroiditis are associated with choroidal arterial inflammation (46).

A retinopathy is perhaps the most common ocular manifestation of polyarteritis. It may be secondary to coexistent hypertension but may occasionally be due to a primary retinal vasculitis. Cotton-wool spots, irregular arteriolar narrowing, and vascular occlusion involving the central retinal artery may occur. Subhyaloid and retinal hemorrhages, retinal edema, and hard exudates have also been described (36, 110). Optic nerve involvement including papillitis and papilledema have been reported (36, 64).

Exophthalmos, diplopia, visual field defects, amaurosis fugax, Horner's syndrome, nystagmus, and cranial nerve palsies have also

been described (36). Intermittent choroidal vascular insufficiency may lead to visual field constriction with sparing of central vision (85). Exudative retinal detachment associated with a severe scleritis may develop and may lead to blindness (63).

Treatment

No satisfactory treatment is available for polyarteritis nodosa. Systemic prednisone 60–80 mg/day is the usual treatment of choice for systemic polyarteritis nodosa. Cytotoxic agents, including cyclophosphamide and azathioprine, have been used for patients who do not respond to corticosteroids, but experience with these drugs is limited. Sound general medical management is essential for problems such as renal failure, hypertension, and heart failure. Topical steroid drops should be used with care in the ocular disease when corneal involvement is present since steroids may enhance melting of the cornea.

ALLERGIC GRANULOMATOUS ANGIITIS

Several types of vasculitis resemble polyarteritis nodosa but may have a granulomatous component. Allergic granulomatous angiitis is a disseminated vasculitis associated with prominent pulmonary manifestations, including asthma. Patients also have blood eosinophilia, weight loss, fever, anemia, and extravascular granulomas (16). The cardiovascular system, kidneys, subcutaneous tissues, and gastrointestinal tract may be involved. A case involving the eye has been reported in which episcleritis and uveitis developed, with subsequent papilledema and atrophy of the globe (27). The histopathologic findings were consistent with allergic granulomatous angiitis.

WEGENER'S GRANULOMATOSIS

Wegener's granulomatosis is generally described as a triad of findings, including 1) necrotizing granulomas of the respiratory tract, 2) disseminated vasculitis involving the small and medium-sized arteries and veins, and 3) glomerulonephritis. It occurs mainly in young and middle-aged individuals and ocular involvement is frequently present. A limited form of Wegener's granulomatosis has been described in which pulmonary lesions identical to those of Wegener's granulomatosis occur but lesions elsewhere are limited or absent. Midline granuloma is sometimes included in the classification of Wegener's granulomatosis; however, the validity of this association has been questioned.

Immunopathology

Wegener's granulomatosis is a necrotizing vasculitis with features of an autoimmune disorder. Circulating autoantibodies to smooth muscle have been demonstrated, as well as circulating immune complexes and decreased levels of serum complement. Increased levels of serum IgA, IgE (22), and C3 have also been reported.

Complement and immunoglobulins have been detected in the vascular lesions of skin and kidneys (56). IgG and C3 have been demonstrated in the glomeruli of one patient and suggest an immune-complex deposition (35). IgG, C3, and fibrin have been detected in the glomerular vessels of another patient (94).

Decreased delayed cutaneous hypersensitivity has been found with various antigens, including mumps, streptokinase–streptodornase (SKSD), purified protein derivative of tuberculin (PPD), and keyhole-limpet hemocyanin (KLH). Decreased lymphocyte responses to mitogens have also been documented. However, some of these studies were done on patients being treated with immunosuppressive agents.

Clinical Features

General. Necrotizing granulomas involving the nose, nasopharynx, sinuses, trachea, and bronchi are prominent features. Focal necrotizing vasculitis involving both the arteries and veins may lead to involvement of many organ systems. Glomerulonephritis with thrombosis of glomerular capillaries is seen and leads to renal failure unless treatment is instituted.

Patients may present with symptoms related to upper or lower respiratory tract involvement. Rhinitis, sinusitis, septal perforation, tracheobronchitis, asthma, or pneumonia may be found. Widespread vasculitis can lead to arthralgias, polyneuropathy, parotitis, myocarditis or pericarditis, prostatitis, skin involvement, or ocular disease. Constitutional symptoms including fever, weight loss, and musculoskeletal pain may also develop. A leukocytosis is common and eosinophilia is seen in more than 50% of patients. The sedimentation rate is usually increased and is a good indicator of active disease.

Limited Wegener's granulomatosis is distinguished by the presence of respiratory tract lesions without evidence of glomerulonephritis. However, extraglomerular lesions of the kidney as well as other extrapulmonary lesions may be seen in this form of the disease. It is slightly more common in females than in males. Cough, fever, dyspnea, and lower lung field lesions may be seen. Involvement of the skin and central nervous system is not uncommon.

The term **lethal midline granuloma** has been used to describe three clinical entities: 1) midline malignant reticulosis, 2) Wegener's granulomatosis, and 3) malignant lymphoma of one of the accepted histologic types. While

conversion of midline granuloma to Wegener's granulomatosis has been documented
(14), some studies indicate that these two diseases represent distinct and separate clinical
entities (104).

Ocular Findings. Ocular involvement was
found in 19 of 44 patients with Wegener's
granulomatosis (115). Orbital lesions may be
continuous with lesions in adjacent respiratory
passages or, alternatively, focal disease without contiguity may occur. Exophthalmos is the
most frequent sign of orbital encroachment.
This may result in proptosis, edema of the
eyelid and conjunctiva, exposure keratitis, and
limitation of extraocular movements. Congestion of the retinal vessels, papilledema, optic
atrophy, and visual loss may result (15). Nasolacrimal duct involvement may lead to epi-
phora, dacryocystitis, or draining fistulas (51).
Conjunctival involvement has been reported
as an initial finding (43). Scleritis, episcleritis,
and corneal ring ulcers are frequent findings in
Wegener's granulomatosis and may occur
prior to systemic manifestations of the disease.
Patients with furrow degeneration of the cornea have been followed up for several months
before a diagnosis of Wegener's granulomatosis was finally made. Uveitis may sometimes
occur. It can be bilateral and can involve both
anterior and posterior segments. Retinal
periphlebitis, retinal and vitreous hemorrhages, cotton-wool spots, rubeosis iridis, and
neovascular glaucoma may occur and eventually can result in blindness (24).

Treatment

The prognosis for Wegener's granulomatosis
has improved dramatically since the advent of
treatment with cytotoxic drugs. Cyclophosphamide or azathioprine given alone or with
corticosteroids is the current treatment of
choice (104). The drugs are administered until
there is a clinical response or until signs of toxicity occur. The limited form of Wegener's
granulomatosis may be treated with corticosteroids alone; however, lack of response to
this therapy is an indication for immunosuppressive agents. Treatment for midline granuloma must be individualized and may include

corticosteroids, immunosuppressive agents, or
irradiation. Regression of a necrotizing, granulomatous sclerouveitis has been seen following
treatment with cyclophosphamide and prednisone (11).

GIANT-CELL ARTERITIS

Giant-cell arteritis is a term used to describe a
group of vasculitides in which epithelioid or
giant cells infiltrate the walls of vessels. While
temporal arteritis is the most important to the
ophthalmologist, other related diseases include polymyalgia rheumatica and aortic arch
syndrome, or Takayasu's disease. Temporal
arteritis ranks as one of the prime medical
emergencies in ophthalmology. Rapid recognition of this disease and early institution of
therapy are essential for the preservation of
vision in affected patients.

Immunopathology

The hallmark of temporal arteritis is granulomatous inflammation which selectively involves the temporal arteries (1). The presence
of epithelioid or giant cells is characteristic.
Destruction of the internal elastic lamina is a
common but not diagnostic feature of the
disease.

Immunofluorescent studies have shown IgG,
IgA, IgM, and complement deposition in the
cytoplasm of cells and along the elastic tissue
within vessel walls (40). Antinuclear antibodies directed against the nuclei of cells within
vessel walls may be seen in patients who have
antinuclear antibodies in their serum. Nonspecific increases in α_2-globulin and fibrinogen
levels in plasma have also been noted. These
may account for the elevated erythrocyte sedimentation rate in patients with giant-cell arteritis, since these proteins reduce the
electronegative charge on circulating red blood
cells and promote rouleau formation (91).
While immunoglobulin abnormalities are
generally not observed, an increase in serum
IgM has been noted in a number of patients
(91). Lymphocytes from patients with polymyalgia rheumatica undergo lymphoblastic
transformation *in vitro* with arterial antigens

(50) or with homogenates of whole muscle which may be contaminated with vascular antigens (40).

There has been speculation that viral antigens may be involved in giant-cell arteritis and polymyalgia rheumatica. Cytoplasmic inclusion bodies have recently been found in temporal artery biopsy specimens (79). The meningoencephalitis caused by varicella virus has been reported as having histologic features similar to those of giant-cell arteritis (96). Others have found selective involvement of the central nervous system vessels by varicella virus (72). Segmental artery involvement has also been reported to occur shortly after herpes zoster ophthalmicus (123). Perhaps viruses or other infectious agents are capable of altering vascular antigens and producing an autoallergic inflammation.

Takayasu's disease is associated with an elevation of serum IgG, IgA, and IgM (37). An immunologic abnormality in this disease may also be basic.

Clinical Features

General. The clinical presentation of temporal arteritis evolves in three stages: initial headache, ocular manifestations, and systemic disease. Headache is frequently unilateral and often associated with tenderness in the region of the temporal arteries. Pain may be boring or throbbing, and may be localized to the retrobulbar or temporal regions. Tenderness is sometimes so severe that it is impossible for the patient to wear a hat, lie on a pillow, or brush his hair. Frequently, pain with chewing is noted. The temporal arteries should be palpated and may demonstrate nodules or loss of pulsations. Vascular ischemia may result in cerebral vascular accidents, myocardial infarctions, vertigo, deafness, ear pain, abdominal pain and tenderness, meningismus, peripheral neuritis, or intermittent claudication. Skin lesions, including necrotic ulcers and gangrene, may be due to ischemia. Constitutional symptoms are often seen, including general malaise, anorexia, fever, and weight loss. The sedimentation rate is nearly always elevated, usually to levels of 80–100 mm/h or higher.

Temporal arteritis is a disease of older adults and is rare before the age of 50.

Takayasu's disease affects the aortic arch and the thoracic aorta. This produces a pulseless disease which is most common in young Oriental women. Arterial pulsations are absent in the head, neck, and upper extremities. Clinical findings include seizures, confusional states, coronary insufficiency, headaches, visual disturbances, muscle weakness, and paresthesias. Treatment involves the use of moderately high doses of corticosteroids. The prognosis in this syndrome is guarded.

Ocular Findings. Visual disturbances are said to occur in up to 50% of patients with temporal arteritis. These may develop in the absence of systemic disease, a condition referred to as **occult temporal arteritis.** Loss of vision is the most common ocular manifestation and is due to arteritis involving the ophthalmic or ciliary arteries. Most frequently, an ischemic optic neuritis is the cause of visual loss. Central retinal artery occlusion occurs less commonly but produces a typical picture of an ischemic retina with a cherry-red spot. Occasionally, cranial nerve involvement may be seen and may present as diplopia or ptosis. Episcleritis, scleritis, and iritis have also been reported. Occasionally, branch artery occlusion, or rubeosis iridis, with secondary glaucoma, may be seen. Scintillating scotomas, photophobia, and ocular or periorbital pain have also been described. Involvement of the second eye occurs in 35% of patients (25) and blindness, which is largely irreversible, occurs in 27% (12).

Diagnosis and Treatment

If a diagnosis of temporal arteritis is suspected, an erythrocyte sedimentation rate should be obtained. If this is elevated, and the history and clinical findings are suggestive of temporal arteritis, a temporal artery biopsy should be carried out, since this is the most useful test in confirming a diagnosis of temporal arteritis. It has been stated that a pattern of inflammation characteristic of temporal arteritis can be found continuously throughout such biopsies (19). Others, however, feel that the presence of "skip areas" make it possible for an entire biopsy specimen to lack evidence of granulomatous inflammation (1).

Immediate treatment is with corticosteroids, and usually 60–100 mg prednisone is given daily. Treatment is frequently continued for 4–6 months or even for several years; the dose may be tapered as the sedimentation rate decreases. Repeated evaluation of the sedimentation rate should be carried out, and if it increases or if clinical symptoms recur, steroid dosage should be immediately increased. Visual loss is generally permanent; however, the rapid institution of corticosteroid therapy may prevent further visual loss. Improvement of visual acuity after beginning therapy has occasionally been reported (18). Temporal arteritis is best managed by the ophthalmologist in conjunction with the patient's neurologist or internist.

POLYMYOSITIS AND DERMATOMYOSITIS

Polymyositis and dermatomyositis encompass a wide spectrum of related disorders characterized by inflammation and degeneration of varying amounts of skeletal muscle. They are multisystem diseases which have features of the rheumatic disorders and may occur in association with malignancy. Ocular manifestations, although not frequently reported, do occur. Five categories of polymyositis and dermatomyositis have been recognized: 1) idiopathic polymyositis, 2) idiopathic dermatomyositis, 3) polymyositis or dermatomyositis associated with malignancy, 4) childhood polymyositis or dermatomyositis, and 5) polymyositis or dermatomyositis associated with other rheumatoid diseases.

Immunopathology

The etiology of the disorders is currently unknown. Features of both humoral and cellular immunity have been recognized in patients with polymyositis or dermatomyositis, and there has been speculation that a virus may play an etiologic role. Viruslike particles of various structural types have been identified

by electron microscopy in the myocytes of patients with polymyositis.

Circulating antibodies to muscle may be found after any muscle injury. Local deposits of IgG, IgM, and complement have been found within the vessel walls of involved skin and muscle in polymyositis (128). These deposits, detectable mainly in children with diffuse vasculitis, suggest the possibility of an immune-complex disorder. Polyclonal hypergammaglobulinemia is commonly seen in patients with polymyositis or dermatomyositis, and both rheumatoid factor and antinuclear antibodies are seen in 20% of cases. Patients with agammaglobulinemia can develop polymyositis, suggesting that immunoglobulins alone are not invloved in all cases (30). Dermatomyositis has been reported in association with a deficiency of the complement component C2, indicating that the classic pathway of complement activation is not always required (70). Deficiencies of the complement system have been reported in a number of rheumatic abnormalities, suggesting an increased susceptibility among these patients to immunologic injury.

There is evidence that cellular immunity is involved in the development of polymositis and dermatomyositis. Lymphocytes from patients with active myositis induce cytotoxic changes in autologous or chick muscle cells in tissue culture (29). Muscle-cell injury is thought to be due to the lymphokine known as lymphotoxin which is produced by T cells. The lymphocytes from affected patients may sometimes respond to their own muscle antigens as though they were foreign (Fig. 8-16). This could be due to an altered membrane antigen on the muscle cells, induced perhaps by a virus. Alternatively, there may be a primary defect in antigen recognition by lymphocytes or cross reactivity between muscle antigen and an unidentified foreign antigen. Presumably, the cellular response would occur at the site of the instigating antigen, and lymphotoxin could diffuse through the tissues and injure the remote muscle fibers.

While the etiology of these disorders remains speculative, a combination of viral and immunologic abnormalities is suggested by current available evidence. Histologic findings

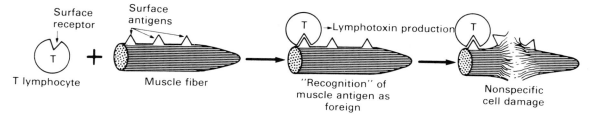

FIG. 8-16. Defective recognition of muscle antigen in polymyositis. (Reproduced with permission from Fye K: Rheumatic Diseases. In Fudenberg H H et al: Basic and Clinical Immunology, Los Altos, Lange, 1976, p. 377)

show a focal or diffuse lymphocytic infiltration of muscle cells. Necrosis, degeneration, and regeneration of muscle cells is typically seen.

Clinical Features

General. Polymyositis and dermatomyositis are twice as common in women as in men. They may occur at any age and there is no racial preponderance. Weakness of the proximal muscles is the most common manifestation. The extremities and neck are commonly involved. Dysphagia may occur as a result of involvement of the posterior pharyngeal muscles. Facial and extraocular muscle involvement is rare. Pain, tenderness, and edema are sometimes present in acutely involved muscles but rarely in chronic cases. The diseases have an insidious onset and constitutional manifestations are relatively rare.

Skin involvement in polymyositis and dermatomyositis is common. The typical rash, a dusky eruption over the malar and periorbital regions, is seen in 40% of cases. Hyperemic patches, which may be raised and scaly, are found over the elbows, knuckles, and malleoli. These are known as **Gottron's papules.** Their appearance may be precipitated by exposure to the sun and they may represent the presenting sign of dermatomyositis, occurring several years before muscle weakness develops. Subcuticular telangiectasias are sometimes seen but are felt to be less specific. They are best observed through a drop of oil with an ophthalmoscope set at plus 20 to plus 40 diopters. The cuticles of the nail may be reddened, roughened, irregular, and hyperkeratotic.

Raynaud's phenomenon and arthritis are sometimes seen but are more likely to occur when other rheumatic diseases are present concomitantly. Sjögren's syndrome is seen in 5%–7% of cases. Rarely, gastrointestinal ulcerations and interstitial pneumonia are observed.

An increased incidence of malignancies has frequently been associated with polymyositis and dermatomyositis. The incidence of tumors is usually considered to be about 20%, but may be as high as 40%–50% in males over the age of 40. The myositis usually precedes the tumor by several years. Carcinomas of the lung, prostate, ovary, uterus, breast, and large intestine are most frequently seen. The stomach, gallbladder, and parotid gland are less frequently involved. Excision of the tumor sometimes results in dramatic improvement of the myositis.

Ocular Findings. The most common ocular manifestation is a heliotrope rash and periorbital edema involving the eyelids. The rash is especially common in children with dermatomyositis (53). A nonspecific conjunctivitis may be present and keratoconjunctivitis sicca may be seen if Sjögren's syndrome is present. Episcleritis, iritis, exophthalmos, extraocular muscle paresis, and nystagmus have all been reported. Myositis involving the extraocular muscles is uncommon and may be due to a coexistent myasthenia gravis (117)

Retinal changes are not common. However, cotton-wool spots are the most frequent finding, as in most other connective tissue disorders. These are found principally at the posterior pole and require 6–8 weeks to resolve. Venous engorgement, deep and superficial retinal hemorrhages, retinal edema, and exudates may be present (48, 81). Papilledema, optic atrophy, and pigmentary disturbances of the posterior pole have also been described (86).

Diagnosis and Treatment

The erythrocyte sedimentation rate is generally elevated in active disease. Serum enzymes, especially creatine phosphokinase, may be elevated in as many as 80% of cases. Aldolase and transaminase are sometimes measured but are considered to be less specific. The urine creatine concentration is felt to be the most sensitive laboratory test for muscle damage and is the first detectable laboratory abnormality in relapses. Muscle biopsy is diagnostic in 50%–80% of cases. Electromyography demonstrates characteristic findings in 70%–80% of patients when involved muscles are examined. Half of the patients have elevated α_2- and γ-globulins on serum protein electrophoresis. Myoglobulinemia and myoglobinuria may also be present.

Systemic corticosteroids are the treatment of choice and will generally induce a remission. Usually prednisone 60–80 mg/day is begun and is tapered slowly, with monitoring of both laboratory and clinical signs. Urine creatine concentration is the most sensitive index of disease activity. An immunosuppressive agent, such as methotrexate, is indicated when patients do not respond to corticosteroids. Usually 25–50 mg methotrexate intravenously is given per week.

PROGRESSIVE SYSTEMIC SCLEROSIS (SCLERODERMA)

Progressive systemic sclerosis is a connective tissue disease that affects various organ systems, especially the skin, lungs, and gastrointestinal tract. For many years it was considered primarily a dermatologic condition; however, the systemic nature of the disease is now well recognized. The main pathologic feature in progressive systemic sclerosis is the increased collagen deposition in the affected organs.

Ocular findings are only occasionally observed; however, a wide spectrum of eye abnormalities has been reported.

Immunopathology

The etiology of progressive systemic sclerosis is unknown. Although many facts are known about progressive systemic sclerosis, a unified workable hypothesis to account for the various clinical findings has not as yet been put forth. Three possible pathogenic mechanisms may contribute to the development of this disease: an immunologic abnormality, an autonomic nervous system problem, and a primary connective tissue defect.

Several immunologic abnormalities have been detected in patients with progressive systemic sclerosis. Most patients have a hypergammaglobulinemia of the polyclonal type, and rheumatoid factor is found in about 35%. Occasionally, positive LE cell tests and false-positive serologic tests for syphilis are found. Antinuclear antibodies are present in at least 60% of patients. These are usually of the coarse, speckled nuclear pattern (97) and do not correlate with the clinical severity of the disease. Recently, a new antinuclear antibody marker system has been found in progressive systemic sclerosis, with a concentrated tissue extract used as antigen (118). This antinuclear antibody seems to be specific for progressive systemic sclerosis since it is not found in other connective tissue diseases.

Antinucleolar antibodies and antibodies to ribonucleoprotein are also found in progressive systemic sclerosis. A mixed cryoglobulin has been found in 50% of patients (57). This protein contains IgG and IgM, and is usually associated with antigammaglobulin activity in serum. This finding suggests the possibility of circulating immune complexes, but their role in the etiology of the disease is at present uncertain. There is still relatively little evidence to suggest that the vascular abnormalities associated with this disorder have an immunologic basis.

Some evidence for the participation of cellular immune mechanisms also exists in progressive systemic sclerosis. Lymphocytes from patients with the disease can destroy embryonic fibroblasts in tissue culture. Cellular infiltration of involved tissues, however, is sparse, except in the synovium.

The importance of an autonomic nervous system component in progressive systemic sclerosis has also been emphasized (20). The high incidence of Raynaud's phenomenon and esophageal abnormalities, their reversal by reserpine and methacholine, and an impaired response to gastrin I and edrophonium have all suggested an autonomic abnormality. The latter two drugs require an intact autonomic nervous system in order to be effective.

A primary defect in collagen has been suggested as contributing to progressive systemic sclerosis. An increase in collagen biosynthesis in tissue culture (71) and abnormalities in the conversion of proline to hydroxyproline (120) have been detected.

Histologically, sclerosis and fibrosis are seen in various tissues. Blood vessels may show intimal fibrosis, endothelial proliferation, and hyperplasia of the media. An interstitial fibrosis is almost always found at autopsy.

Clinical Features

General. Progressive systemic sclerosis is two to three times more common in females than in males and is usually seen between ages 30 and 50. The disease usually has an insidious onset characterized by edema and atrophy of the skin and often, Raynaud's phenomenon. The course is progressive, disabling, and often fatal.

Skin involvement occurs in three stages. The first stage is characterized by nonpitting edema which begins in the hands and feet and which eventually affects the arms, chest, abdomen, back, and face. The skin becomes tight, smooth, and waxy during the sclerotic phase and the face develops a stretched masklike appearance with thin lips and a "pinched" nose. Finally, pigmentary changes, subcutaneous calcifications, telangiectasias, and ulcerations of the fingertips may be seen. Raynaud's phenomenon occurs in about 30% of patients. A relatively benign variant of progressive systemic sclerosis is known as the CRST syndrome. It includes calcinosis, Raynaud's phenomenon, sclerodactyly, and telangiectasias, and may be confined to the skin for prolonged periods of time.

Systemic involvement may affect various body systems. Arthritis is common in progressive systemic sclerosis and usually involves the small joints of the hands and feet. Muscle involvement may be indistinguishable from that seen in polymyositis. Patients may have dyspnea, orthopnea, hemoptysis, chest pain, hoarseness, and pleurisy. There is a high incidence of alveolar-cell carcinoma in patients with progressive systemic sclerosis. Myocardial fibrosis and pericarditis are sometimes seen. Renal involvement is uncommon but may be life-threatening. Gastrointestinal lesions are common, with esophageal sclerosis, dysphagia, and reflux esophagitis present in about 80% of patients. Hypomotility of the gastrointestinal tract leads to bacterial overgrowth and malabsorption. Biliary cirrhosis and mononeuropathy are sometimes seen.

Progressive systemic sclerosis may be a component of other connective tissue disease syndromes. A recently described entity known as **mixed connective tissue disease syndrome** combines features of progressive systemic sclerosis, SLE, and polymyositis (108). Patients usually have abnormal esophageal motility, Raynaud's phenomenon, arthritis, myositis, lymphadenopathy, and hypergammaglobulinemia. They also have in their serum an antibody to an extractable nuclear antigen which is probably a ribonucleoprotein.

A second syndrome with features of scleroderma is the so-called **eosinophilic fasciitis** (95). Patients have inflammation and thickening of the fascia between the subcutis and muscle, associated with the skin and serologic abnormalities characteristic of progressive systemic sclerosis. Eosinophils are found in large numbers in the blood and in the inflammatory reaction.

Ocular Findings. Skin involvement of the eyelids is common in progressive systemic sclerosis. Early findings include a brawny nonpitting edema followed by tightness of the lids and a woody hardness. Blepharophimosis and lagophthalmos may develop. Telangiectasias may appear over the eyelids as over other areas of the face. Keratoconjunctivitis sicca is reported in 5%–7% of cases and decreased tear secretion is seen in 30%–50% (54). Conjunctival fornices may become shallow. A chronic, nonspecific conjunctivitis and a filamentary keratitis have also been reported (66, 116). An increased incidence of cataracts has been mentioned occasionally in scleroderma; however, controlled studies have indicated no such increased incidence (54). Fundus lesions are uncommon in scleroderma; cotton-wool spots, retinal hemorrhages, and edema have been reported (74). Often these are associated with systemic hypertension or renal failure, but they have been observed in patients with normal blood pressure (75). Disc edema and localized retinal detachments are sometimes seen (6). Ocular motility disturbances, including incomplete external ophthalmoplegia, have been reported (121). Recently, iridocyclitis and focal chorioretinitis have been noted in association with a case of sclerodemra (28).

Treatment

No effective therapy is currently available for progressive systemic sclerosis. Neither corticosteroids nor immunosuppressive agents appear to alter the progressive course of the disease. Chlorambucil has been reported to diminish skin contractions and limit pulmonary fibrosis in a small group of patients. Supportive measures have been useful, including antihypertensive agents, antibiotics for intercurrent infection, physiotherapy, esophageal dilation, and protection from the cold. Systemic and subconjunctival steroids have been used with apparent success in the treatment of the chorioretinal lesions (28).

The usual course of the disease is one of relentless progression with widespread visceral and dermal involvement. The five-year survival rate is approximately 40%; death may be due to aspiration pneumonia, esophageal dysfunction, or renal failure.

REFERENCES

1. Albert DM, Ruchman MC, Keltner JL: Skip areas in temporal arteritis. Arch Ophthalmol 94:2072, 1976

2. Amor B, Kahan A, Lecoq F, Delbarre F: Le test de transformation lymphoblastique par les antigenes bedsoniens (TTL Bedsonien). Rev Rheum Mal Osteoartic 39:671, 1972

3. Anderson LG, Cummings NA, Asofsky R et al: Salivary gland immunoglobulin and rheumatoid factor synthesis in Sjögren's syndrome: natural history and response to treatment. Am J Med 53:456, 1972

4. Andrianakos AA, Sharp JT, Person DA et al: Cell-mediated immunity in rheumatoid arthritis. Ann Rheum Dis 36:13, 1977

5. Andriopoulos NA, Mestecky J, Miller EJ, Bennett JC: Antibodies to human native and denatured collagens in synovial fluids of patients with rheumatoid arthritis. Clin Immunol Immunopathol 6:209, 1976

6. Ashton N, Coomes EN, Garner A, Oliver DO: Retinopathy due to progressive systemic sclerosis. J Pathol 96:259, 1968

7. Bell C, Talal N, Schur PH: Antibodies to DNA in patients with rheumatoid arthritis and juvenile rheumatoid arthritis. Arth Rheum 18:535, 1975

8. Bloch KJ, Buchanan WW, Wohl MJ, Bunim JJ: Sjögren's syndrome, a clinical, pathological and serological study of sixty-two cases. Medicine 44:187, 1965

9. Bøyum A: Separation of leukocytes from blood and bone marrow. Scand J Clin Lab Invest [Suppl] 21 (97): 1968

10. Brewerton DA, Caffrey M, Hart FD et al: Ankylosing spondylitis and HL–A27. Lancet 1:904, 1973

11. Brubaker R, Font RL, Shepard EM: Granulomatous sclerouveitis: regression of ocular lesions with cyclophosphamide and prednisone. Arch Ophthalmol 86:517, 1971

12. Bruce GM: Temporal arteritis as a cause of blindness. Review of the literature and report of a case. Trans Am Ophthalmol Soc 47:300, 1949

13. Buc M, Nyulassy S, Stefanovic J et al: HL–A system and juvenile rheumatoid arthritis. Tissue Antigens 4:395, 1974

14. Byrd LJ, Shear MA, Tu WH: Relationship of lethal midline granuloma to Wegener's granulomatosis. Arth Rheum 12:247, 1969

15. Cassen SM, Divertie MG, Hollenhorst RW, Harrison EG: Pseudotumor of the orbit and limited Wegener's granulomatosis. Ann Intern Med 72:687, 1970

16. Churg J, Strauss L: Allergic granulomatous, allergic angiitis, and periarteritis nodosa. Am J Pathol 27:277, 1951

17. Cogan DG: Corneoscleral lesions in periarteritis nodosa and Wegener's granulomatosis, Trans Am Ophthalmol Soc 53:321, 1955

18. Cohen DN: Temporal arteritis: improvement in visual prognosis and management with repeated biopsies. Trans Am Acad Ophthalmol Otolaryngol 77:74, 1973

19. Cohen DN, Smith TR: Skip areas in temporal arteritis: myth versus fact. Trans Am Acad Ophthalmol Otolaryngol 78:OP-722, 1974

20. Cohen S, Fisher R, Lipshutz W et al: The pathogenesis of esophageal dysfunction in scleroderma and Raynaud's disease. J Clin Invest 51:2663, 1972

21. Cole BC, Taylor MB, Ward JR: Studies on the infectious etiology of human rheumatoid arthritis. II. Search for humoral and cell-bound antibodies against mycoplasmal antigens. Arth Rheum 18:435, 1975

22. Conn DL, Gleich GJ, DeRemee RA, McDonald TJ: Raised serum immunoglobulin E in Wegener's granulomatosis. Ann Rheum Dis 35:377, 1976

23. Coppeto J, Lessell S: Retinopathy in systemic lupus erythematosus. Arch Ophthalmol 95:794, 1977

24. Coutu RE, Klein M, Lessell S et al: Limited form of Wegener's granulomatosis: eye involvement as a major sign. JAMA 233:868, 1975

25. Cullen JF: Ischemic optic neuropathy. Trans Ophthalmol Soc UK 87:759, 1967

26. Cummings NA, Schall GL, Asofsky R et al: Sjögren's syndrome-newer aspects of research, diagnosis and therapy. Ann Intern Med 75:937, 1971

27. Cury D, Breakey AS, Payne BF: Allergic, granulomatous angiitis associated with uveoscleritis and papilledema. Arch Ophthalmol 55:261, 1956

28. David R, Ivry M: Focal choroiditis and iridocyclitis associated with scleroderma. Ann Ophthalmol 8:199, 1976

29. Dawkins RL, Mastaglia FL: Cell-mediated cytoxicity to muscle in polymyositis. N Engl J Med 288:434, 1973

30. Dermatomyositis—Medical Staff Conference. University of California, San Francisco. West J Med 124:316, 1976

31. Douglass MC, Lamberg SI, Lorincz AI et al: Lupus erythematosus-like syndrome with a familial deficiency of C2. Arch Dermatol 112:671, 1976

32. Editorial: Lancet 2:79, 1976

33. Emery AEH, Lawrence JS: Genetics of ankylosing spondylitis. J Med Genet 4:239, 1967

34. Epstein WV, Tan M, Easterbrook M: Serum antibody to double-stranded RNA and DNA in patients with idiopathic and secondary uveitis. N Engl J Med 285:1502, 1971

35. Fauci AS, Wolff SM: Wegener's granulomatosis: studies in eighteen patients and a review of the literature. Medicine 52:535, 1973

36. Ford RG, Siekart RG: Central nervous system manifestations of periarteritis nodosa. Neurology 15:114, 1965

37. Fraga A, Mintz G, Valle L et al: Takayasu's arteritis: frequency of systemic manifestations (study of 22 patients) and favorable response to maintenance steroid therapy with adrenocorticosteroids (12 patients). Arth Rheum 15:617, 1972

38. Friou GJ: Antinuclear antibodies: diagnostic significance and methods. Arth Rheum 10:151, 1967

39. Froland SS, Natvig JB, Wisloff F, Munthe E: Lymphocyte reactions in rheumatoid arthritis. In Beers RF Jr, Bassett EG (eds): The Role of Immunological Factors in Infectious, Allergic, and Autoimmune Processes. New York, Raven Press, 1976, p 289

40. Fye K, Moutsopoulos H, Talal N: Rheumatoid diseases. In Fudenberg HH et al (eds): Basic and Clinical Immunology. Los Altos, Lange, 1976, p 379

41. Gilbert WS, Talbot FJ: Cogan's syndrome. Signs of periarteritis nodosa and cerebral venous sinus thrombosis. Arch Ophthalmol 82:633, 1969

42. Gocke DJ, Hsu K, Morgan C et al: Vasculitis in association with Australia antigen. J Exp Med 134:330S, 1971

43. Goder G, Dolter J: Wegener's granulomatosis of conjunctival origin. Ophthalmologica 162:321, 1971

44. Gofton JP, Bennett PH, Smythe HA et al: Sacroiliitis and ankylosing spondylitis in North American Indians. Ann Rheum Dis 31:474, 1972

45. Gofton JP, Lawrence JS, Bennett PH et al: Sacroiliitis in eight populations. Ann Rheum Dis 25:528, 1966

46. Goldstein I, Wexler D: Bilateral atrophy of the optic nerve in periarteritis nodosa. Arch Ophthalmol 18:767, 1937

47. Good AE, Schultz JS: Reiter's syndrome following Shigella flexneri 2a. Arth Rheum 20:100, 1977

48. Harrison SM, Frenkel M, Grossman BJ, Matalon R: Retinopathy in childhood dermatomyositis. Am J Ophthalmol 76:786, 1973

49. Hawkins D: Diffuse connective tissue diseases. I. Systemic lupus erythematosus and related disorders. In Freedman SO, Gold P (eds): Clinical Immunology, 2nd ed. Hagerstown, Harper & Row, 1976, pp 256–294

50. Hazelman BC, MacLennan ICM, Esiri MM: Lymphocyte proliferation to artery antigen as a positive diagnostic test in polymyalgia rheumatica. Ann Rheum Dis 34:122, 1975

51. Henkind P, Gold DH: Ocular manifestations of rheumatic disorders. Rheumatology 4:13, 1973

52. Hepburn B, McDuffie FC, Ritts RE Jr: Impaired blastogenic response of lymphocytes from synovial fluid and peripheral blood of patients with rheumatoid arthritis. J Rheum 3:118, 1975

53. Hill RH, Woods WS: Juvenile dermatomyositis. Can Med Assoc J 103:1152, 1970

54. Horen EC: Ophthalmic manifestations of

progressive systemic sclerosis. Br J Ophthalmol 53:388, 1969

55. Horwitz JA, Worthen DM: Episcleral nodule in systemic vasculitis. Ann Ophthalmol 4:482, 1972

56. Hu C-H, O'Laughlin S, Winkelman RK: Cutaneous manifestation of Wegener Granulomatosis. Arch Derm 113:175, 1977

57. Husson JM, Druet P, Contet A et al: Systemic sclerosis and cryoglobulinemaia. Clin Immunol Immunopathol 6:77, 1976

58. Jansson E, Mäkisara P, Tuuri S: Mycoplasma antibodies in rheumatoid arthritis. Scand J Rheum 4:165, 1975

59. Johnson PM, Watkins J, Holborow EJ: Antiglobulin production to altered IgG in rheumatoid arthritis. Lancet 1:611, 1975

60. Julkunen H: Rheumatoid spondylitis: clinical and laboratory studies of 149 cases compared with 182 cases of rheumatoid arthritis. Acta Rheum Scand [Suppl] 4:4, 1962

61. Juvenile rheumatoid arthritis—a viral disease (editorial). Br Med J 2:901, 1976

62. Key S, Kimura SJ: Iridocyclitis associated with juvenile rheumatoid arthritis. Am J Ophthalmol 80:425, 1975

63. Kielar RA: Exudative retinal detachment and scleritis in polyarteritis. Am J Ophthalmol 82:694, 1976

64. Kimbrell OC Jr, Wheliss JA: Polyarteritis nodosa complicated by bilateral optic neuropathy. JAMA 201:61, 1967

65. Kimura S, Hogan M, O'Connor GR, Epstein WV: Uveitis and joint disease. A review of 191 cases. Trans Am Ophthalmol Soc 64:301, 1966

66. Kirkham TH: Scleroderma and Sjögren's syndrome. Br J Ophthalmol 53:131, 1969

67. Krachmer JH, Laibson PR: Corneal thinning and perforation in Sjögren's syndrome. Am J Ophthalmol 78:917, 1974

68. Laitinen H, Peltola P, Sarajas-Kyllonen S: Spondylarthritis ankylopoietica associated with iritis. Ann Med Intern Fenniae 48:48, 1959

69. Landry M: Phagocyte function and cell-mediated immunity in systemic lupus erythematosus. Arch Dermatol 113:147, 1977

70. Leddy JP, Griggs RC, Klemperer MR: Hereditary C2 deficiency and dermatomyositis. Am J Med 58:83, 1975

71. LeRoy EC: Connective tissue synthesis by scleroderma skin fibroblasts in cell culture. J Exp Med 135:1351, 1972

72. Lie JT, Gordon LP, Titus JL: Juvenile temporal arteritis: biopsy study of four cases. JAMA 234:496, 1975

73. Lockshin MD, Fotino M, Gough WW, Litwin S: Ankylosing spondylitis and HL-A. A genetic disease plus? Am J Med 58:695, 1975

74. Maclean H, Guthrie W: Retinopathy in scleroderma. Trans Ophthalmol Soc UK 89:209, 1969

75. Manshot WA: Generalized scleroderma with ocular symptoms. Ophthalmologica 149:131, 1965

76. McGavin DDM, Williamson J, Forrester JV et al: Episcleritis and scleritis. A study of their clinical manifestations and association with rheumatoid arthritis. Br J Ophthalmol 60:192, 1976

77. Millard LG, Rowell NR: Primary amyloidosis and myelomatosis associated with excessive fibrinolytic activity. Br J Dermatol 94:569, 1976

78. Millard LG, Rowell NR, Rajah SM: Histocompatibility antigens in discoid and systemic lupus erythematosus. Br J Dermatol 96:139, 1977

79. Mitschek G, Auböck L, Berthier G: La découverte d'inclusions cytoplasmiques d'allure virale dans l'artérite temporale. Ann Anat Pathol 18:449, 1973

80. Mitsui H, Juji T, Sonozaki H et al: Distribution of HLA-B27 in patients with juvenile rheumatoid arthritis. Ann Rheum Dis 36:86, 1977

81. Munro S: Fundus appearance in a case of acute dermatomyositis. Br J Ophthalmol 43:548, 1959

82. Munthe E, Natvig JB: Complement fixing intracellular complexes of IgG rheumatoid factor in rheumatoid plasma cells. Scand J Immunol 1:217, 1972

83. Natvig JB, Munthe E, Pahle J: Evidence for intracellular complement fixing complexes of IgG rheumatoid factor in rheumatoid plasma cells. Rheumatology 6:167, 1975

84. Natvig JB, Winchester RJ: Complement in rheumatoid inflammation. Acta Rheum Scand 15:161, 1969

85. Newman NM, Hoyt WF, Spencer WH: Macula-sparing monocular blackouts: clinical and pathological investigations of intermittent choroidal vascular insufficiency in a case of periarteritis nodosa. Arch Ophthalmol 91:367, 1974

86. Nutt AB: Ophthalmic manifestations in pediatric practice. Trans Ophthalmol Soc UK 79:315, 1959

87. Ohno S, Char D, Kimura SJ, O'Connor GR: HLA antigens and antinuclear antibody titres in juvenile chronic iridocyclitis. Br J Ophthalmol 61:59, 1977

88. Ostler HB, Schachter J, Dawson CR: Ocular infection of rabbits with a Bedsonia isolated from a patient with Reiter's Syndrome. Invest Ophthalmol 9:256, 1970

89. Person DA Sharp JT, Lidsky MD: Cytotoxicity of leukocytes and lymphocytes from patients with rheumatoid arthritis for synovial cells. J Clin Invest 58:690, 1976

90. Rachelefsky G, Terasaki PI, Katz R, Stiehm ER: Increased prevalence of W27 in juvenile rheumatoid arthritis. N Engl J Med 290:892, 1974

91. Rahi AHS, Garner A: Immunopathology of the Eye. Oxford, Blackwell, 1976, pp 303–304

92. Recent clinical and experimental developments in Sjögren's syndrome—Medical Staff Conference. University of California, San Francisco. West J Med 122:50, 1975

93. Reeves JA: Keratopathy associated with systemic lupus erythematosus. Arch Ophthalmol 74:159, 1965

94. Roback SA, Herdman RC, Hoyer J et al: Wegener's granulomatosis in a child: observations on pathogenesis and treatment. Am J Dis Child 112:587, 1966

95. Rodnan GP, DiBartolomeo AG, Medsger TA Jr et al: Eosinophilic faciitis—report of seven cases of a newly recognized scleroderma-like syndrome (abstr). New York, American Rheumatism Association Annual Meeting, 1975, p 50

96. Rosenblum WZ, Hadfield MG: Granulomatous angiitis of the nervous system in cases of herpes zoster and lymphosarcoma. Neurology (Minneap) 22:348, 1972

97. Rothfield NF, Rodnan GP: Serum antinuclear factors in progressive systemic sclerosis (scleroderma). Arthritis 11:607, 1968

98. Russell AS, Lentle BC, Percy JS: Investigation of saroiliac disease: comparative evaluation of radiological and radionuclide techniques. J Rheum 2:45, 1975

99. Russell AS, Lentle BC, Percy JS, Jackson FI: Scintigraphy of sacroiliac joints in acute anterior uveitis. A study of thirty patients. Ann Intern Med 85:606, 1976

100. Santos R, Barojas E, Alarcón-Segovia D, Ibanez G: Retinal microangiopathy in systemic lupus erythematosus. Am J Ophthalmol 80:249, 1975

101. Schachter J: Isolation of Bedsoniae from human arthritis and abortion tissues. Am J Ophthalmol 63:1082, 1967

102. Schaller JG, Johnson GD, Holborow EJ et al: The association of antinuclear antibodies with the chronic iridocyclitis of juvenile rheumatoid arthritis (Still's Disease). Arth Rheum 17:409, 1974

103. Schaller JG, Wedgwood RJ: Is juvenile rheumatoid arthritis a single disease? A review article. Pediatrics 50:940, 1972

104. Schecter SL, Bole GG, Walker SE: Midline granuloma and Wegener's granulomatosis: clinical and therapeutic considerations. J Rheumatol 3:241, 1976

105. Scherbel AL, Mackenzie AH, Nousek JE, Atdjian M: Ocular lesions in rheumatoid arthritis and related disorders with particular reference to retinopathy. N Engl J Med 273:360, 1965

106. Schlosstein L, Terasaki PI, Bluestone R et al: High association of an HL–A antigen, W27, with ankylosing spondylitis. N Engl J Med 288:704, 1973

107. Semon H, Wolff E: Acute lupus erythematosus with fundus lesions. Proc R Soc Med 27:153, 1933

108. Sharp GG, Irvin WS, Tan EM et al: Mixed connective tissue disease—an apparently distinct rheumatic disease syndrome associated with a specific antibody to an extractable nuclear antigen (ENA). Am J Med 52:148, 1972

109. Shearn MA: Sjögren's syndrome. Semin Arth Reum 2:165, 1972

110. Sheehan B, Harriman DGF, Bradshaw JPP: Polyarteritis nodosa with ophthalmic and neurological complications. Arch Ophthalmol 60:357, 1958

111. Shore RN, Faricelli JA: Borderline and reactive FTA–ABS. Results in lupus erythematosus. Arch Dermatol 113:37, 1977

112. Smiley WK: Ocular involvement in juvenile rheumatoid arthritis (Still's Disease). Proc R Soc Med 66:1163, 1973

113. Smiley WK: The eye in juvenile rheumatoid arthritis. Trans Ophthalmol Soc UK 94:817, 1974

114. Spaeth GL: Corneal staining in systemic lupus erythematosus. N Engl J Med 276:1168, 1967

115. Straatsma B: Ocular manifestations of Wegener's granulomatosis. Am J Ophthalmol 44:789, 1957

116. Stucchi CA, Geiser JD: Manifestations oculaires de la sclérodermie generalisée (Points communs avec le syndrome de Sjögren). Doc Ophthalmol 22:72, 1967

117. Susac JO, Garcia-Mullen R, Glaser JS: Ophthalmoplegia in dermatomyositis. Neurology (Minneap) 23:305, 1973

118. Tan EM, Rodnan GP: Profile of antinuclear antibodies in progressive systemic sclerosis (PSS) (abstr). New York, American Rheumatism Association Annual Meeting, 1975, p 41

119. Thonar EJ-MA, Sweet MBE: Cellular hypersensitivity in rheumatoid arthritis, ankylosing spondylitis, and anterior nongranulomatous uveitis. Arth Rheum 19:539, 1976

120. Uitto J, Helin G, Helin P et al: Connective tissue in scleroderma. Acta Derm Venereol (Stockh) 51:401, 1971

121. Walsh FB: Scleroderma (progressive systemic sclerosis). In Walsh FB, Hoyt W (eds) Clinical Neuroophthalmology, Vol 2. Baltimore, Williams & Wilkins, 1969

122. Walsh FB, Hoyt WF: Clinical Neuro-Ophthalmology. Baltimore, Williams & Wilkins, 1969, p 1167

123. Walker RJ, El Gammal T, Allen MB: Cranial arteritis associated with herpes zoster. Radiology 107:109, 1973

124. Watson PG, Hayreh SS: Scleritis and episcleritis. Br J Ophthalmol 60:163, 1976

125. Weisbart RH, Bluestone R, Goldberg LS: Cellular immunity to autologous IgG in rheumatoid arthritis and rheumatoid-like disorders. Clin Exp Immunol 20:409, 1975

126. Williams RC Jr, Debord JR, Mellbye OJ et al: Studies of B and T lymphocytes in patients with connective tissue diseases. J Clin Invest 58:690, 1976

127. Winfield JB, Winchester RJ, Wernet P, Kunkel H: Antibodies to lymphocytes and the estimation of B and T cells in the connective tissue disorders. In Beers RF, Bassett EG (eds): The Role of Immunological Factors in Infectious, Allergic, and Autoimmune Processes. New York, Raven Press, 1976, p 137

128. Witaker JN, Engel WK: Vascular deposits of immunoglobulin and complement in inflammatory myopathy. N Engl J Med 286:333, 1972

129. Zeek PM: Periarteritis nodosa: a critical review. Am J Clin Pathol 22:777, 1952

130. Zvaifler NJ: The immunopathology of joint inflammation in rheumatoid arthritis. Adv Immunol 16:265, 1973

allergic and multisystem diseases

Immunologic mechanisms appear to play a major role in the pathogenesis of a wide variety of systemic diseases in which the etiology is uncertain. An abnormal immune response may be manifested in a variety of different organ systems. Because of certain anatomic, physiologic, or antigenic factors, the eye may be incidentally or preferentially involved in systemic immunologic diseases. Frequently, the uveal tract or the limbal area of the cornea is affected. This chapter will deal with ocular manifestations of several systemic diseases with immunologic properties and the possible mechanisms for their pathogenesis.

HAY FEVER

Conjunctivitis is the chief ocular manifestation of many allergies to common airborne substances. Pollens of trees, grasses, and weeds; house dust; animal dander; and molds have been implicated in these recurrent and often seasonal allergies. Such reactions are a manifestation of type I hypersensitivity and are mediated by immunoglobulin E (IgE). Mucous membranes, including the nasal mucosa and conjunctiva, are generally affected.

Immunopathology

Hay fever, or allergic rhinitis, is an immediate hypersensitivity reaction to environmental antigens. Common allergens which cause allergic rhinitis are listed in Table 9-1. Most of these substances are chemically complex and are derived from plants or animals. The allergens which produce hay fever vary from one geo-graphic area to another, but in many parts of the country, ragweed is the most frequently encountered allergen. It pollenates between July and mid-October. Grass and tree pollens, molds, house dust, animal danders, industrial chemicals, and certain foods may also be allergenic. While symptoms related to these allergens may occur year-round, most pollens and molds have characteristic seasonal peaks. It is important for the clinician to know the common allergens in his particular region of the country, and the time of year when various trees, grasses, and weeds pollenate. Air sampling devices for identifying and quantitating pollen are available.

The mechanism by which allergens produce symptoms is known as type I hypersensitivity (see Atopic or Anaphylactic Reactions, Ch. 2). The allergen comes into direct contact with the nasal mucosa or conjunctiva, and interacts with IgE that is bound to tissue mast cells. This results in the release of mediators including histamine, slow-reacting substance of anaphylaxis (SRS-A), eosinophil chemotactic factor of anaphylaxis (ECF-A), and platelet activating factor (PAF). These mediators have an effect on local blood vessels, smooth muscle, and secretory glands, which in turn leads to the clinical manifestations of allergy. The combination of allergen with mast-cell–bound IgE molecules causes a change in the Fc portion of the IgE molecule attached to the cell membrane. This in turn activates a serine esterase and initiates a chain of intracellular biochemical events leading to the physiologic release of mediators. The release of mediators is inhibited by the elevation of intracellular cyclic AMP (cAMP). Levels of cAMP may be in-

TABLE 9–1. ALLERGENS THAT CAUSE ASTHMA AND RHINITIS

Pollens
    Ragweed, timothy grass, orchard grass, sweet vernal grass, redtop grass, rye grass, Bermuda grass, elm, oak, birch, maple, poplar, ash, alder, hazel, cedar, cypress, juniper
Molds
    Alternaria, Hormodendrum, Aspergillus, Penicillium, Mucor, Candida, Fusarium, smuts
Indoor allergens
    Dust mites, cat, dog, horse, rabbit, mouse, rat, cattle, guinea pig, gerbil, hamster, feathers, wool, cottonseed, kapokseed
Insects
    Caddis fly, Hymenoptera emanations
Industrial organic dusts
    Green coffee dust, wood dusts, tannic acid, castor bean, cottonseed, flours, grain dust, enzyme detergents, hog trypsin, psyllium powder
Industrial chemicals
    Platinum salts, nickel salts, phenylmercuric compounds, toluene diisocyanate, paraphenylenediamine, piperazine, penicillin
Foods
    Most commonly fish, shellfish, nuts

(Freedman SO, Gold P (eds): Clinical Immunology, 2nd ed. Hagerstown, Harper & Row, 1976, p 95)

creased by β-adrenergic stimulation, by prostaglandins, and by histamine. Release of histamine and other mediators is facilitated by cholinergic stimulation.

In allergic rhinitis, the chief mediator appears to be histamine. In asthma, SRS-A plays a major role. ECF-A is probably responsible for the influx of the large number of eosinophils in type I hypersensitivity reactions. The role of the eosinophil itself is uncertain but recent studies indicate that it may inactivate products of basophil or mast cell secretion (49).

Although all individuals in a particular environment may be exposed to the same allergens, only the atopic individuals develop clinical allergy. The reasons for this variation in response to allergens is not entirely clear. It has been suggested that the nasal mucosa of allergic individuals may be more permeable to allergens than that of normal subjects (17). This increased permeability is probably due to local edema, vasodilation, and epithelial hyperplasia. There is also a striking association between IgA deficiency states in children and the development of allergic disease (61). The reason for this association is not clear. One

possibility is that the absence of IgA at the mucosal surface reduces the opsonization and phagocytosis of allergens. These antigens may then become available for stimulation of IgG-producing lymphoid tissues (49).

It has long been known that genetic factors play a role in allergic sensitization (24). An association has been shown between HLA-A7 and the IgE response to ragweed antigen Ra_s (82). Genes which control the immune response may govern the recognition of antigen by T cells and may also account for impaired production of IgA. The absence of local defense mechanisms may allow for an increased penetration of allergenic substances and trigger an overproduction of specific IgE antibodies. Thus, genetic influences may be one factor contributing to the development of an allergic state.

Overproduction of IgE antibody is felt to be due to excessive T helper cell activity and an impaired T suppressor cell population (64). Locally synthesized IgE concentrates on mast cells and basophils in numbers ranging from 10,000 to 40,000. The percentage of occupied receptors per cell is higher in the allergic individual than in the nonallergic one. The serum levels of IgE are somewhat higher in allergic patients than in normal persons, but there is no direct correlation between cell-bound IgE and serum IgE.

Although uveitis has been linked with allergy, a clear association has not been shown. An acute iridocyclitis has been associated with ingestion of lobster, and a recurrent iritis has been seen in hay fever (108), but Van Metre (125) found no association between allergy and uveitis in 556 patients. Daily instillation of an antigen into the conjunctival sac, however, may eventually result in an iritis (4). Allergy to epinephrine was studied by Aronson and Yamamoto (5) and antibodies to epinephrine were found in the serum of several patients. Granulomatous iridocyclitis has also been reported in association with allergy to cat dander (127).

Clinical Features

A typical attack of allergic rhinitis consists of watery rhinorrhea, sneezing, and nasal obstruction. Itching of the nose and eyes is common. Attacks are usually seasonal; however, with perennial allergens such as house dust, the symptoms may occur year-round.

The conjunctiva is edematous and appears pale and boggy. The lids may also be edematous and hyperemic. Instillation of the offending pollen into the conjunctival sac produces typical signs of hay fever conjunctivitis.

Diagnosis

A series of cutaneous tests may be utilized to establish the antigens causing a patient's hypersensitivity. Scratch or prick tests may be applied to the lower surface of the forearm. An immediate wheel-and-flare reaction indicates sensitivity. In questionable or negative cutaneous tests, intracutaneous injections can be given. These are usually administered in limited numbers and in lower dilutions since systemic reactions are more likely to develop.

A scraping of the nasal mucosa or conjunctiva may be helpful if a diagnosis of hay fever is in question. A Giemsa-stained scraping will reveal many eosinophils.

Treatment

Antihistamines may be given systemically to relieve allergic symptoms. Some of the popular ones are diphenhydramine, tripelennamine, and chlorpheniramine maleate. Antihistamines are competitive inhibitors of histamine and must be used repeatedly and regularly to be effective. They also have sedative and anticholinergic effects. Topically applied preparations such as Vasocon-A drops often contain both an antihistamine and a vasoconstrictor. For severe conjunctival edema, epinephrine drops may be instilled in the conjunctival sac, since this helps to reduce edema quickly. Corticosteroids may be extremely effective in relieving symptoms of allergic rhinitis but since the disease is a chronic, recurrent, benign condition, these drugs should only be used in extreme situations. Instillation of 2%–4% cromolyn into the conjunctival sac may be effective in reducing sneezing, rhinorrhea, nasal congestion, and ocular irritation in ragweed hay fever (45).

Hyposensitization therapy appears to be useful in certain types of allergic rhinitis. Repeated injections of increasing concentrations of the offending allergen result in the production of blocking antibodies of the IgG class which prevent the interaction of antigen with cell-bound IgE. The cells also lose their capacity to release histamine in response to a particular allergen and sometimes in response to unrelated allergens. Immunotherapy is especially effective in allergy due to ragweed, grass, and possibly house dust. However, the potential danger of serious systemic reactions such as anaphylaxis must be kept in mind during this type of therapy.

DRUG ALLERGY

Drug reactions are among the most commonly encountered problems in medical practice, including ophthalmology. With frequent use of topical medications, it is often difficult to separate the toxic from the allergic side effects of a particular drug. Drug allergy may be caused by a heterogeneous group of immunologic mechanisms. Any of the four hypersensitivity mechanisms may be responsible for a drug-induced allergy. Type IV or delayed hypersensitivity reactions are among the most common.

Immunopathology

Type I or anaphylactic hypersensitivity reactions are the most serious reactions and are often potentially fatal. They occur within moments after the administration of a drug. These reactions are mediated by IgE, and complement is not involved. The typical clinical manifestations include urticaria and morbilliform eruptions, which may involve the skin of the eyelids. Other manifestations include hypotension, shock, asthma, and laryngeal edema. Anaphylactic reactions may occur in response to aspirin, antibiotics such as penicillin and streptomycin or foreign serums. Penicillin can also cause adverse side effects through type II, type III, and type IV hypersensitivity mechanisms.

Type II or cytotoxic hypersensitivity occurs when antibody interacts with antigen attached to a target cell. These reactions are complement-dependent. Usually a complex containing drug, antibody, and complement becomes fixed to the cell membrane. This leads to lysis of the target cells, which may include leukocytes or platelets. Type II reactions can be induced by penicillin, methyldopa, sulfonamides, quinidine, or incompatible blood transfusions.

Type III hypersensitivity drug reactions may lead to urticaria, serum sickness, or a multisystem complement-dependent vasculitis. Immune complexes are deposited within tissues, including blood vessels, and the complement pathways are activated, resulting in local inflammatory foci. Bilateral iritis has been described in a patient who developed serum sickness following a series of injections of equine antipneumococcal serum for pneumonia (121) and after injection of tetanus antiserum. A similar type of uveitis has been produced experimentally in the rabbit.

Type IV hypersensitivity reactions are commonly encountered in the form of contact allergy to topical medications. In ophthalmology, drug allergies of this type occur with various topical antibiotics, anesthetics, and dilating agents, and with certain preservatives. These reactions are discussed more thoroughly in Chapter 6.

The β-adrenergic blocker practolol may be associated with various adverse side effects, including skin rashes, a lupuslike syndrome, and a sclerosing peritonitis. Recently, an oculomucocutaneous syndrome has been reported with practolol (135). Affected patients present with skin rashes, dry eyes, distinctive corneal and conjunctival signs, secretory otitis, and fibrinous thickening of serous membranes leading to small bowel obstruction (31). This syndrome does not appear to be related to toxicity but does have several immunologic features. Patients have an increased incidence of autoantibodies, including antinuclear antibodies and thyroid cytoplasmic antibodies (53). They demonstrate cutaneous anergy to candida and SKSD (streptokinase–streptodornase) antigens, and depressed lymphocyte function *in vitro*.

The conjunctival lesions associated with practolol administration include loss of goblet cells and subepithelial fibrosis. An inflammatory reaction involving the conjunctiva, lacrimal gland, iris, and ciliary body are sometimes found at autopsy. An interesting feature is the deposition of IgG and IgM between the epithelial cells of the conjunctiva. A similar finding is commonly seen in pemphigoid. Complement has not been demonstrated in these tissues, suggesting that complement activation does not occur and that the antibodies are probably not cytotoxic. The formation of autoantibodies is more likely to be secondary to epithelial damage (103). While T cell responses have been observed, recent studies have found lymphocyte transformation in patients with eye damage due to practolol to be within normal limits.

Allergic keratitis associated with chlordiazepoxide (Librium) has been reported as an extremely rare side effect of this medication (32). Apparently the keratitis was related to edema of bilateral pterygia.

Clinical Features

Taking the history is the most important step in the diagnosis of drug reactions. Careful questioning about medications, including those which the patient does not himself consider actual drugs, is required. Patients frequently do not regard aspirin, analgesics, anovulatory agents, or vitamins as drugs.

While the clinical manifestations of drug reactions are protean, skin reactions are among the more frequently encountered. These include urticaria (penicillin), exanthematous eruptions (ampicillin), exfoliative dermatitis (barbiturates, heavy metals, sulfonamides), bullae (iodides, bromides), erythema multiforme (sulfonamides, barbiturates), lichenoid eruptions (gold salts, thiazides, and antimalarials), and fixed drug eruptions (phenolphthalein, barbiturates, and sulfonamides).

One problem peculiar to ophthalmology is that of the drug reaction which occurs following intravenous fluorescein administration (117). A variety of seemingly allergic reactions have been reported with this diagnostic drug. These include urticarial reactions, wheezing, respiratory arrest, pruritus, shock, laryngeal edema, and exanthems. Skin testing and antibody studies have not convincingly identified the mechanism by which these reactions occur. They do, however, seem to be allergic in nature, and precautions should be taken when fluorescein is administered. A small indwelling catheter has been recommended to keep the vein open in case a reaction should develop. An emergency tray should also be available, with epinephrine 1:1000, diphenhydramine (Benadryl), aminophylline, metaraminol bitartrate (Aramine), hydrocortisone sodium succinate (Solu-Cortef), parenteral fluids with intravenous adaptors, syringes, needles, an airway, and oxygen.

Diagnosis and Treatment

Many *in vitro* tests are available for the diagnosis of drug allergy, including the basophil degranulation test, lymphocyte activation test, radioallergosorbent test (RAST), and others. The practicality and usefulness of these assays remain to be seen.

Treatment of drug allergies requires the discontinuation of the suspected drug. An alternative drug which does not cross react should be substituted when necessary. Symptomatic and supportive treatment should be administered when appropriate.

SERUM SICKNESS

Serum sickness is a type III hypersensitivity reaction in which immune complexes are deposited in various tissues. The immunologic mechanisms are discussed in Chapter 2. Serum sickness usually follows the injection of a heterologous protein. Antitoxins, such as those for diphtheria, rabies, snake venom, and botulism, may produce this type of reaction. Certain drugs, including penicillin and sulfonamides, have also been implicated. Signs and symptoms appear 1–2 weeks after the injection of the foreign protein. Findings include arthritis, fever, urticaria, lymphadenopathy, and splenomegaly. Rarely, glomerulonephritis and laryngeal edema may be seen. Ocular involvement has been reported (48, 121): immune complexes are thought to be deposited in the uveal tract, as in the kidney and synovial

membranes. These complexes presumably fix complement and attract inflammatory cells. Clinical findings include a bilateral anterior uveitis characterized by inflammatory cells in the anterior chamber and by keratic precipitates. Serum sickness iritis has been reported following the injection of equine antipneumococcal serum and after the injection of tetanus antiserum. The patient described by Theodore and Lewson (121) developed bilateral iritis in association with generalized serum sickness on two occasions 9 days and 30 days after a series of inoculations with equine antipneumococcal serum for pneumococal pneumonia. Experimental uveitis, similar to that described in serum sickness, has been produced in the rabbit by Wong *et al* (133).

Laboratory abnormalities in serum sickness include an elevated sedimentation rate, leukocytosis, hematuria, proteinuria, and decreased levels of serum complement. Usually the disease is self-limited and free of complications. The urticaria may be treated with epinephrine and antihistamines. The arthritis generally responds well to salicylates. If the patient is severely ill, a short course of systemic corticosteroids can be given. The uveitis seems to respond well to treatment with topical corticosteroids and dilating drops.

SARCOIDOSIS

Sarcoidosis is a multisystem disease of unknown etiology which is characterized by a number of immunologic abnormalities. The disease primarily affects the lungs and lymph nodes; however, almost any organ can be involved. Ocular findings are seen in about 25% of cases. An ocular syndrome having the characteristic findings of sarcoidosis but lacking systemic disease may also be seen.

Immunopathology

Various etiologic agents have been implicated in sarcoidosis, including mycobacteria, pine pollen, organic dusts, beryllium, fungi, and viruses. The cause, however, remains unknown. Sarcoidosis is frequently classified as an immunologic disorder because of the characteristic alterations in cell-mediated immunity (55, 60, 90), but whether sarcoidosis is the result of an immunologic disturbance, or whether the immunologic disturbances are secondary to widespread inflammation of lymph nodes, is unclear. A slow virus remains an etiologic possibility; however, attempts to culture a virus have thus far been unsuccessful (118). Recently, a transmissible agent has been isolated from human sarcoid tissue homogenates which produced epithelioid and giant-cell granulomas in the foot pads of mice (89). The ability to produce granulomas was destroyed when the homogenates were autoclaved. This hypothetic agent could represent either a mycobacterium or a virus.

The immunologic abnormalities in sarcoidosis can be classified into three main areas: 1) depression of delayed hypersensitivity, 2) lymphoproliferation with increased serum γ-globulins, and 3) granulomatous reactions, such as the Kveim test.

Depression of delayed hypersensitivity is a well-known feature of sarcoidosis. Skin test reactivity to a variety of antigens, including mumps, tuberculin, dinitrochlorobenzene (DNCB), pertussis, and keyhole-limpet hemocyanin (KLH), is depressed or absent (55). The tuberculin skin test is negative in two-thirds of patients with sarcoidosis. However, it may become positive when the disease resolves, whereas most patients cannot be sensitized to either DNCB or KLH (55). This suggests a T-lymphocyte–mediated anergy and impaired cellular immunity, but whether the impaired delayed hypersensitivity is due to an abnormality of circulating T lymphocytes or to circulating serum inhibitors is still unknown.

In vitro studies in sarcoidosis have usually revealed a depression of T cell activity and an overaction of B cell function (27, 55). Lymph node involvement in sarcoidosis may impair the recirculation of T lymphocytes and contribute to lower T cell counts (104). Lymphocytes from patients with sarcoidosis respond less actively to the mitogen phytohemagglutinin (47). During remission, this mitogenic response is restored. Lymphocytes from patients with sarcoidosis also show an enhanced spontaneous blastogenic response *in vitro* (18), especially after the lymphocytes are cultivated

for 5–7 days. This phenomenon is associated with the release of lymphokines, and recently migration inhibition factor (MIF) activity has been demonstrated in the serum of patients with sarcoidosis (124). Attempts have been made to establish an *in vitro* test for sarcoidosis based on the production of MIF (8). Although inhibition can be demonstrated using spleen tissue from a sarcoidosis patient as an antigen, the lymphocytes of some controls also give a positive result. Other attempts to produce lymphocyte MIF, using lymphocytes from patients with sarcoidosis and Kveim antigens, have met with mixed results; positive responses in patients with Hodgkin's disease and tuberculosis may limit their clinical usefulness (57).

In contrast to the depressed cellular immunity in sarcoidosis, antibody production is overly active. Elevated levels of IgG, IgA, and IgM have been described. Clinical improvement results in decreased levels of IgG and IgM, but, IgA usually remains elevated. Increased levels of circulating antibody to Epstein–Barr virus and to herpes simplex, rubella, measles, and parainfluenza viruses have been reported (20, 126). False-positive serologic tests for syphilis and increased antibody responses to mismatched blood have also been described (109). IgD levels in serum have been either normal or increased (39); however, in middle-aged sarcoidosis patients they may be depressed (19). Serum IgE has been found to be significantly elevated (10). Immunoglobulin levels in bronchial secretions of sarcoidosis patients are increased but similar increases have also been noted in various other diseases. There is no evidence that patients with sarcoidosis have any particular HLA type.

Immune complexes have been detected in the serum of patients with sarcoidosis (1, 46). Some of these patients have had erythema nodosum and one had acute iritis (1). Increased complement activity has also been found in the serum of patients with active sarcoidosis (18).

Circulating immune complexes are considered to be responsible for some of the clinical symptoms in sarcoidosis patients. These complexes may nonspecifically attach to lymphocytes via their Fc receptors and may lead to inaccurate quantitation of T and B cells. B lymphocytes bearing complement receptors are increased in sarcoidosis patients. The frequency of autoantibodies does not appear to be different in sarcoidosis patients as compared with the normal population.

The Kveim test for sarcoidosis is positive in four-fifths of patients with this multisystem disorder and is negative in all but 2% of control patients. The test is performed by intradermally injecting an extract of spleen tissue from a patient with active sarcoidosis. The site is observed for 6 weeks to note development of a nodule. Any nodule that appears is biopsied and examined for the formation of a sarcoid granuloma. Some disadvantages of the Kveim test should be noted. In atypical cases, in which a specific test would be most useful, the Kveim reactions may be negative. The Kveim antigen is not readily available, and some authors feel that the test is sufficiently complicated and difficult to make it impractical for the diagnosis of sarcoidosis (55).

Clinical Features

General. Sarcoidosis has a worldwide distribution but is especially common in Scandinavia and among blacks in the United states. The disease is most frequent in the third and fourth decades of life and also has a higher incidence during pregnancy and lactation. Two clinical forms are recognized. The acute form of the disease is characterized by prominent hilar lymphadenopathy, erythema nodosum, and slow resolution over a period of 2 years. The chronic form is marked by involvement of the lung parenchyma and skin, and has a poorer prognosis.

Constitutional symptoms include fever, malaise, anorexia, and weight loss. Many cases, however, are asymptomatic. Lymphadenopathy, especially in the hilar region, is the most common manifestation of sarcoidosis. Involvement of the lungs produces the most frequent presenting symptoms and leads to disability later in the course of the disease. Symptoms include cough, dyspnea, chest pain, and hemoptysis. Chest x-ray may show hilar or mediastinal adenopathy, parenchymal lung

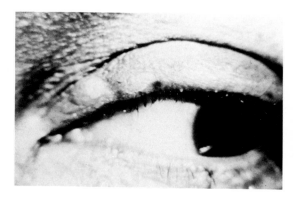

FIG. 9-1. Skin nodules of eyelid in sarcoidosis. (Courtesy of F. I. Proctor Foundation)

disease, cavitary lesions, pneumothorax, pleural effusion, or emphysema. It is generally felt that adenopathy represents an early stage of sarcoidosis, while pulmonary fibrosis is associated with chronic disease of greater than 2 years' duration.

The skin and mucous membranes are involved in one-third of patients with sarcoidosis. Small skin nodules may be present around the face, nose, eyes, and mouth and on the back of the neck (Fig. 9-1). Lesions may be erythematous and raised or nondescript plaques and papules. The mucous membranes, including the nasal mucosa, palate, larynx, and conjunctiva, may be involved (Fig. 9-2). Erythema nodosum is common in sarcoidosis, although not specifically related to

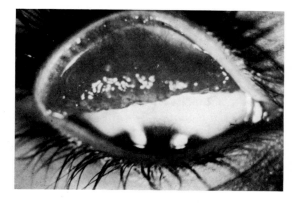

FIG. 9-2. Conjunctival involvement in sarcoidosis. (Courtesy of F. I. Proctor Foundation)

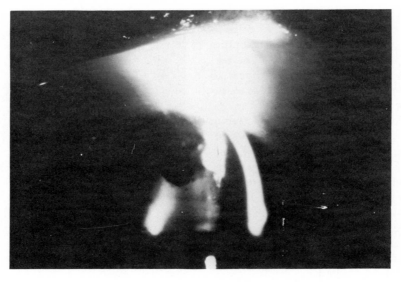

FIG. 9-3. Granuloma of iris in sarcoidosis. (Courtesy of Dr. R. Weinberg)

this disease. Transient erythematous nodules generally occur on the pretibial surfaces.

Hepatic tubercles are present in 75% of autopsy cases, and liver biopsy is frequently used for diagnostic purposes in sarcoidosis. Splenomegaly occurs in 20% of cases. "Punched-out" bone lesions are present in 10% of cases and arthritis may also be seen. The parotid and other salivary glands may be enlarged. Cranial nerve palsies, especially seventh nerve palsy, may be seen. The heart, kidneys, gatrointestinal tract, and skeletal muscles are sometimes involved.

Ocular Findings. About one-fourth of patients with sarcoidosis have ocular manifestations (54). Estimates, however, range from 8.7%–64%. Virtually any tissue of the eye may be involved. Small "millet-seed" nodules may be seen on the eyelids as on the skin elsewhere. Conjunctival nodules are frequently present on the palpebral conjunctiva and these may be biopsied to confirm the diagnosis. Yellowish sarcoid nodules are sometimes seen on the episclera, especially over the insertion of the rectus muscles. Scleral plaques are sometimes observed. The most common corneal manifestation of sarcoidosis is band keratopathy. This has been observed in sarcoidosis

patients with normal as well as high levels of serum calcium. Nummular keratitis and interstitial keratitis may also be seen (30).

Iridocyclitis is probably the most frequent ocular manifestation of sarcoidosis. Acute iridocyclitis is characterized by ciliary congestion and "mutton-fat" keratic precipitates. Koeppe and Busacca nodules may be seen on the surface of the iris. In chronic iridocyclitis there is a tendency to form anterior and posterior synechiae, and cataracts and secondary glaucoma may develop during the course of chronic inflammation. Granulomas on the iris (Fig. 9-3) may sometimes be large and have been mistaken for tumors. The ciliary body is frequently affected in sarcoidosis. Chronic cyclitis may occur, with membrane formation on the pars plana or exudation into the vitreous or peripheral preretinal region. Glaucoma may develop as a result of peripheral anterior synechiae or extensive posterior synechiae with iris bombé. Steroid glaucoma and cataracts may be sequelae of treatment. Impairment of aqueous outflow due to nodular infiltration of the trabecular meshwork can occur and may account for the rise in intraocular pressure seen in some cases (52). Uveoparotid fever (Heerfordt's disease), which is characterized by uveitis and enlargement of the parotid or submaxillary glands, may be a presenting feature of sarcoidosis.

A nonspecific chorioretinitis may develop and may lead to scarring, chorioretinal atrophy, and pigment clumping. Scattered discrete exudates may be seen along the veins. Vitreous opacities and preretinal infiltrates are seen in 30%. Eighty percent of patients with fundus lesions have some systemic involvement (40). Central nervous system involvement occurs in 35% of sarcoidosis patients with fundus lesions as opposed to 2% of all cases of sarcoidosis.

Retinal lesions are common in sarcoidosis and consist of the characteristic "candle-wax drippings" or *en taches de bougie* (Fig. 9-4). Small greyish white or yellow masses may be seen along the retinal vessels, especially the veins. Hemorrhages, vascular constriction, thrombosis, and granulomatous masses arising from the retina may also be present. Irregular pigmentation of the macula or macular edema may occur. Retinal periphlebitis and recurrent vitreous hemorrhages are occasionally seen in sarcoidosis. Newly formed blood vessels may develop in a fanlike pattern in the peripheral retina, similiar to the vascularization seen in sickle cell anemia (77). The optic nerve head may be involved directly with a sarcoid granuloma (36, 68). Optic nerve edema, enlargement of the optic foramen on x-ray, and a visual field loss may be seen. Other cranial nerves, including the facial nerve, may be affected. Unilateral internal ophthalmoplegia has also been reported (123).

Orbital involvement in sarcoidosis is rare but when it occurs may produce an exophthalmos (86). Lacrimal gland involvement is frequent and can be associated with the keratitis sicca syndrome (75).

Diagnosis

Characteristic x-ray features, including bilateral hilar adenopathy, are helpful in the diagnosis of systemic sarcoidosis. If characteristic x-ray changes are lacking, a biopsy is very useful. The presence of an epithelioid granuloma in a single lymph node or in a liver biopsy does not prove the diagnosis of sarcoidosis: 5% of all cases of Hodgkin's dis-

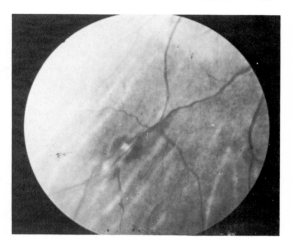

FIG. 9-4. "Candle wax" exudates of retina and vasculitis in sarcoidosis. (Courtesy of Dr. R. Weinberg)

ease will have similar findings on liver biopsy (57). Conjunctival biopsy (Fig. 9-5) is a useful diagnostic technique, being positive in 33% of patients with sarcoidosis but not in other disease processes (63). It is said to be diagnostically useful even in the absence of ophthalmologic symptoms or conjunctival lesions. The Kveim skin test is positive in 80% of patients with sarcoidosis and the incidence of false-positives is only 2%. The Kveim test antigen is extracted from sarcoid tissue and is not commercially available.

An increase in IgG, IgM, and IgA is usually present in sarcoidosis. Hypercalcemia occurs in about 15% of patients. Other approaches to diagnosis include the measurement of serum lysozyme (129) and angiotensin-converting enzyme (74), and gallium scans (51). However, serum lysozyme levels are elevated not only in patients with active uveitis and systemic sarcoidosis, but also in patients with active uveitis without an established diagnosis of sarcoidosis (129).

Treatment

The mainstay of treatment in sarcoidosis is the use of systemic corticosteroids. There is some controversy about when corticosteroids should be administered. Most clinicians feel that corticosterioids should be given to pa-

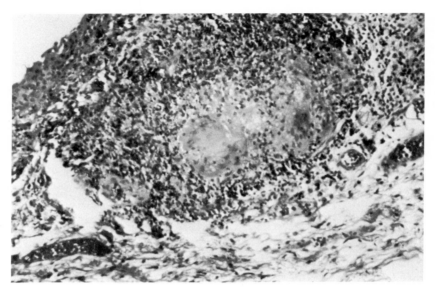

FIG. 9-5. Conjunctival biopsy in sarcoidosis showing granuloma formation. (Courtesy of Dr. R. Weinberg)

tients who are disabled or ill with respiratory or systemic sarcoidosis, including those with persistent hypercalcemia or with central nervous system, myocardial, ocular, or disfiguring cutaneous involvement (50). On the other hand, patients with only hilar or mediastinal adenopathy and with no symptoms or impairment of pulmonary function should not be treated with steroids. Some investigators feel that severe sarcoidosis progresses despite the use of corticosteroids and that most patients with sarcoidosis improve irrespective of treatment. Others feel that corticosteroid therapy decreases clinical symptoms and prevents extensive fibrotic changes.

Steroid therapy may be given topically and subconjunctivally or under Tenon's capsule in addition to the systemic treatment. The prognosis is usually good; however, in certain cases, especially in blacks, the ocular disease may be severe and progressive and lead to significant visual loss.

BEHÇET'S DISEASE

Behçet's disease is a chronic recurrent inflammatory disease with widespread clinical mani-festations. It affects adults of both sexes, and is found especially in Mediterranean countries and in Japan. Classically, Behçet's disease consists of the triad of relapsing iritis and recurrent oral and gential ulcers (9). Other common features include vasculitis, skin lesions, arthritis, meningomyelitis, and inflammatory bowel disease. Loss of vision is one of the most frequent and serious manifestations of Behçet's disease. In Japan, Behçet's disease is said to be responsible for one-third of all cases of uveitis. The etiology of Behçet's disease is unknown, but viral, immunologic, and hereditary factors have all been im plicated.

Immunopathology

Behçet was the first to propose a viral etiology for this disease, having described inclusion bodies in the smears of ulcer exudates (9). Others claim to have isolated a virus from the blood of patients with aphthae and to have produced the disease in mice and rabbits by inoculation (93, 111). In addition to culturing a virus, Evans *et al* showed the presence of neutralizing antibodies in the serum of patients with Behçet's disease (34). The validity of these findings has been questioned by some authors (29), and recent attempts to isolate a virus from body fluids have been unsuccessful (114). The possibility of a viral etiology in this disease therefore remains in question.

The importance of autoimmune mechanisms in the pathogenesis of Behçet's disease has been investigated in recent years (99, 112). Elevation of serum globulin, especially the α_2 fraction, has been demonstrated (25). Autoantibodies to oral mucosa have been detected (70, 94, 99); however, some authors believe that these antibodies result from nonspecific destruction of the mucosa, especially since no correlation has been found between antibody titer and the activity of the disease (42). Moreover, these antibodies have been found with the same frequency in patients suffering from aphthous stomatitis (69). It has been suggested that the characteristic skin hyperactivity seen in Behçet's disease represents an Arthus-like reaction (26). However, no local immunoglobulin or complement deposits have been found in these skin lesions, suggesting that local humoral factors may not be relevant (42).

Elevated levels of total hemolytic complement activity have been reported in Behçet's disease (65), and a marked increase in levels of complement component C9 has also been demonstrated (62). The significance of these observations in the pathogenesis of Behçet's disease is still unclear. C3 levels have been reported as being normal (42).

Cell-mediated immune mechanisms have also been studied in patients with Behçet's disease. Lymphocyte transformation in response to mucosal antigens has been demonstrated (71), as well as cytotoxic effects of lymphocytes on oral mucosa (28, 107). Delayed hypersensitivity reactions to skin homogenates have been observed, and the skin reactions are characterized histologically by intense lymphocytic infiltration (23a). None of these findings proves a cellular immune etiology for Behçet's disease. Lymphocyte sensitization following tissue injury may explain some of the findings, while lymphocyte skin reactions can certainly be caused by nonimmunologic factors such as trauma. Still, cell-mediated immunity has been correlated with the activity of Behçet's disease (72), and a possible impairment of the regulatory mechanism which controls T cell proliferation has been suggested (42).

Increased numbers of mast cells have been reported in the cellular infiltrates of the recurrent ulcers and in the skin lesions of Behçet's disease (42, 73). Mast cells are found in decreased numbers in nonspecific ulcers of the mouth and may conceivably play a role in the skin and mucosal lesions of Behçet's disease.

A number of patients with Behçet's disease have reported exacerbations of their symptoms after ingestion of certain foods, especially walnuts, chocolate, and tomatoes. Extracts of English walnuts were cultured with lymphocytes from normal subjects and from patients with Behçet's syndrome; this resulted in increased incorporation of tritiated thymidine (81). Within 2 days of ingestion of walnuts by normal subjects and those with Behçet's syndrome, the *in vitro* lymphocyte reactivity to walnut extract and candida antigens was significantly decreased in both groups. This depression lasted longer in the patients with Behçet's syndrome than in the normal subjects. The mitogenic and subsequent depressive effect of English walnuts in Behçet's disease, although nonspecific, may have deleterious effects on the course of the disease.

An increased incidence of HLA-B5 has been found in Japanese patients with Behçet's disease (98). The latter antigen is known to be closely related to HLA-B5, Bw35, and B18. Other investigators have shown no significant increase of any HLA antigen (95). The presence of familial Behçet's syndrome in four generations has been reported and strengthens the argument for genetic transmission of susceptibility in Behçet's disease (38).

Clinical Features

General. Behçet's disease has a world-wide distribution, although it has a particularly high incidence in the Mediterranean basin, the Middle East, and Japan. The mean age at onset is during the 20s, but the syndrome may even appear in childhood. The most frequent initial manifestation is oral ulceration. However, patients often do not seek medical help until they develop ocular symptoms. The classic triad of oral–genital–ocular disease has broadened with the recognition of multiple organ system involvement. In general, the longer the follow-up of cases, the greater is the chance of additional systems becoming involved.

Nearly all patients with Behçet's disease have recurrent aphthous ulcers of the oropharynx. These ulcers are painful and may occur in the oral cavity or on the lips. They are larger than common aphthae, appear in crops, and heal without scarring (25).

Genital ulcers also tend to be recurrent and are mostly single in the male but multiple in the female. They may involve the scrotum and penis, or labia and vagina. They are circular, erythematous with a whitish core, and up to 3 or 4 cm in diameter; they heal slowly in 3–4 weeks, leaving a distinct scar.

Skin lesions are variable and are observed in a majority of patients. Erythema nodosum is seen in approximately one-third of patients. Other skin lesions include erythema multiforme, maculopapular eruptions and pyodermatous lesions. An interesting phenomenon in patients with Behçet's disease is the hyperreactivity of the skin to any intracutaneous injection or needle prick. This phenomenon, known as **pathergy,** is manifested clinically by erythematous induration at the site of trauma and the development of a small pustule containing sterile pus (14). The reaction is maximal at 48 h and often progresses to frank ulcer formation. Pathergy is a unique feature of Behçet's disease and is currently unexplained. The reaction is not specific and occurs with the injection of autologous plasma, saline, or a simple venipuncture. It is characterized histologically by a perivascular round-cell infiltrate. Although it was believed at one time to represent an Arthus phenomenon (26), recent studies have been unable to confirm this (116). Pathergy is said to occur in 37% of patients with Behçet's disease.

Joint involvement is common in Behçet's disease and is characterized by arthralgias and an inflammatory arthritis. It does not lead to permanent joint deformation. Vascular lesions consist of recurrent superficial or deep migratory thrombophlebitis. This affects the lower limbs especially, but the inferior or superior vena cava may be involved, and intracranial venous thrombosis may occur and may lead to papilledema (83). Aortic and peripheral artery aneurysms have also been reported.

Central nervous system involvement in Behçet's disease occurs in 4%–42% of patients, with a mean of 18% (22). The clinical picture varies and may include a meningoencephalitis, increased intracranial pressure, brain stem lesions, cranial nerve palsies, cerebellar and extrapyramidal signs, or spinal cord and peripheral nerve lesions.

The gastrointestinal tract may be involved, producing an ulcerative colitis syndrome. Liver involvement is uncommon but may occur. Other clinical manifestations include pulmonary and cardiac lesions, epididymitis, and orchitis. Kidney involvement is rare but acute glomerulonephritis has recently been reported (59).

Ocular Findings. Ocular lesions are common, occurring in approximately 75% of patients (22). The usual presenting sign is an iridocyclitis with a hypopyon (Fig. 9-6). This may be associated with pain and redness; however, at times the eye is uninflamed. The hypopyon lasts for 3–8 days and resolves with or without treatment. The uveitis is often bilateral either at onset or within one year. Other ocular manifestations include choroiditis, and retinal phlebitis and arteritis. An occlusive retinal vasculitis is frequently seen. Optic nerve involvement has also been reported (22). Optic papillitis (Fig. 9-7), papilledema, and optic atrophy have all been seen. Prior to the onset of iridocyclitis, a hyperfluorescence of the disc may appear, suggesting vascular involvement and increased permeability around the optic nerve (105). Inflammatory cells and hemorrhages may be seen in the vitreous. The conjunctiva may be injected and chemotic, and may exhibit hemorrhages. The cornea may show a punctate keratitis, stromal opacities, edema, and ulcerations (41).

Ocular complications include cataract and glaucoma, and blindness is not uncommon. Patients with only anterior segment involvement tend to have a better prognosis. Complications are more closely related to posterior involvement and to the duration of the dis-

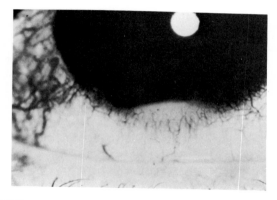

FIG. 9-6. Hypopyon iritis in Behçet's disease. (Courtesy of Dr. K. Yamaguchi)

ease. Blindness has been reported in 44% of patients with posterior segment involvement after 4–8 years (22).

Treatment

No satisfactory treatment currently exists for Behçet's disease. Topical administration of corticosteroids to the aphthous ulcers may or may not have an immediate ameliorative effect. Systemic administration of corticosteroids has been widely used for the systemic disease and may cause remission of central

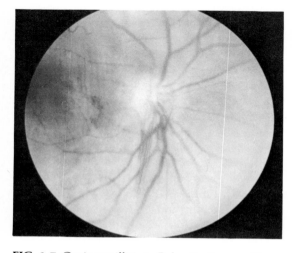

FIG. 9-7. Optic papillitis in Behçet's disease. (Courtesy of Dr. G. Mintsioulis)

nervous system involvement. It is difficult to evaluate treatment in Behçet's disease because of the natural exacerbations and remissions and the considerable variability among patients.

Recently, treatment with immunosuppressive agents in this disease has been encouraging. Chlorambucil appears to be one of the most useful drugs of this type in the treatment of Behçet's disease. It has been associated with long-lasting remissions in some patients with uveitis (79, 115, 122). Chlorambucil may be used in conjunction with small doses of corticosteroids. Beneficial effects have also been obtained from plasma or blood transfusions, and with fibrinolytic agents in the treatment of mucocutaneous or vascular disease. Systemic corticosteroids and immunosuppressive treatment should probably be reserved only for patients whose clinical disease threatens life or sight.

VOGT–KOYANAGI–HARADA SYNDROME

The Vogt–Koyanagi–Harada (VKH) syndrome is a chronic bilateral exudative uveitis associated with whitening of the hair and eyelashes, vitiligo, and meningeal irritation. The syndrome encompasses two overlapping diseases. Vogt-Koyanagi syndrome consists of severe anterior segment inflammation associated with dysacousia, vitiligo, alopecia, and poliosis. In Harada's disease uveal inflammation is mainly posterior, with serous retinal detachments, disc hyperemia, meningeal inflammation, and a lesser incidence of skin and hair changes. The significant overlap in symptoms and the similiar histopathologic features of both diseases has led to the combining of these two syndromes into a single disease entity.

Immunopathology

Although it has not been satisfactorily confirmed, a viral etiology has been suggested for VKH syndrome. Vitreous from a patient with posterior segment involvement was found to produce a uveitis and optic neuritis when injected into the cerebrospinal fluid in rabbits (120). Others have injected cerebrospinal fluid from affected patients into the eyes of experimental animals to demonstrate the transmissibility of the disease (35, 106). Inclusion bodies within phagocytic cells have been demonstrated (91, 132), although viral cultures have been negative.

Antibodies to uveal pigment have been demonstrated in patients with VKH syndrome (58), as have delayed hypersensitivity skin reactions to uveal pigment (58, 95). Lymphocytes sensitized to melanin have been found in the peripheral blood of patients with VKH syndrome (43), and leukocyte migration is inhibited when lymphocytes from VKH patients are cultured in the presence of uveal pigment (44). Bovine uveal antigen was found to inhibit leukocyte migration in eight of twelve patients with Harada's disease (110). Cellular hypersensitivity to uveal pigment has also been demonstrated in sympathetic ophthalmia by means of lymphocyte transformation and leukocyte migration inhibition assays (43, 44). Circulating antimelanin antibodies are found in vitiligo, one of the clinical signs commonly associated with VKH syndrome.

The significance of heightened cellular and humoral reactivity to uveal antigens is unclear. Whether these findings indicate that pigment hypersensitivity is important in the development of the disease or whether cellular reactivity to uveal antigens is secondary to uveal inflammation is still unknown. Recently, a decreased number of T lymphocytes in the peripheral blood has been demonstrated in patients with VKH syndrome using two types of rosette assays (23). While it is unclear whether the diminished T lymphocytes represent all T cells, or suppressor cells or other subpopulations of lymphocytes, these findings strengthen the concept that immune factors are important in the development of VKH syndrome. Increased levels of complement, and especially of C3, may be detected during the early course of the disease.

Recent interest has been shown in HLA typing of patients with VKH syndrome. An increase in HLA-Bw22J has been shown in Japanese patients with VKH syndrome (119). This antigen is found in 43% of VKH patients and in 13% of controls. In another series, however, none of 9 patients with VKH syndrome had HLA-Bw22J although a number of these patients were Oriental (96).

Histopathologically, VKH syndrome produces a granulomatous uveitis. Its appearance is similiar to sympathetic ophthalmia, although a greater amount of chorioretinal scarring is generally seen in VKH syndrome (134). A nongranulomatous uveitis has been observed in some VKH patients (102). Plasma cell infiltration of the uveal tract, hyperplasia of the retinal pigment epithelium, and pigment phagocytosis may be seen in VKH syndrome, as in sympathetic ophthalmia.

Clinical Features

VKH syndrome most commonly occurs between the ages of 20 and 40. Males and females are equally affected. The disease is especially common in Japan, where it is the third most frequent cause of uveitis (3). No correlation seems to exist, however, between race and the course of the disease (97). The clinical manifestations of VKH syndrome are varied and the complete syndrome may not be present in a particular case. While the systemic manifestations of the disease may be variably present, the ocular findings are usually the same. For convenience, patients may be classified into three groups: those with type 1 disease show characteristic ocular signs and symptoms without evidence of skin or ear involvement; those with type 2 disease have typical ocular findings and at least one manifestation of skin or ear involvement; and those with type 3 disease have ocular involvement accompanied by two or more skin, ear, or hair changes (97). In more than 70% of patients with type 1 and 2 disease, the duration of the illness is less than 1 year. In two-thirds of those with type 3 involvement, the active disease lasts longer than 1 year.

Characteristic ocular findings in VKH syndrome consist of exudative retinal detachments and chorioretinal scars which suggest prior retinal detachment. Keratic precipitates,

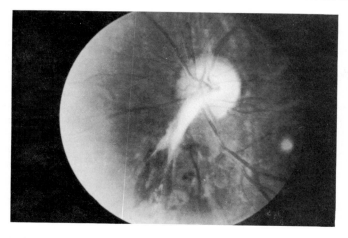

FIG. 9-8. Posterior involvement in Vogt–Koyanagi–Harada syndrome with pigmentary changes and scarring. (Courtesy of Dr. R. Weinberg)

posterior synechiae, and iris nodules may all be present. Keratic precipitates can be either small or the large, mutton-fat type. Koeppe or Busacca nodules may be seen on the iris. The ocular findings in VKH syndrome are usually bilateral, and both eyes are generally affected simultaneously. If the disease is not bilateral at onset, the second eye is usually affected within 1 month of the first. Figure 9-8 shows the posterior involvement of VKH syndrome, with pigmentary changes and scarring.

Two-thirds of patients have ocular symptoms without evidence of ear or skin involvement (97). In these patients, with type 1 disease, the diagnosis is presumptive. However, because of the characteristic ocular findings of exudative retinal detachment and bilateral diffuse granulomatous uveitis, the diagnosis of VKH syndrome seems reasonable.

The systemic manifestations of VKH syndrome are variable. Central nervous system involvement occurs in about 30%, and most such patients have a cerebrospinal fluid pleocytosis and clinical signs of meningeal irritation. The cerebrospinal fluid from patients with VKH syndrome may show increased numbers of mononuclear cells and elevated protein in the early stages of the disease. Alopecia, poliosis (Fig. 9-9), dysacousia, tinnitus, and vitiligo are seen with variable frequency.

Alopecia and poliosis may occur 3 weeks to 6 years after the onset of the disease. Vitiligo has been reported to occur 5 years before and up to 3 years after the eye symptoms. Poliosis and alopecia have appeared as long as 6 years after the onset of uveitis.

The optic nerve is often hyperemic and it may be necessary to rule out a brain tumor when low degrees of papilledema are present (Fig. 9-10). Disc edema may be an early finding in VKH syndrome. Fluorescein angiography shows numerous fluorescent dots at the level of the retinal pigment epithelium in the early choroidal phase. These dots slowly enlarge in many cases as the transit of fluorescein progresses. Increased permeability of the disc capillaries may be seen during a later phase of fluorescein transit.

The visual prognosis is best in patients with type 1 involvement: 50% of these patients recover a visual acuity of at least 20/50 in the better eye and only 25% become legally blind (97).

Treatment

The early systemic administration of corticosteroids may prevent progression of the disease, lessen its duration, and prevent systemic manifestations such as ear, skin, or hair lesions that usually appear 1–2 months after the eye

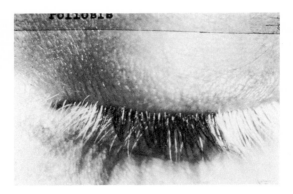

FIG. 9-9. Poliosis in Vogt–Koyanagi–Harada syndrome. (Courtesy of F. I. Proctor Foundation)

lesions (97). Some patients show a striking clinical remission after the use of immunosuppressive agents such as chlorambucil. Treatment of the ocular disease in VKH syndrome should reduce the inflammatory reaction and also avoid secondary glaucoma. Hypertonic mannitol solution has been given during the first 5 days of the disease to normalize the permeability of Bruch's membrane (84). Retrobulbar steroids have also been used with reported good results in treating the posterior pole inflammation (80). Steroid maintenance is generally required for several months after the onset of the disease. If oral corticosteroids are given in VKH syndrome, it is preferable to use

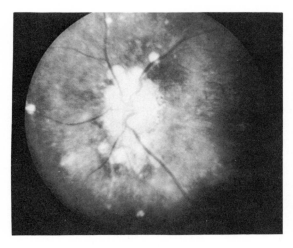

FIG. 9-10. Optic nerve involvement in Vogt–Koyanagi–Harada syndrome. (Courtesy of Dr. R. Weinberg)

an alternate-day regimen to avoid adrenal suppression.

INFLAMMATORY BOWEL DISEASE

Ulcerative colitis (UC) and Crohn's disease (CD) are inflammatory diseases of unknown etiology that primarily affect the gastrointestinal tract but also having accompanying extraintestinal manifestations. Because of the many similarities in these two disorders, and because of the strong view in recent years that they represent polar ends of a spectrum, both diseases are sometimes included in the term inflammatory bowel disease (IBD). A variety of etiologic factors has been suggested, including infectious, autoimmune, psychogenic, and toxic processes. Ocular manifestations may accompany IBD, with uveitis being the most frequent finding. A high incidence of arthritis and sacroiliitis is also known to occur.

Immunopathology

The possibility of an infectious etiology in IBD has received much attention. It has been possible to transmit a condition similiar to Crohn's disease to mice (88) and rabbits (21), using filtrates of human ileum from patients with the disease. The transmissible agent may be a virus (37) or an aberrant bacterium (100). Similar lesions have been induced in mice using homogenates taken from the colon of ulcerative colitis patients.

A dietary allergy to milk has been suggested as a possible etiology for ulcerative colitis (2). Although exclusion of cow's milk or other proteins from the diet may be beneficial in some patients, milk allergy is no longer considered an important cause of most IBD. Still, some indirect evidence does favor a type I hypersensitivity reaction in ulcerative colitis. Some patients have increased numbers of eosinophils in the blood and rectal mucosa, increased circulating basophils, increased numbers of mast cells in the lamina propria, and a high histamine content in rectal biopsy tissue (12). These features are generally absent in patients with Crohn's disease.

Humoral immune mechanisms have been investigated in some depth in patients with IBD. No consistent differences in circulating immunoglobulins are found. Autoantibodies, however, have been demonstrated in the serum of children with ulcerative colitis, suggesting the possibility of an autoimmune disease (16, 130). These antibodies to colonic tissue are true autoantibodies since they react with autologous as well as heterologous rectal biopsy tissue. They may belong to any of the three major immunoglobulin classes and cannot be related to the extent of severity of clinical disease. They persist after colectomy, and are not cytotoxic for colon cells in tissue culture. It is presently considered unlikely that they are pathogenic in IBD. It has been suggested that bacterial antigens, particularly *Escherichia coli*, may stimulate the production of antibodies which then cross react with endogenous colonic tissue (130). Antibody titers to *E. coli*, however, do not differ in IBD and control patients, and although it is an attractive hypothesis, this mechanism has not been proven.

Other circulating autoantibodies have been demonstrated in patients with IBD. These include antinuclear factors, rheumatoid factor, precipitins to pancreatic homogenates, and antibodies to erythrocytes, gastric and small intestinal mucosa, gastric parietal cells, thyroglobulin, adrenal tissue, extracts of liver or kidney, and reticulin (67). Autoimmune disorders have frequently been associated with ulcerative colitis and less frequently with Crohn's disease. Those autoimmune disorders associated with colitis include systemic lupus erythematosus, chronic active hepatitis, autoimmune hemolytic anemia, Hashimoto's thyroiditis, myasthenia gravis, and pernicious anemia. These associations may, however, be coincidental.

Immune complexes have been demonstrated in the serum of some patients with ulcerative colitis. While the nature of the antigen has not been determined, the antibody appears to be an IgG (7). These complexes could account for some of the extraintestinal manifestations of IBD. Serum complement levels are usually normal.

Cellular immunity has been studied in IBD

with great interest, using skin testing and *in vitro* assays. Several studies have demonstrated anergy using tuberculin or dinitrochlorobenzene (DNCB) (13, 56). Anergy to DNCB and decreased numbers of circulating T lymphocytes have been demonstrated in both ulcerative colitis and Crohn's disease (87). Delayed cutaneous hypersensitivity responses to DNA have been found in one-third of patients with colitis, and positive Kveim tests have been reported in Crohn's disease. The significance of these findings and a possible relationship to sarcoidosis await further investigtion.

Transformation of lymphocytes by plant mitogens and assays for migration inhibition factor have been inconclusive in proving a cellular immune component in IBD. Both normal and reduced responses have been seen with phytohemagglutinin (131). Leukocyte migration inhibition has, however, been demonstrated in ulcerative colitis and Crohn's disease using extracts of gastrointestinal tissue (131).

Leukocytes from patients with colitis have been shown to be cytotoxic for human fetal colon cells (101). Cytotoxicity for autologous or allogeneic adult human colon cells has been demonstrated in both colitis and Crohn's disease (113). Normal lymphocytes can also be made cytotoxic by incubating them for 4 days with serum from patients with ulcerative colitis or Crohn's disease; or with *E. coli* lipopolysaccharide. This effect is lost ten days after colectomy. The cytotoxic factor seems to be contained in lymphocytes derived from patients with IBD, which suggests a lymphotoxin-mediated destruction of target cells (128). These findings suggest either that sensitized T cells bind to epithelial cells through specific surface receptors or that killer cells coated with immune complexes recognize target colonic epithelial cells. These findings suggest that IBD is a consequence of a lymphocyte-mediated hypersensitivity reaction to bacterial antigens that are normally present in the lower gastrointestinal tract.

Histocompatibility antigens have been investigated in IBD. An increased frequency of HLA-A11 and B7 has been found (6), as well as an increased frequency of HLA-A2, HLA-Bw35, and HLA-Bw40, and a decrease in HLA-A10 (92). Other studies report no significant difference in antigen frequency between patients and controls, although HLA-B27 is increased in IBD patients who also have ankylosing spondylitis or sacroiliitis (78).

Clinical Features

General. Inflammatory bowel disease is characterized by diarrhea, colic, and malabsorption, with weight loss and consequent nutritional deficiencies. Intestinal bleeding is more common in ulcerative colitis than in Crohn's disease, while fistula formation is more common in Crohn's disease. Crohn's disease more often affects young people between ages 11 and 40, and has an equal incidence in both sexes. The terminal ileum is the most common site of involvement; however, colonic inflammation is frequently recognized. Inflammation is more segmental in Crohn's disease and "skip areas" are characteristic. Carcinoma is seen with increased frequency in ulcerative colitis but not in Crohn's disease.

Extracolonic manifestations are similar in both conditions. These include spondylitis and peripheral arthritis, erythema nodosum, aphthous ulcers, pyoderma gangrenosum, and amyloidosis. Arthritis is seen in up to 20% of all patients and is usually a migratory monoarthritis or ankylosing spondylitis. The incidence is somewhat higher in ulcerative colitis than in Crohn's disease.

Ankylosing spondylitis is found twenty times more commonly in patients with Crohn's disease than in the general population. In contrast to the peripheral arthritis, ankylosing spondylitis is not related to the extent or severity of the bowel disease. Other extraintestinal manifestations of IBD which are related to pathophysiology of the small bowel, but not to colitic activity, included malabsorption of vitamin B_{12}, bile salts, and other substances, gallstones, obstructive hydronephrosis, kidney stones, and renal amyloid deposition.

Ocular Findings. The most common ocular complication of IBD is uveitis. It is said to occur in 0.5%–12% of patients with ulcerative colitis and in approximately 50% of those with accompanying sacroiliitis (15). Inflammation is usually bilateral and nongranulomatous, and is frequently unrelated to acute flare-ups of colitis. Those patients with iritis also have symptoms of joint involvement (11). It has been stated that uveitis is unlikely to recur after colectomy (66); however, the recurrent nature of the iritis makes it difficult to evaluate.

A keratopathy with subepithelial thickening and white opacification just inside the limbus may also be seen in Crohn's disease. Other ocular changes include recurrent conjunctivitis, marginal corneal ulcers, Sjögren's syndrome, scleritis, episcleritis, myositis, serous retinitis, orbital and lid edema, optic neuritis, and neuroretinitis (76).

Treatment

Treatment of IBD remains quite unsatisfactory. Initial therapy consists of corticosteroids, sulfasalazine, and, at times, azathioprine. Azathioprine may be useful in allowing reduction of the corticosteroid dosage; it has been associated with some toxicity, especially pancreatitis. Surgery is not curative but may be necessary to relieve the complications of obstruction and fistula formation. Recently, BCG has been given intradermally in order to stimulate the immune system nonspecifically. Intravenous hyperalimentation has been used to correct nutritional deficiencies and is considered a supportive measure in IBD.

Ocular disease may be transient and self-limited. A persistent uveitis can frequently be managed with topical corticosteroids and dilating agents (33). Uveitis is unlikely to recur after colectomy; however, it is rarely a sufficient indication for surgery (66). Marginal corneal infiltrates respond well to topical steroids, but these should be used with caution, especially if peripheral corneal thinning is present. Neuroretinitis appears to respond to systemic corticosteroid therapy (76).

REFERENCES

1. Agnello V, Winchester RJ, Kunkel HG: Precipitin reaction of the C1q component of complement with aggregated γ-globulin and

immune complexes in gel diffusion. Immunology 19:909, 1970

2. Andresen AFR: Gastro-intestinal manifestations of food allergy. Med J Rec 122:271, 1925

3. Araki Y: The epidemiology and present status on ocular involvement of Behçet's disease in Japan. Saishin Igaku 26:458, 1971

4. Aronson SB, Goodner EK, Yamamoto E, Foreman M: Mechanisms of the host response in the eye. I. Changes in the anterior eye following immunization to a heterologous antigen. Arch Ophthalmol 73:402, 1965

5. Aronson SB, Yamamoto EA: Ocular hypersensitivity to epinephrine. Invest Ophthalmol 5:75, 1966

6. Asquith P, Mackintosh P, Stokes PL et al: Histocompatibility antigens in patients with inflammatory bowel disease. Lancet 1:113, 1974

7. Ballard J, Shiner M: Evidence of cytotoxicity in ulcerative colitis from immunofluorescent staining of the rectal mucosa. Lancet 1:1014, 1974

8. Becker FW, Krul P, Deicher H, Kalden JR: The leukocyte migration test in sarcoidosis. Lancet 1:120, 1972

9. Behçet H: Über die rezidivierende Aphthose durch ein Virus verursachte Geschwüre am Mund, am Auge und an den Genitalien. Derm Wochenschr 105:1152, 1937

10. Bergmann Von K-Ch, Zausmell I, Lachman B: IgE konzentratione im serum von patienten mit sarkoidose und lungentuberkulose. Dtsch Gesindheitsw 27:1774, 1972

11. Billson FA, DeDombal FT, Watkinson G, Goligher JC: Ocular complications of ulcerative colitis. Gut 8:102, 1967

12. Binder V, Hvidberg E: Histamine content of rectal mucosa in ulcerative colitis. Gut 8:24, 1967

13. Blackburn G, Hadfield G, Hunt AH: Regional ileitis. St. Bartholomew's Hospital Reports 72:181, 1939

14. Blobner F: Zur rezidivierenden Hypopyoniritis. Z Augenheilk 91:129, 1937

15. Bloch RS: Gastrointestinal and nutritional diseases. In Duane TD: Clinical Immunology. Hagerstown, Harper & Row, 1976

16. Broberger O, Perlmann P: Autoantibodies in human ulcerative colitis. J Exp Med 110:657, 1959

17. Buckley CE, Cohen AB: Nasal mucosal hyperpermeability to macromolecules in atopic rhinitis and extrinsic asthma. J Allergy Clin Immunol 55:213, 1975

18. Buckley CE, Nagaya H, Sieker HO: Altered immunologic activity in sarcoidosis. Ann Intern Med 64:508, 1966

19. Buckley CE, Trayer HR: Serum IgD concentrations in sarcoidosis and tuberculosis. Clin Exp Immunol 10:257, 1972

20. Byrne EB, Evans AS, Fouts DW, Israel HL: A sero-epidemiological study of Epstein-Barr virus and other viral antigens in sarcoidosis. Am J Epidemiol 97:355, 1973

21. Cave DR, Mitchell DN, Kane SP et al: Further animal evidence of a transmissible agent in Crohn's disease. Lancet 2:1120, 1973

22. Chajek T, Fainaru M: Behçet's disease. Report of 41 cases and a review of the literature. Medicine 54:179, 1975

23. Char DH, Brunn J, West W: Thymus-derived lymphocytes in the Vogt-Koyanagi-Harada syndrome. Invest Ophthalmol 16:179, 1977

23a. Coe JE, Feldman JD, Lee S: Immunologic competence of thoracic duct cells. I. Delayed hypersensitivity. J Exp Med 123:267, 1966

24. Cooke RA, Veer VA: Human sensitization. J Immunol 1:201, 1916

25. Cooper DA, Penny R: Behçet's syndrome: clinical, immunological and therapeutic evaluation of 17 patients. Aust NZ J Med 4:585, 1974

26. Cooper DA, Penny R, Fiddes P: Autologous-plasma sensitisation in Behçet's disease. Lancet 1:910, 1971

27. Cummiskey JM, McLaughlin H, Keelan P: T and B lymphocytes in sarcoidosis: a clinical correlation. Thorax 31:665, 1976

28. Dolby AE: Recurrent aphthous ulceration: effect of sera and peripheral blood lymphocytes upon oral epithelial tissue culture cells. Immunology 17:709, 1967

29. Dowling GB: Behçet's disease. Proc R Soc Med 54:101, 1961

30. Duke-Elder S: System of Ophthalmology, Vol VIII, Part I, Diseases of the Outer Eye. St Louis, Mosby, 1965, pp 561–567

31. Editorial: Beta-blockers and the eye. Br J Ophthalmol 60:311, 1976

32. Efet VA: About allergic keratitis in patients treated with librium. Oftalmol Zh 28:108, 1973

33. Ellis PP, Gentry JH: Ocular complications of ulcerative colitis. Am J Ophthalmol 58:779, 1964

34. Evans AD, Pallis CA, Spillane JD: Involvement of the nervous system in Behçet's syndrome: report of three cases and isolation of virus. Lancet 2:349, 1957

35. Friedenwald JS, McKee EM: A filter-passing agent as a cause in endophthalmitis. Am J Ophthalmol 21:723, 1938

36. Gass JDM, Olson CL: Sarcoidosis with optic nerve involvement. Arch Ophthalmol 94:945, 1976

37. Gitnik GL, Rosen VJ: Electron microscopic studies of viral agents in Crohn's disease. Lancet 2:217, 1976

38. Goolamli SK, Comaish JS, Hassanyeh F: Familial Behçet's syndrome. Br J Dermatol 95:637, 1976

39. Goldstein RA, Israel HA, Janicki BW, Yo-

koyami M: Serum immunoglobulin D levels in sarcoidosis. Proceedings of the VIth International Conference on Sarcoidosis, Tokyo University Press, 1974, p 196

40. Gould H, Kaufman HE: Sarcoid of the fundus. Arch Ophthalmol 65:453, 1961

41. Grayson M, Keates RH: Manual of Diseases of the Cornea. Boston, Little, Brown, 1969, p 125

42. Haim S, Sobel JD, Friedman-Birnbaum R, Lichtig C: Histological and direct immunofluorescence study of cutaneous hyperactivity in Behçet's disease. Br J Dermatol 95:631, 1976

43. Hammer H: Lymphocyte transformation test in sympathetic ophthalmitis and Vogt-Koyanagi-Harada syndrome. Br J Ophthalmol 55:850, 1971

44. Hammer H: Cellular hypersensitivity to uveal pigment confirmed by leucocyte migration tests in sympathetic ophthalmitis and the Vogt-Koyanagi-Harada syndrome. Br J Ophthalmol 58:773, 1974

45. Handelman NI, Friday GA, Schwartz HJ et al: Cromolyn sodium nasal solution in the prophylactic treatment of pollen-induced seasonal allergic rhinitis. J Allergy Clin Immunol 59:237, 1977

46. Hedfors E, Norberg R: Evidence for circulating immune complexes in sarcoidosis. Clin Exp Immunol 16:493, 1974

47. Hirschorn K, Schreibman RR, Bach FH, Siltzbach LE: In vitro studies of lymphocytes from patients with sarcoidosis and lymphoproliferative disease. Lancet 2:842, 1964

48. Hoover RE: Nongranulomatous uveitis, a complication of serum sickness. Am J Ophthalmol 41:534, 1956

49. Hubscher TT: Immune and biochemical mechanisms in the allergic disease of the upper respiratory tract: role of antibodies, target cells, mediators and eosinophils. Ann Allergy 38:83, 1977

50. Israel HL: Some controversial aspects of sarcoidosis. Ann Allergy 38:112, 1977

51. Israel HL, Parks CH, Mansfield CM: Gallium scanning in sarcoidosis. Proc Seventh Int Conf on Sarcoidosis. Ann NY Acad Sci 278:514, 1976

52. Iwata K, Nanba K, Sobue K, Abe H: Ocular sarcoidosis: evaluation of intraocular findings. Ann NY Acad Sci 278:445, 1976

53. Jachuk SJ, Bird T, Stephenson J, Jackson FS, Clark F: Practolol-induced autoantibodies and their relation to oculo-cutaneous complications. Postgrad Med J 53:75, 1977

54. James DG, Anderson R, Langley D et al: Ocular sarcoidosis. Br J Ophthalmol 48:461, 1964

55. James DG, Neville E, Walker A: Immunology of sarcoidosis. Am J Med 59:388, 1975

56. Jones JV, Housley J, Ashurst PM, Hawkins CF: Development of delayed hypersensitivity to dinitrochlorbenzene in patients with Crohn's disease. Gut 10:52, 1969

57. Kadin MD, Donaldson SS, Dorfman RF: Isolated granulomas in Hodgkin's disease. N Engl J Med 283:859, 1970

58. Kahan A, Sztanojevits A, Szabados T et al: Pigment-autoaggression in der Pathogenese des Vogt-Koyanagi-Harada syndrome. Albrecht V Graefes Arch Klin Ophthalmol 167:246, 1964

59. Kansu E, Deglin S, Cantor RI et al: The expanding spectrum of Behçet's syndrome. A case with renal involvement. JAMA 237:1855, 1977

60. Kataria VP: Sarcoidosis. An overview. Clin Notes Resp Dis 14:2, 1975

61. Kaufman HS, Hobbs JR: Immunoglobulin deficiencies in atopic population. Lancet 2:1061, 1970

62. Kawachi-Takahashi S, Takahashi M, Kogure M, Kawashima M: Elevation of C9 level associated with Behçet's disease. Jpn J Exp Med 44:488, 1974

63. Khan F, Wessely Z, Chazin SR, Seriff NS: Conjunctival biopsy in sarcoidosis: a simple safe and specific diagnostic procedure. Ann Ophthalmol 9:671, 1977

64. Kisimoto T, Ishizaka K: Regulation of antibody response in vitro. 6. Carrier specific helper cells for IgG and IgE antibody response. J Immunol 111:720, 1973

65. Kogure M, Shimada K, Hara HG: Complement titer in patients with Behçet's disease. Acta Soc Ophthalmol Jpn 75:1260, 1971

66. Korelitz BI, Coles RS: Uveitis (iritis) associated with ulcerative granulomatous colitis. Gastroenterology 52:78, 1967

67. Kraft SC, Kirsner JB: The immunology of ulcerative colitis and Crohn's disease: clinical and humoral aspects. In Kirsner JB, Shorter RG: Inflammatory Bowel Disease. Philadelphia, Lea & Febiger, 1975, pp 72–73

68. Laties A. Scheie HG: Sarcoid granuloma of the optic disc: evolution of multiple small tumors. Trans Am Ophthalmol Soc 68:219, 1970

69. Lehner T: Immunological aspects of recurrent oral ulcers. Lancet 2:80, 1964

70. Lehner T: Behçet's syndrome and autoimmunity. Br Med J 1:465, 1967

71. Lehner T: Stimulation of lymphoctye transformation by tissue homogenate in recurrent oral ulceration. Immunology 13:159, 1967

72. Lehner T: Characterization of mucosal antibodies in recurrent aphthous ulceration and Behçet's syndrome. Arch Oral Biol 14:843, 1969

73. Lehner T: Pathology of recurrent oral ulceration and oral ulceration in Behçet's syndrome. Light electron and fluorescence microscopy. J Pathol 97:481, 1969

74. Lieberman J: Elevation of serum angiotensin

converting enzyme level in sarcoidosis. Am J Med 59:365, 1975

75. Lorentzen SE: Keratoconjunctivitis sicca in sarcoidosis. Acta Ophthalmol 38:235, 1960

76. Macoul KL: Ocular changes in granulomatous ileocolitis. Arch Ophthalmol 84:95, 1970

77. Madigan JC, Gragoudas ES, Schwartz PL, Lapus JV: Peripheral retinal neovascularization in sarcoidosis and sickle cell anemia. Am J Ophthalmol 83:387, 1977

78. Mallas, EG, Mackintosh P, Asquith P, Cooke WT: Histocompatibility antigens in inflammatory bowel disease. Gut 17:906, 1976

79. Mamo J: Treatment of Behçet's disease with chlorambucil. A follow-up report. Arch Ophthalmol 94:580, 1976

80. Manor RS: Particular aspects of the Vogt-Koyanagi-Harada syndrome. Ophthalmologica 165:425, 1972

81. Marquardt JL, Snyderman R, Oppenheim JJ: Depression of lymphocyte transformation and exacerbation of Behçet's syndrome by ingestion of English walnuts. Cell Immunol 9:263, 1973

82. Marsh DG, Bias WB, Hsu SH, Goodfriend L: Association of an HL-A7 cross-reacting group with a specific reaginic antibody response in allergic man. Science 179:691, 1973

83. Masheter HC: Behçet's syndrome complicated by intracranial thrombophlebitis. Proc R Soc Med 52:1039, 1959

84. Masuda K, Tanijima T: Harada's disease—new therapeutic approach. Jpn J Clin Ophthalmol 23:4, 1969

85. McPherson SD, Woods AC: The significance of the intracutaneous test for hypersensitivity to uveal pigment. Am J Ophthalmol 31:35, 1948

86. Melmon KL, Goldberg JS: Sarcoidosis with bilateral exophthalmos as the initial symptom. Am J Med 33:158, 1962

87. Meyers S, Sachar DB, Taub RN, Janowitz HD: Anergy to dinitrochlorbenzene and depression of T-lymphocytes in Crohn's disease and ulcerative colitis. Gut 17:911, 1976

88. Mitchell DN, Rees RJW: Agent transmissible from Crohn's disease tissue. Lancet 2:168, 1970

89. Mitchell DN, Rees RJW, Goswami KKA: Transmissible agents from human sarcoid and Crohn's disease tissues. Lancet 2:761, 1976

90. Mitchell DN, Scadding JG: Sarcoidosis. Am Rev Resp Dis 110:774, 1974

91. Morris RW, Schlaegel TF: Virus-like inclusion bodies in subretinal fluid in uveoencephalitis. Am J Ophthalmol 58:940, 1964

92. Nahir M, Gideoni O, Eidelman S, Barzilai A: HLA antigens in ulcerative colitis. Lancet 2:573, 1976

93. Noyan B. Gursky G, Aktiu E: Inoculation of cerebrospinal fluid of a neuro-Behçet patient into mice. Acta Neuropathol (Berl) 12:195, 1969

94. O'Duffey JD, Carney JA: Behçet's disease: report of 10 cases, 3 with new manifestations. Ann Intern Med 75:561, 1971

95. O'Duffey JD, Taswell HF, Elvebeck LR: HL-A antigens in Behçet's disease. J Rheumatol 3:1, 1976

96. Ohno S, Char DH, Kimura SJ, O'Connor GR: HLA and Vogt-Koyanagi-Harada syndrome. N Engl J Med 295:788, 1976

97. Ohno S, Char DH, Kimura SJ, O'Connor GR: Vogt-Koyanagi-Harada syndrome. Am J Ophthalmol 83:735, 1977

98. Ohno S, Nakayama E, Suguira S et al: Specific histocompatibility antigens associated with Behçet's disease. Am J Ophthalmol 80:636, 1975

99. Oshima Y, Shimizu T, Yokohari R et al: Clinical studies on Behçet's syndrome. Ann Rheum Dis 22:36, 1963

100. Parent K, Mitchell P: Cultivation of viral agents from Crohn's disease. Lancet 2:576, 1976

101. Perlmann P, Broberger O: In vitro studies of ulcerative colitis. Cytotoxic action of white blood cells from patients on human fetal colon cells. J Exp Med 117:717, 1963

102. Perry HD, Font RL: Clinical and histopathologic observations in severe Vogt-Koyanagi-Harada syndrome. Am J Ophthalmol 83:242, 1977

103. Rahi AHS, Chapman CM, Garner A, Wright P: Pathology of practolol-induced ocular toxicity. Br J Ophthalmol 60:312, 1976

104. Ramachandar K, Douglas SD, Siltzbach LE: Peripheral blood lymphocyte subpopulations in sarcoidosis. Cell Immunol 16:442, 1975

105. Ramalho PS, D'Almeida F, Magalhães A: Behçet's disease: clinical endocrinological and immunological aspects. Trans Ophthalmol Soc UK 94:614, 1974

106. Remky H: Beitrag zur Kenntnis schwerer Foremen der Uveoencephalitis. Klin Monatsbl Augenheilkd 123:166, 1953

107. Rogers RS, Sams WM, Shorter RG: Lymphocytotoxicity in recurrent aphthous stomatitis: lymphototoxcity for oral epithelial cells in recurrent aphthous stomatitis and Behçet's syndrome. Arch Dermatol 109:361, 1974

108. Ruedemann AD: Ocular manifestations of allergy. In Thomas JW (ed): Allergy in Clinical Practice. Philadelphia, Lippincott, 1961, pp 256–274

109. Sands JH, Palmer PP, Maycock RL: Evidence for serologic hyper-reactivity in sarcoidosis. Am J Med 19:401, 1955

110. Sanefuji M: Cell-mediated immunity in uveitis. 2. Leukocyte migration inhibition test in Harada Disease. Acta Soc Ophthalmol Jpn 78:306, 1974

111. Sezer N: Further investigations on the virus of Behçet's disease. Am J Ophthalmol 41:41, 1956

112. Shimizu T, Katsuta Y, Oshima Y: Immunological studies on Behçet's syndrome. Ann Rheum Dis 24:494, 1965

113. Shorter RG, Cardoza M, Spencer RJ, Huizenga KA: Further studies of in vitro cytotoxicity of lymphocytes from patients with ulcerative and granulomatous colitis for allogeneic colonic epithelial cells including the effects of colectomy. Gastroenterology 56:304, 1969

114. Sigel N, Larson R: Behçet's syndrome: a case with benign pericarditis and recurrent neurologic involvement treated with adrenal steroids. Arch Intern Med 115:203, 1965

115. Smulders FM, Oosterhuis JA: Treatment of Behçet's disease with chlorambucil. Ophthalmologica 171:347, 1975

116. Sobel J, Haim S, Shafir A, Gellei B: Cutaneous hyperreactivity in Behçet's disease. Dermatologica 146:350, 1973

117. Stein MR, Parker CW: Reactions following intravenous fluorescein. Am J Ophthalmol 72:861, 1971

118. Steplewski Z, Israel HL: The search for viruses in sarcoidosis. Proc Seventh Int Conf on Sarcoidosis. Ann NY Acad Sci 278:260, 1976

119. Tagawa Y, Suegiura S, Yakura H: HLA and Vogt-Koyanagi-Harada syndrome. N Engl J Med 295:788, 1976

120. Takahashi M: Clinical and experimental studies on the nature of idiopathic, bilateral, severe uveitis. Acta Soc Ophthalmol Jpn 34:506, 1930

121. Theodore FH, Lewson AC: Bilateral iritis complicating serum sickness. Arch Ophthalmol 21:828, 1939

122. Tricoulis D: Treatment of Behçet's disease with chlorambucil. Br J Ophthalmol 60:55, 1976

123. Turner RG, James DG, Friedmann AI et al: Neuroophthalmic sarcoidosis. Br J Ophthalmol 59:657, 1975

124. Umbert P, Belcher RW, Winkelmann RK: Lymphokines (MIF) in the serum of patients with sarcoidosis and cutaneous granuloma annulare. Br J Dermatol 95:481, 1976

125. Van Metre TE: Role of the allergist in diagnosis and management of patients with uveitis. JAMA 195:105, 1966

126. Wahren B, Carlens E, Espmark A et al: Antibodies to various herpes viruses in sera from patient with sarcoidosis. J Natl Cancer Inst 47:747, 1971

127. Walker V: Allergy in ophthalmology. Proc R Soc Med 40:582, 1947

128. Watson DW, Shorter RG: The immunology of ulcerative colitis and Crohn's disease: cell-mediated immune responses. In Kirsner JB, Shorter RG: Inflammatory Bowel Disease. Philadelphia, Lea & Febiger, 1975, p 61

129. Weinberg RS, Tessler HH: Serum lysozyme in sarcoid uveitis. Am J Ophthalmol 82:105, 1976

130. Weinstein L: Bacterial aspects of ulcerative colitis. Gastroenterology 40:323, 1961

131. Whorwell PJ, Wright R: Immunological aspects of inflammatory bowel disease. Clin Gastroenterol 5:303, 1976

132. Wilczek M, Feltynowski A: Study of sympathetic ophthalmia by electron microscopy. Klin Oczna 25:77, 1956

133. Wong VG, Anderson RR, McMaster PRB: Endogenous immune uveitis. Arch Ophthalmol 85:93, 1971

134. Woods AC: Endogenous Uveitis. Baltimore, Williams & Wilkins, 1958, p 267

135. Wright P: Untoward effects associated with practolol administration. Br Med J 1:595, 1975

TEN TEN TEN neurologic and endocrine diseases

Immunologic mechanisms in neurologic and endocrine diseases have become the focus of increased interest and investigation. In multiple sclerosis, for example, an infectious agent may trigger an immune response which attacks the tissues of the nervous system. In other disorders, auto-antibodies or immune cells may interact with and destroy host tissues. While the entire pathogenesis of these diseases is not known, new methods of diagnosis and treatment have been established that are based on immunologic findings.

MULTIPLE SCLEROSIS

Multiple sclerosis (MS) is the commonest neurologic disease affecting young adults in temperate climates. It is mainly a disease of Caucasians, especially those of European descent. The disease is characterized pathologically by an inflammatory demyelination of the central nervous system. Clinically, affected individuals develop debilitating symptoms lasting for many years which are associated with remissions and exacerbations. The eyes are frequently affected, and optic neuritis or extraocular muscle disturbances may be early findings. Although the etiology is unknown, a number of studies have implicated viral, immunologic, and genetic factors.

Immunopathology

The initial impression that MS might be related to an early viral infection came from epidemiologic investigations. Multiple sclerosis is a disease closely associated with geographic factors. The prevalence of MS increases with increasing latitude, both north and south of the equator. The distribution closely follows the classic pattern associated with viral infections whose effects are delayed for some time after the initial infection. The risk of developing MS seems to be determined by some event which takes place in early childhood. When adults move from a high-risk to a low-risk area, their chances of developing MS are associated with the original environment. If an individual migrates before the age of 15, however, the risk becomes that of the new environment.

Increased titers of antibodies to measles virus have been demonstrated in the serum and cerebrospinal fluid of patients with MS (32, 54). In addition, measles virus has been isolated from the brains of some patients who died from MS (44). High concentrations of antibodies to other viruses have been demonstrated in MS patients, including antibodies to vaccinia, rubella, and herpes simplex. It has been suggested that MS patients have an inborn defect in their immune system which allows viruses to proliferate in the central nervous system. Utermohlen and Zabriskie have reported that cellular immune responses to measles virus are selectively suppressed in patients with MS (73). Other investigators, however, have reported conflicting results (15), suggesting that these findings depend on the particular preparation of measles antigen used. The serum of patients with MS may contain a blocking factor which prevents leukocytes from destroying cells infected with measles virus (44). This blocking factor appears to be specific in that it does not prevent leukocytes from attacking cells infected with other viruses. It is, however, found in subacute sclerosing panencephalitis (SSPE), a fatal demyelinating disease thought to be caused by persistent measles virus (see Rubella, Ch. 7).

Recently, an *in vitro* blood test for MS was developed that uses measles-virus–infected tissue culture cells (39). Lymphocytes from MS patients show marked rosetting activity when cultured *in vitro* with epithelial cells that are infected with measles virus. This test is not affected by the severity, duration, or activity of the disease and may prove to be a useful blood test for the diagnosis of MS. Measles virus antigen has been detected recently in the jejunal mucosa of MS patients by fluorescent antibody techniques (57). This appears to be the first demonstration of measles antigen in MS. If these findings are confirmed, they would support the concept that persistent measles infection is associated with the development of MS. As indicated previously and in Chapter 7, SSPE appears to be another demyelinating disease which may be associated with persistent measles virus (14).

Defective cell-mediated immunity to measles virus has been detected in MS patients by the leukocyte migration inhibition test (73). This abnormal immune response may lead to a failure to eliminate the virus completely from the body. The persistence of the virus may lead to continued antigenic stimulation and high levels of antibody. Continued antibody production may further depress the cellular response to measles antigen, a phenomenon observed in immune responses to other microbial antigens (21). Depression of cellular immunity may or may not be demonstrable with respect to other viruses.

Other viruses have been suggested as possible etiologic agents in MS. Those receiving the greatest attention are members of the paramyxovirus group, especially parainfluenza-1 and a recently described transmissible agent known as the multiple-sclerosis–associated agent (MSAA) (13). Parainfluenza-1 has been isolated from the brains of two patients with MS (71); however, no further such isolations have been reported and the relationship of this virus to MS must be considered unproven. Recently, much attention has been given to MSAA. This agent, although ill-defined, produces depression of neutrophils in the blood of mice injected with extracts of brain, spleen, blood, or cerebrospinal fluid from MS patients. This effect suggests a viral infection of some sort. The depressive effect on neutrophils can be transmitted to other mice by inoculation with brain homogenates.

One of the most helpful diagnostic tests for MS is the finding of an elevated titer of IgG in the cerebrospinal fluid (CSF). This abnormality is found in 66%–94% of cases, depending on the assay used (41). Elevated IgA is found in the CSF of 10%–30% of MS patients. IgG and IgA synthesis has been demonstrated in lymphocytes obtained from the CSF of patients with MS (15), and nervous tissue lesions also contain increased proportions of immunoglobulins. About 50% of MS patients have a twofold increase in the ratio of κ to λ light chains in the immunoglobulins of their CSF, although their serum has a normal 1:1 ratio (43). These antibody studies in MS patients suggest a local synthesis of antibodies to an unknown antigen within the central nervous system.

Cellular hypersensitivity to central nervous system protein has been demonstrated by the leukocyte migration inhibition test (68). Studies using lymphoblastic transformation as a measure of cellular hypersensitivity have, however, given variable results. Transfer factor has been used in the treatment of MS without definite improvement; however, further studies using higher doses and longer observation periods are necessary to permit definite conclusions. Both serum and lymphocytes of patients with MS have been shown to be toxic for glial cells and for myelin (11).

Much of the evidence that the immune system is involved in MS comes from the study of an experimental model of the disease known as **experimental allergic encephalitis (EAE).** A demyelinating encephalitis now known to be this disease was first recognized about 40 years ago in humans who were given rabies vaccine containing rabbit brain cells. EAE has been produced in a variety of laboratory animals by injection of central nervous system tissues in complete Freund's adjuvant. Within 2 weeks after the injection, the animals begin to lose weight, then develop paralysis and ultimately die. EAE is mediated by T lymphocytes and can be transferred passively with lymph node cells containing sensitized T cells. The protein responsible for sensitization is known as **myelin basic protein.** Some investigators have been able to identify leukocytes sensitized to myelin basic protein in MS patients. Interestingly, myelin basic protein not only can initiate EAE but can also prevent the disease and can alleviate or even stop its symptoms after the disease has begun. Myelin basic protein has even been used to treat a few carefully selected cases of MS. The question of whether EAE is a good model for MS, however, remains controversial.

A number of studies have been carried out to determine the role of genetic factors in MS. HLA-A3 and B7 are found significantly more often in MS patients than in the general population (10), and HLA-Dw2 is present in more than 70% of MS patients in Denmark, compared with only 16% of healthy individuals. In addition, typing of antigens on the surface of human bone-marrow–derived B lymphocytes has shown that 83% of MS patients possess a certain marker (BT101), compared with 33% of controls (17).

Clinical Features

General. The initial episode in MS and subsequent relapses may follow trauma, acute infection, vaccination, pregnancy, or other types of stress. The patient may develop slurred speech, intention tremor, incontinence, spastic paralysis, increased deep tendon reflexes, and bilateral extensor plantar responses. Secondary infections of the bladder and kidney are common. Late in the disease, euphoria may be seen.

The course of MS is varied and unpredictable. Remissions may last several months or even years. A clinical course covering 10–20 years is not uncommon, and the average survival after the onset of the disease has been estimated at 27 years.

Key features in making a clinical diagnosis are 1) that clinical findings indicate the presence of central nervous system lesions in two or more areas of white matter, and cannot be explained by a single abnormality; and 2) that signs and symptoms are subject to repeated remissions and exacerbations. The finding of increased γ-globulin in the CSF is a helpful diagnostic test. Some patients, however, show no pathologic alteration in the CSF. Pathologic findings include grey patches of degeneration in the brain and spinal cord which vary in size from a few millimeters to several centimeters.

Ocular Findings. Double vision is the first symptom in 11% of MS patients (77). A history of diplopia at some time during the disease can be obtained in more than 40% of patients. Good visual acuity is maintained in most cases during the entire course of the disease; however, visual field defects at some point in the disease are a common finding.

Nystagmus, internuclear ophthalmoplegia, pupillary inequality, and abnormal responses to light are often seen. Nystagmus of the abducting eye may be accentuated by fatigue. Impairment of smooth following movements of the eye or slowing of adduction relative to abduction in conjugate gaze may be the only clinical evidence of brain stem lesions.

Uveitis may be seen with an increased frequency, and in one survey was present at some time in 15% of MS patients (60). Sheathing of the retinal veins has been described in patients with MS. Some observers, however, have doubted the association between MS, uveitis, and retinal vein sheathing.

Optic neuritis (discussed subsequently) may be a presenting sign in 28% of patients with MS (77). Optic nerve pallor may sometimes be seen, especially temporally. Pallor may be difficult to interpret and frequently the optic neuritis is retrobulbar. Visual field testing may reveal an enlarged blind spot or a central or paracentral scotoma. A uniocular color defect is good evidence of optic nerve damage. Nerve fiber bundle defects may be recognized ophthalmoscopically with a very bright, red-free light.

Treatment

No specific medical treatment exists for MS. Corticosteroid therapy and vasodilators have been advocated for the treatment of acute relapses but results in the treatment of chronic disease with these agents have been poor. Although their value has not been established, therapeutic claims have been made for tolbutamide, isoniazid, vitamin B$_{12}$, procaine, blood transfusions, and fat-free diets.

Levamisole has been used in the treatment of MS patients (20); however, five out of seven patients deteriorated while taking this medication. Although levamisole has had a beneficial effect in some chronic viral infections, perhaps in MS the increased inflammatory reaction impinged upon normal tissue in an already compromised neurologic system. Transfer factor has also been tried in some MS patients; however, results have been variable and this mode of therapy is currently difficult to assess (28, 65).

OPTIC NEURITIS

Acute optic neuritis is more frequently associated with multiple sclerosis than with any other disease entity (45). The reported incidence of this association, however, varies widely. Several years after the onset of optic neuritis, multiple sclerosis has been reported in 13% (37) to 85% of cases (40). Different criteria for classifying these conditions accounts to some extent for this apparent discrepancy. Other causes for optic neuritis besides multiple sclerosis include the Guillain–Barré syndrome (8), infectious mononucleosis (58), and subacute sclerosing panencephalitis.

Immunopathology

Oligoclonal IgG can be demonstrated in the cerebrospinal fluid in about one-third of patients with optic neuritis (70). These patients have elevated titers of measles antibody in

their serum (42) and about one-half of them have evidence of a measles virus antibody response within the central nervous system. Many optic neuritis patients with measles-virus–specific IgG in their serum will eventually develop multiple sclerosis (34). Increased titers of antibody to rubella, parainfluenza, and the Epstein–Barr virus may be detected in the cerebrospinal fluid of patients with optic neuritis (53). An abnormally high ratio of κ to λ light chain can be found in the cerebrospinal fluid IgG of these patients (70).

The histocompatibility antigens HLA-A3, A7, and Dw2 are reported to be increased in optic neuritis as well as in multiple sclerosis (59). Others have found no significant difference in HLA distribution between patients with optic neuritis and controls (4, 70). Such discrepancies are probably due to the use of different criteria in the diagnosis of optic neuritis.

In the Guillain–Barré syndrome, *in vitro* cellular immunity to central and peripheral nervous tissue myelin has been demonstrated using the macrophage migration inhibition test.

An experimental allergic optic neuritis can be produced by immunizing guinea pigs with an isogeneic spinal cord emulsion in complete Freund's adjuvant (61). The animals develop a retrobulbar neuritis with infiltration of the optic nerve, chiasm, or brain by mononuclear cells. Focal demyelination of the nerve and a neuroretinitis may also be seen. This experimental model may be useful in future studies of optic neuritis.

Clinical Features

Women account for 73% of patients with optic neuritis (33). The age at onset ranges from 14 to 59, but 74% of cases occur between the ages of 20 and 50. The median age at onset is 29 years. The attack rate tends to be highest from April to July and lowest from August to November. Some 57% of cases are unilateral and 19% are bilateral; 24% are recurrent. The onset of visual symptoms may be sudden or gradual and progressive. Pain, especially associated with movement of the globe, is present in over three-fourths of patients. Visual acuity may be minimally reduced or markedly impaired. Patients with recurrent attacks tend to have poor visual acuity. The disc is usually described as normal; however, it may be blurred, edematous, or pale.

The probability that patients with optic neuritis will develop multiple sclerosis appears to increase with longer follow-up periods. Patients with bilateral optic neuritis or with recurrent disease seem to be at a greater risk of developing multiple sclerosis (33).

MYASTHENIA GRAVIS

Myasthenia gravis (MG) is a chronic disease characterized by abnormal fatigability of striated muscle. The disease may last for many years and include several remissions. The disease may be generalized or a single muscle group may be involved. Severe wasting and weakening may eventually develop and death may occur as a result of respiratory muscle involvement. Ptosis and extraocular muscle abnormalities are frequently seen in MG. The ocular muscles may even be the first muscles to be affected. Recent investigations have suggested that autoimmune factors are important in the pathogenesis of MG. Antibodies against muscle end-plate protein and immune complexes localized to the motor end-plate can be demonstrated in patients with MG.

Immunopathology

In 1960, Simpson (69) suggested an autoimmune basis for MG because of its association with a number of other autoimmune disorders, including systemic lupus erythematosus, rheumatoid arthritis, pemphigus, pernicious anemia, thyrotoxicosis, and myxedema. Subsequently, antibodies were demonstrated against acetylcholine receptor protein in the serum of as many as 87% of patients with MG (7). Serum from myasthenic patients injected into mice can produce clinical or electrophysiologic changes characteristic of MG (72). The active fraction in the serum has been identified

as IgG and its effect can be enhanced by the third component of complement (C3). Immune complexes containing IgG and C3 have been localized to the motor end-plate in patients with MG, further suggesting the importance of an autoimmune mechanism (25). This and other experiments suggest that MG involves an antibody-mediated autoimmune attack on acetylcholine receptors at the neuromuscular junction. Antibody might permit access of macrophages and possibly of cytotoxic lymphocytes to the motor end-plate by a complement-mediated toxic effect. Other humoral antibodies have been recognized which are directed against the A band of muscle but these are probably not relevant in the pathogenesis of MG (23). Antibodies to striated muscle cross react with epithelial cells of the thymus and may be associated with the thymic abnormalities that occur in MG. Antinuclear and antithyroid antibodies have also been demonstrated in MG.

While abnormalities of the humoral immune system are probably more important in MG, the role of cellular immunity has also been under investigation. Peripheral lymphocytes from myasthenic patients show stimulation when exposed to purified acetylcholine receptors in vitro (62). Delayed hypersensitivity to muscle and thymic antigens occurs frequently in patients with MG (31). Approximately half of myasthenic patients have evidence of cellular immunity to myelin basic protein (35). Lymphocytes from patients with myasthenia have been found to be cytotoxic for fetal muscle tissues when stimulated with phytohemagglutinin (3). Such investigations show the possible importance of cellular immunity in MG. Cellular immunity may be more important pathogenically in older people who develop MG.

Thymic abnormalities are present in 80% of myasthenic patients. Some 70% have thymic hyperplasia with increased numbers of germinal centers, and 10% have true thymomas. These hyperplastic thymuses contain increased numbers of B lymphocytes. Two-thirds of patients who undergo thymectomy have complete or partial remission of MG suggesting that the thymus may be a site for production of a neuromuscular blocking agent. Soluble fractions of thymus gland show immunologic cross reactivity with acetylcholine receptor protein.

HLA typing in MG shows an increased incidence of HLA-B8 (29). This association is most prevalent in females with early onset of the disease and is correlated with the presence of thymic follicular lymphoid hyperplasia. HLA-A3 was increased in males with late-onset MG and was common among myasthenics with thymomas.

Clinical Features

General. Myasthenia gravis is characterized by muscle weakness and easy fatigability. Muscles innervated by the bulbar nuclei (face, neck, tongue, throat, and eyes) are preferentially involved. Symptoms are generally worse later in the day. The disease is most common in women between the ages of 20 and 40; however, it may occur in either sex during any decade of life. The disease may remit spontaneously in 25% of cases within the first 2 years. Some patients, however, have a downhill course with eventual respiratory impairment and complicating diseases.

The presence of circulating antimuscle antibodies in patients suspected of having MG may aid in diagnosis. In addition, abnormalities in neuromuscular transmission may be determined by electromyography. In the edrophonium (Tensilion) test, an anticholinesterase agent is given intravenously, which temporarily improves myasthenic weakness, and aids in making a correct diagnosis.

Ocular Findings. Weakness may first be noted in the extraocular and lid muscles and the patient may present with diplopia or ptosis. A compensatory wrinkling of the brow is absent; however, a myasthenic pupil and paresis of accommodation may be present. Convergence insufficiency may occur secondary to involvement of the medial recti and may lead to a spasm of accommodation and pseudo myopia. A twitch in the ptotic lid may be observed after the patient blinks or on attempted upward gaze and is considered to be typical of myasthenia.

Treatment

Anticholinesterase drugs such as pyridostigmine (Mestinon) or neostigmine are given initially. Atropine can be given concomitantly to prevent a cholinergic crisis. Pyridostigmine is probably the most satisfactory drug in newly discovered myasthenic patients. The usual dose is 60–100 mg/day in divided doses.

In keeping with the probable autoimmune etiology of MG, ACTH and corticosteroids have been found to be useful. High-dose, alternate-day prednisone therapy has produced encouraging results, especially in older male patients with far advanced disease which does not respond to coventional therapy (26). The usual dose of 100 mg prednisone every other day is supplemented with potassium, antacids, and a high-protein, low-carbohydrate diet providing 2 g sodium. This treatment does not completely eradicate the disease and symptoms may recur within a few months of discontinuing the medication (30). Therefore, a 5- to 10-mg maintenance dose of prednisone every other day is generally used. Immunosuppressive treatment with azathioprine has been introduced recently for patients who do not respond to corticosteroids.

Beneficial effects from thymectomy are seen in the majority of cases of MG, and all patients, except those with ocular myasthenia or very mild, non disabling symptoms, are candidates for thymectomy. The best results are seen in young women who have had the disease for 5 years or less and show distinct abnormalities of the thymus. In these cases clinical improvement may be expected in about 85% of patients undergoing thymectomy; complete and permanent remission occurs in one-third of these patients (16). Thymectomy appears to be better than irradiation of the thymus. Patients with thymomas rarely achieve remission after thymectomy. The usual approach to treatment of MG is with anticholinesterase drugs initially, followed by thymectomy in all patients who do not respond adequately. In those who still do not respond, corticosteroids are given, and if this approach fails, immunosuppresive and cytotoxic agents may be used.

The prognosis in MG is variable. A remission rate of 25% can be expected during the first 2 years. A chronic persistent course is routine in other cases and a 20%–30% fatality rate has been reported. Drug therapy must be handled judiciously since cholinergic crises with severe weakness may result from an overdose of anticholinesterase drugs.

DIABETES MELLITUS

Recent studies have suggested that some forms of diabetes mellitus are associated with autoimmunity. At present it is impossible to determine how important immunologic factors are in the development of diabetes. Immunologic abnormalities in diabetes may be associated with the presence of antibodies to insulin and with a variety of autoantibodies.

Immunopathology

Diabetic patients have an increased incidence of autoimmune disease involving the thyroid, adrenals, and gastric mucosa (pernicious anemia). Thyroid microsomal antibody and gastric parietal cell antibody are found in 20% and 16%, respectively, of patients with diabetes mellitus (51). These antibodies and antibodies to pancreatic islet cells are particularly common in patients with juvenile diabetes mellitus of recent onset. The finding of islet cell antibodies may precede the onset of diabetes by several years. Whether these antibodies and other autoantibodies are involved in the genesis of diabetes or are a cause of diabetogenic islet cell damage is presently uncertain. Antibodies to pancreatic islet cells are of the IgG immunoglobulin class and can be demonstrated by indirect immunofluorescence in patients with insulin-dependent diabetes (46).

Delayed hypersensitivity to crude pancreatic islet antigen can be demonstrated in diabetic patients by use of macrophage inhibition (50). Transient impairment of glucose tolerance occurs when mice are immunized with mouse pancreatic extract. Immunized animals exhibit delayed hypersensitivity skin test reactions and inhibition of macrophage migration with pancreatic islet antigen.

The histocompatibility antigen HLA-B8 is found with increased frequency in insulin-dependent diabetes, Graves' disease, and Addison's disease (52). An increased incidence of HLA-Bw15 has also been demonstrated in insulin-dependent diabetics (19).

Insulin preparations are foreign proteins and are therefore capable of evoking an antibody response. Repeated injections of insulin into humans can give rise to antibody formation (9). Beef insulin is felt to be more antigenic for man than pork insulin. An immunologic response to insulin may take the form of an allergic reaction or of increasing resistance to the effects of insulin. The allergic reaction is usually a generalized urticaria presumably mediated by IgE. Chronic insulin resistance seems to be due to insulin-binding IgG antibodies (9). Insulin resistance and allergy rarely occur in the same patient. Insulin antibody levels tend to be lower in pregnant patients (27).

Recently the vasoproliferative effects of insulin have been studied by Shabo and associates (66, 67). They suggest that vascular proliferation may be due to the immunogenic nature of insulin in addition to an intrinsic vascular abnormality in diabetics. Insulin injected intravitreally into sensitized monkeys causes proliferation of preretinal vessels and connective tissue, rubeosis iridis, vascular hemorrhages, and tortuosity and beading of vessels. Inflammation may be a significant factor in the development of this experimental neovascularization.

Clinical Features

The effects of diabetes mellitus on the visual apparatus are numerous. Xanthelasma is said to occur slightly more frequently in diabetic patients than in normal individuals. Conjunctival blood vessels have been noted to show dilation with a diurnal variation, and vasoconstriction and microaneurysms have been noted. Extraocular muscle palsies may occur owing to third or sixth nerve involvement in diabetic neuropathy; however, the pupil is generally spared. Fine wrinkles may develop in the central portion of Descemet's membrane in diabetics. Ectropion uveae and rubeosis iridis are well-known clinical signs.

Cataracts seem to be more frequent and to occur at an earlier age in diabetic patients. A "true" or juvenile diabetic cataract may occur bilaterally in younger patients. Myopic lens changes are associated with an increase in blood sugar, while hyperopic changes occur when the blood glucose is decreased. The basement membrane of the ciliary body is thicker in diabetic patients; however the significance of this finding is unknown. Asteroid hyalitis is said to occur with greater frequency in diabetic patients, although some investigators deny this. Orbital complications of diabetes mellitus are uncommon; however, mucormycosis, when it occurs, can be devastating.

Diabetic retinopathy is the most significant and disabling ocular complication of diabetes mellitus. It is characterized by microaneurysms, hemorrhages, exudates, and neovascularization. Cotton-wool spots, macular edema, and large areas of capillary nonperfusion can be demonstrated in many patients who have only mild or moderate retinopathy.

GRAVES' DISEASE

Graves' disease was described 150 years ago, but it has only been in the past 15 years that we have begun to understand the mechanism of this disorder. Abnormalities in both the humoral and cellular immune systems have now been recognized in Graves' disease and in Hashimoto's thyroiditis. In addition to immunologic phenomena, hormonal and genetic factors contribute to the exophthalmos of Graves' disease.

Immunopathology

Many lines of evidence point to the importance of autoimmunity in the pathogenesis of Graves' disease. Thyroid antibodies are present in virtually all patients with the disease and in 50% of their relatives (6, 75). Other autoantibodies and certain autoimmune disorders may be found as well. Various immunoglobulins are found within the stroma of the thyroid gland in Graves' disease, and lymphocytes and plasma cells infiltrate the thyroid gland and retroorbital tissues.

Early studies of autoimmune thyroiditis

suggested that thyroglobulin was a secluded antigen during fetal life and therefore individuals did not develop tolerance to it. If the thyroid gland was damaged by trauma or infection, however, cytotoxic thyroid antibodies could be formed. This theory is no longer tenable since circulating thyroglobulin has been demonstrated in 60% of normal individuals (63), but thyroglobulin antibodies are rarely found in patients without thyroid disease. Experimental thyroiditis can be produced by immunizing animals with thyroid tissue emulsified in Freund's adjuvant. The disease may be transferred passively with immune serum (49) or lymphocytes, the latter suggesting a possible role for cell-mediated hypersensitivity in the development of experimental thyroiditis.

The most compelling evidence for an immunologic basis for hyperthyroidism comes from the studies on long-acting thyroid stimulator (LATS). When the serum of patients with diffuse thyroid hyperplasia is injected into mice or guinea pigs, a prolonged stimulation of the animals' thyroid glands occurs. LATS, the substance which is responsible for this phenomenon, can be isolated in the γ-globulin fraction of human serum. It is precipitated and neutralized by anti-IgG, and it has been suggested that LATS is either an immunoglobulin or a soluble complex of thyrotropin and its antibody. LATS is found in 50%–80% of patients with Graves' disease (47).

Other immunoglobulin-containing substances have also been identified in the serum of patients with Graves' disease. One such substance, known as LATS protector (LATS-p), can block the binding of LATS to a human thyroid protein fraction (1). Another human thyroid-stimulating substance, stimulates the formation of intracellular colloid droplets in human thyroid slices and is found in virtually all LATS-negative patients with Graves' disease (56). Complement-fixing antibodies to thyroid microsomes are frequently found in hyperthyroidism. These antibodies may increase the function of thyroid cells. Antibodies to thyroglobulin, predominantly of the IgG and IgA class, may also be demonstrated.

The role of cell-mediated immunity may also be important in thyroid disorders. Lymphocytes from patients with Graves' disease undergo blast transformation (24) and produce migration inhibition factor (MIF) in response to human thyroid antigen (38). During a remission of thyroid disease, MIF production cannot be demonstrated. MIF is also produced in response to liver mitochondrial antigens in patients with Graves' disease or Hashimoto's thyroiditis (75). This may be due to cross reactivity between the thyroid and liver or the presence of more than one population of sensitized T lymphocytes.

Production of MIF in response to retroorbital muscle antigen can be demonstrated in patients with exophthalmos who have no evidence of thyroid disease or cellular immunity to thyroid antigens (48). Therefore, it would appear that antigens involved in the production of exophthalmos are separate from those responsible for the thyroid abnormality. Exophthalmos may be a separate autoimmune process that has a considerable overlap with the hyperthyroidism of Graves' disease (74). The cause of exophthalmos in Graves' disease is unknown. However, immune factors may be involved in its pathogenesis. Exophthalmos-producing factor (EPF) is a substance derived from thyrotropin that binds to membrane receptors of retroorbital tissues. This binding affinity is enhanced by serum immunoglobulins from patients with severe degrees of Graves' ophthalmopathy (64). Both thyroglobulin and immune complexes bind to human extraocular muscle membrane (36). Lymphatic connections between the thyroid gland and the orbits may exist so that in Graves' disease exophthalmos could result from stimulation by thyroid glandular antigens or antibodies and their complexes which interact with orbital muscle receptors and produce muscle injury and inflammation (36).

Lymphocytes from patients with Graves' disease can be stimulated by phytohemagglutinin (PHA) to produce thyroid-stimulating immunoglobulins, whereas normal lymphocytes cannot (74). Since PHA stimulates only T lymphocytes, and T lymphocytes cannot produce immunoglobulins, PHA must activate helper T lymphocytes which in turn stimulate B lymphocytes to produce these immunoglobulins. It has been suggested that in Graves' disease a specific "forbidden clone" of helper T lymphocytes exists because there is an in-

herited defect of immunologic control over these T cells. If this clone appears by normal, random mutation it might not be destroyed and would proceed to interact with thyroid antigen. This would stimulate the replication of the forbidden T lymphocytes, which would then cooperate with B lymphocytes in the production of thyroid-stimulating immunoglobulins. Thus both cellular and humoral immune mechanisms would be involved in this hypothetical model (Fig. 10-1).

Certain genetic factors may also be involved in the pathogenesis of Graves' disease. An increased incidence of the histocompatibility antigen HLA-B8 is found among Caucasians and HLA-B40 is increased among Japanese patients (76). The concordance rate in monozygotic twins is high. The incidence of Graves' disease is much higher in women than in men, and possibly the X chromosome or estrogens play a role in the development of the disease.

Clinical Features

General. The signs and symptoms of Graves' disease are due to the overproduction of thyroid hormone. Tissue metabolism is increased and the patient experiences restlessness, heat intolerance, weight loss, and palpitations. The skin is warm, moist, and smooth and sweating is excessive. A diffusely enlarged thyroid gland may be found on physical examination. A fine tremor, tachycardia, wide pulse pressure, and muscle weakness are also characteristic.

LATS or LATS protector, and sometimes both, may be found in the serum of patients with Graves' disease. Antibodies to various thyroid antigens may also be detected by complement fixation or other assays. Protein-bound iodine, thyroxine, and triiodothyronine levels are generally elevated, and radioactive iodine uptake is increased.

Ocular Findings. Ophthalmologic findings in Graves' disease may range from nonexistent to devastating. Half of the patients with hyperthyroidism have no ocular abnormality. A common finding is widening of the palpebral fissures due to retraction of the upper lid. This may be due to the effect of thyroid hormone on Müller's muscle. Since it may also occur in

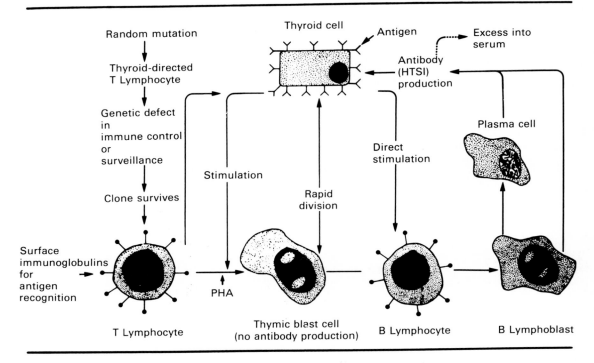

FIG. 10-1. Proposed pathogenesis of Graves' disease. (Volpé R: The pathogenesis of Graves' disease. Comp Ther 2:43, 1976)

euthyroid patients with Graves' disease, perhaps some other mechanism is responsible. About 20% of patients with Graves' disease exhibit proptosis (5). This is thought to reflect retroorbital infiltration and soft tissue swelling. If proptosis and lid retraction are severe enough, an exposure keratitis may result (Fig. 10-2). Diplopia may be an early sign of Graves' disease and is due initially to infiltration of the extraocular muscles and later to fibrosis. The most severe complication associated with Graves' ophthalmopathy is irreversible optic nerve damage due to pressure on the optic nerve or its blood supply. This results in decreased vision, visual field loss, and papilledema.

Treatment

The treatment of hyperthyroidism associated with Graves' disease may involve removal of the thyroid gland, administration of radioactive iodine, or therapy with antithyroid drugs.

Methimazole or propylthiouracil are effective in relieving major symptoms. However, they do not prevent the release of already formed thyroid hormone. They are often given for purposes of control prior to surgical removal of the gland. Radioactive iodine is a β-ray emitter which damages thyroid cells by preferentially localizing in the thyroid gland. Its main disadvantage is the difficulty in determining the proper dose for achieving a euthyroid status.

Mild ophthalmopathy is relatively easy to treat by keeping the cornea well hydrated with lubricants and preventing exposure keratitis. Guanethidine eyes drops may be used for treatment of lid retraction (18); however, they are irritating and produce a superficial punctate keratitis.

In order to prevent irreversible damage to the optic nerve, visual acuity must be checked frequently and decompression of the optic nerve must be carried out at the first sign of compromise.

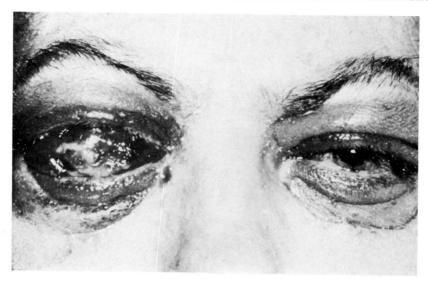

FIG. 10-2. Lid edema and exposure keratitis in Graves' disease. (Courtesy Dr. G. Mintsioulis).

A number of forms of treatment have been recommended for severe ophthalmopathy. These include thyroid hormones, radiation, pituitary ablation, estrogens and androgens, iodine, and azathioprine. Total ablation of the thyroid gland has been suggested for prevention of ophthalmopathy or treatment of established ocular disease (12). Success with this form of treatment has not been confirmed and it is therefore not widely used. Supervoltage irradiation of the retroorbital region has been successful without causing damage to the lens or retina (22). Recent results with this procedure seem encouraging. High doses of systemic corticosteroids have been used to treat malignant exophthalmos. Generally prednisone 60 to 80 mg/day or more is required to achieve some improvement, and treatment should be instituted early in the course of the disease. If there is no improvement within a week, the drug should be tapered and discontinued. Reduction of the upper eyelid retraction and edema, and regression of the exophthalmos, have been reported with steroid treatment (2). Surgical decompression of the orbit is a highly successful treatment for severe ophthalmopathy. Several techniques have been used in the past, including the Krönlein operation and the Naffziger procedure. The transantral approach introduced by Ogura in 1947 currently appears to be the most successful procedure (55).

REFERENCES

1. Adams DD, Kennedy TH: Evidence to suggest that LATS protector stimulates the human thyroid gland. J Clin Endocrinol Metab 33:47, 1971
2. Apers RC, Oosterhuis JA, Bierlaagh JJM: Indications and results of prednisone treatment in thyroid ophthalmopathy. Ophthalmologica 173:163, 1976
3. Armstrong RM, Nowak R, Falk R: Thymic lymphocyte function in myasthenia gravis. Neurology (Minneap) 23:1078, 1973
4. Arnason BGW, Fuller TC, Lehrich JR, Wray SH: Histocompatibility types and measles antibodies in multiple sclerosis and optic neuritis. J Neurol Sci 22:419, 1974
5. Barbosa J, Wong E, Doe RP: Ophthalmopathy of Graves' disease: outcome after treatment with radioactive iodine, surgery or antithyroid drugs. Arch Intern Med 130:111, 1972
6. Bastenie PA, Ermans AM: Thyroiditis and thyroid function: clinical, morphological and physiopathological studies. International Series of Monographs in Pure and Applied Biology, Modern Trends in Physiological Sciences, Vol 36. Oxford, Pergamon Press, 1972
7. Bender AN, Ringel SP, Engel WK et al: Myasthenia gravis: a serum factor blocking

acetylcholine receptors of the human neuro-muscular junction. Lancet 1:607, 1975

8. Behan PO, Lessell S, Roche M: Optic neuritis in the Landry-Guillain-Barre-Strohl syndrome. Br Med J 60:58, 1976

9. Berson SA, Yalow RS: Insulin in blood and insulin antibodies. Am J Med 40:676, 1966

10. Bertrams HJ, Kuwert EK: Association of histo-compatibility haplotype HLA-A3-B7 with multiple sclerosis. J Immunol 117:1906, 1976

11. Bornstein MB, Appel SH: Tissue culture studies of demyelination. Ann NY Acad Sci 122:280, 1965

12. Catz B, Perzik SL: Total thyroidectomy in the management of thyrotoxic and euthyroid Graves' disease. Am J Surg 118:434, 1969

13. Carp RI, Licursi PC, Merz PA et al: Decreased percentage of polymorphonuclear neutrophils in mouse peripheral blood after inoculation with material from multiple sclerosis patients. J Exp Med 136:618, 1972

14. Chen TT, Watanabe I, Zeman W, Mealy J Jr: Subacute sclerosing panencephalitis: propagation of measles virus from brain biopsy in tissue culture. Science 163:1193, 1969

15. Ciongoli AK, Platz P, Dupont B et al: Lack of antigen response to myxoviruses in multiple sclerosis. Lancet 2:1147, 1973

16. Cohn HE, Solit RW, Schatz NJ et al: Surgical treatment in myasthenia gravis: a 27 year experience. J Thorac Cardiovasc Surg 68:876, 1974

17. Compton DAS, Batchelor JR, McDonald WI: B-lymphocyte alloantigens associated with multiple sclerosis. Lancet 2:1261, 1976

18. Crombie AL: Long-term trial of local guanethidine in treatment of eye signs of thyroid dysfunction and idiopathic lid retraction. Br Med J 4:592, 1967

19. Cudworth AG, Gamble DR, White GBB et al: Aetiology of juvenile-onset diabetes. A prospective study. Lancet 1:385, 1977

20. Dau PC, Johnson KP, Spitler LE: The effect of cellular immunity in multiple sclerosis. Clin Exp Immunol 26:302, 1976

21. Derick CL, Hitchcock CH, Swift HF: Reactions to nonhemolytic streptococci. III. A study of modes of sensitization. J Exp Med 52:1, 1930

22. Donaldson SS, Bagshaw MA, Kriss JP: Supervoltage orbital radiotherapy for Graves' ophthalmopathy. J Clin Endocrinol Metab 37:276, 1973

23. Editorial: Human disease transferred to mice: Myasthenia gravis. N Engl J Med 296:168, 1977

24. Ehrenfeld EN, Klein E, Benezra D: Human thyroglobulin and thyroid extract as specific stimulators of sensitized lymphocytes. J Clin Endocrinol Metab 32:115, 1971

25. Engel AG, Lambert EH, Howard FM Jr: Immune complexes (IgG and C3) at the motor end-plate in myasthenia gravis. Ultrastructural and light microscopic localization and electro-physiologic correlations. Mayo Clin Proc 52:267, 1977

26. Engel WK, Festoff BW, Patten BM et al: Myasthenia gravis (NIH Conference). Ann Intern Med 81:225, 1974

27. Exon PD, Dixon K, Malons JM: Insulin antibodies in diabetic pregnancy. Lancet 2:126, 1974

28. Fog T: Transfer factor in multiple sclerosis. Lancet 2:99, 1976

29. Fritze D, Herrman C Jr, Naeim F et al: HL-A antigens in myasthenia gravis. Lancet 1:240, 1974

30. From the NIH. New Prednisone regimen in myasthenia gravis. JAMA 237:635, 1977

31. Ghoust JM, Castaigne A, Moulias R: Delayed hypersensitivity to muscle and thymus in myasthenia gravis and polymyositis. Clin Exp Immunol 18:39, 1974

32. Haire M, Millar JHD, Merrett JD: Measles virus-specific IgG in cerebrospinal fluid in multiple sclerosis. Br Med J 4:192, 1974

33. Hutchinson WM: Acute optic neuritis and the prognosis for multiple sclerosis. J Neurol Neurosurg Psychiatry 39:283, 1976

34. Hutchinson WM, Haire M: Measles-virus-specific IgG in optic neuritis and in multiple sclerosis after optic neuritis. Br Med J 1:64, 1976

35. Kott E, Rule AH: Myasthenia gravis: cellular response to basic myelin protein compared with cellular and humoral immunity to muscle antigens. Neurology (Minneap) 23:745, 1973

36. Kriss JP, Konishi J, Herman M: Studies on the pathogenesis of Graves' ophthalmopathy (with some related observations regarding therapy). Recent Prog Horm Res 31:533, 1975

37. Kurland LT, Beebe GW, Kurtzke JF et al: Studies on the natural history of multiple sclerosis. Acta Neurol Scand [Suppl] 19:157–176, 1966

38. Lamki L, Row VV, Volpé R: Cellular immunity in Graves' disease and Hashimoto's diseases as shown by migration inhibition factor (abstr). Clin Res 20:431, 1972

39. Levy NL, Auerbach PS, Hayes EC: A blood test for multiple sclerosis based on the adherence of lymphocytes to measles-infected cells. N Engl J Med 294:1423, 1976

40. Lynn BH: Retrobulbar neuritis. Trans Ophthalmol Soc UK 79:701, 1959

41. Link H, Muller R: Immunoglobulins in multiple sclerosis and infections of the nervous system. Arch Neurol 25:326, 1971

42. Link H, Norrby E, Olsson J-E: Immunoglobulins and measles antibody in optic neuritis. N Engl J Med 289:1103, 1973

43. Link H, Zetteruall O: Multiple sclerosis: disturbed lambda chain ratio of globulin G in cerebrospinal fluid. Clin Exp Immunol 6:435, 1970

44. Maugh TH: Multiple sclerosis: two or more viruses may be involved. Science 195:768, 1977

45. McAlpine D: Optic (retrobulbar) neuritis. In McAlpine D, Lumsden CE, Acheson ED (eds): Multiple Sclerosis: A Reappraisal. Edinburgh, Churchill-Livingstone, 1972, pp 148–163

46. McCuish AC, Barnes EW, Irvine WJ, Duncan LJP: Antibodies to pancreatic islet cells in insulin-dependent diabetes with co-existent autoimmune disease. Lancet 2:1529, 1974

47. McKenzie JM: Humoral factors in the pathogenesis of Graves' disease. Physiol Rev 48:252, 1968

48. Munro RE, Lamki L, Row VV, Volpé R: Cell-mediated immunity in the exophthalmos of Graves' disease as demonstrated by the migration inhibition factor (MIF) test. J Clin Endocrinol Metab 37:286, 1973

49. Nakamura RM, Weigle WO: Transfer of experimental autoimmune thyroiditis by serum from thyroidectomized donors. J Exp Med 130:263, 1969

50. Nerup J, Anderson OO, Bendixen G et al: Antipancreatic cellular hypersensitivity in diabetes mellitus. Diabetes 20:424, 1971

51. Nerup J, Binder C: Thyroid, gastric and adrenal auto-immunity in diabetes mellitus. Acta Endocrinol (Kbh) 72:279, 1973

52. Nerup J, Platz P, Andersen OO et al: HL-A antigens and diabetes mellitus. Lancet 2:864, 1974

53. Nikoskelainen E, Nikoskelainen J, Salmi AA, Italonen PE: Virus antibody levels in the cerebrospinal fluid from patients with optic neuritis. Acta Neurol Scand 51:347, 1975

54. Norrby E, Link H, Olsson J-E et al: Comparison of antibodies against different viruses in cerebrospinal fluid and serum samples from patients with multiple sclerosis. Infect Immunol 10:688, 1974

55. Ogura JH: Transantral orbital decompression for progressive exophthalmos. A follow-up of 54 cases. Med Clin North Am 52:399, 1968

56. Onaya T, Kotani M, Yamada T, Ochi Y: New in vitro tests to detect the thyroid stimulator in sera from hyperthyroid patients by measuring colloid droplet formation and cyclic AMP in human thyroid slices. J Clin Endocrinol Metab 36:859, 1973

57. Pertschuk LP, Cook AW, Gupta J: Measles antigen in multiple sclerosis: identification in the jejunum. Life Sci 19:1603, 1976

58. Picken S, Sangster G: Retrobulbar neuritis and infectious mononucleosis. Br Med J 4:729, 1975

59. Platz P, Ryder LP, Staub Nielsen L et al: HL-A and idiopathic optic neuritis. Lancet 1:520, 1975

60. Porter R: Uveitis in association with multiple sclerosis. Br J Ophthalmol 58:478, 1972

61. Rao NA, Tso MOM, Zimmerman LE: Experimental allergic optic neuritis in guinea pigs: preliminary report. Invest Ophthalmol Vis Sci 16:338, 1977

62. Richman DP, Patrick J, Arnason BGW: Cellular immunity in myasthenia gravis. N Engl J Med 294:694, 1976

63. Roitt IM, Torrigiani G: Identification and estimation of undegraded thyroglobulin in human serum. Endocrinology 81:421, 1967

64. Rosenberg IN: Euthyroid Graves' disease. N Engl J Med 296:223, 1977

65. Sacks N, Potgieter HJ, Van Rensburg AJ: The use of transfer factor in the treatment of multiple sclerosis. S Afr Med J 50:1556, 1976

66. Shabo AL, Maxwell DS: Insulin-induced immunogenic retinopathy resembling the retinitis proliferans of diabetes. Trans Am Acad Ophthalmol Otolargyngol 81:497, 1976

67. Shabo AL, Maxwell DS, Shintaku IP et al: Experimental immunogenic rubeosis iridis. Invest Ophthalmol Vis Sci 16:343, 1977

68. Sheremata W, Cosgrove JBR, Eylar EH: Cellular hypersensitivity to basic myelin (A1) protein and clinical multiple sclerosis. N Engl J Med 241:14, 1974

69. Simpson JA: Myasthenia gravis. A new hypothesis. Scott Med J 5:419, 1960

70. Stendahl L, Link H, Moller E, Norrby E: Relation between genetic markers and oligoclonal IgG in CSF in optic neuritis. J Neurol Sci 27:93, 1976

71. ter Meulen V, Koprowski H, Iwasaki Y et al: Fusion of cultured multiple sclerosis brain cells with indicator cells: presence of nucleocapsids and virion and isolation of parainfluenza-type virus. Lancet 2:1, 1972

72. Toyka KV, Drachman DB, Griffin DE et al: Myasthenia gravis. Study of humoral immune mechanisms by passive transfer to mice. N Engl J Med 296:125, 1977

73. Utermohlen V, Zabriskie JB: A suppression of cellular immunity in patients with multiple sclerosis. J Exp Med 138:1591, 1973

74. Volpé R: The pathogenesis of Graves' disease. Comp Ther 2:43, 1976

75. Volpé R, Farid NR, Von Westarp C, Row VV: The pathogenesis of Graves' disease in Hashimoto's thyroiditis. Clin Endocrinol 3:239, 1974

76. Weise W, Wenzel KW: Distribution of HLA-antigens in Graves' disease and in autonomous adenoma of the thyroid. Diabete Metab 2:163, 1976

77. Zeller RW: Ocular findings in the remission phase of multiple sclerosis. Am J Ophthalmol 64:771, 1967

ELEVEN
ELEVEN
ELEVEN corneal transplantation

Transplantation of solid tissue allografts is one of the most fundamental and important areas of immunologic study. The mechanisms by which the host recognizes transplanted tissues as being "foreign" or "self" are basic to the understanding of the body's immune system. The cornea has been used by immunologists for many years as a favorite site for the study of transplant rejection. The normal clarity of the cornea, and its so-called "privileged" nature, have made corneal transplantation a popular method of investigating transplantation immunobiology.

Corneal transplantation has become a useful sight-restoring procedure clinically, and represents one of the most commonly encountered basic immunologic phenomena in ophthalmology. A successful corneal transplant is shown in Figure 11-1. An understanding of the mechanisms by which corneal transplants are accepted or rejected is essential for the proper management of patients undergoing corneal transplantation.

TRANSPLANTATION IMMUNOLOGY

In all animals, including man, the most important determinants responsible for graft rejection are products of a closely linked cluster of genes on a single chromosome. This region is called the major histocompatibility complex (MHC), and in man the region has been designated the HLA region (for human leukocyte antigen). These genes determine the presence of histocompatibility antigens which are present on the surface of all nucleated cells.

The HLA region has been partially mapped and at least four major loci, designated HLA-A, HLA-B, HLA-C, and HLA-D, have been identified. (HLA-A was formerly known as the LA locus, HLA-B as the Four locus, HLA-C as the AJ locus, and HLA-D as the LD locus.) Each locus has a number of known antigenic specificities, or alleles (see Table 1-3 in Ch. 1). The first three loci determine antigens which can be defined by serologic methods, and because of this their antigens are sometimes termed serologically defined (SD) antigens. The HLA-D region codes for antigens which are located in lymphocytes and whose presence can be determined by mixed lymphocyte culture (MLC). The lymphocyte-defined (LD) antigens are easily identified on B lymphocytes, but not on T lymphocytes. Specific antiserums have been developed which can identify the specific antigens of the HLA-D locus on B cells. Aside from lymphocytes, HLA-D antigens have also been demonstrated on sperm, macrophages, and skin cells. The HLA-C locus is difficult to identify because it is so closely linked to the HLA-B locus.

HLA antigens are freely movable in the lipid layer of the cell membrane. They are found in association with virtually every type of cell. The one major exception is the mature nonnucleated human red blood cell, where HLA antigens are not found. HLA antigens are, however, present on leukocytes and platelets.

The HLA-D locus was formerly known as

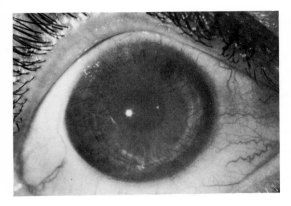

FIG. 11-1. Successful corneal allograft.

the MLC locus, as well as the LD locus. Mixed lymphocyte culture reactions occur when lymphocytes from two different individuals are cultured together. The lymphocytes respond to differences in their cell surface determinants by synthesizing DNA at increased rates and undergoing cell division. The reaction can be measured by the incorporation of tritiated thymidine into DNA: HLA-D differences (between donor and recipient) appear to be necessary for target cell destruction (at least in the recognition phase) and MLC differences are believed to be a major factor in the rejection of organ transplants. The actual killing of target cells is not dependent on MLC differences, but on differences in HLA antigens or products of genes closely linked to the HLA complex.

Since many specificities have been identified for each HLA locus, the potential combinations are numerous. The HLA phenotype of an individual can be determined with antiserums, and matching of HLA antigens can therefore be carried out prior to organ transplantation. There is a good correlation between the degree of HLA matching and the ultimate survival of the transplant. Although it is usually not possible to match all four loci, an attempt is made to achieve the best possible match prior to transplantation. HLA typing has been particularly useful in selecting appropriate donors for kidney transplantation. While these principles probably apply to other types of organ transplants, the number of heart, liver, and bone marrow transplants has

not been sufficient to prove that HLA matching is essential.

TISSUE TYPING IN CORNEAL TRANSPLANTATION

Because of the high rate of acceptance of corneal allografts, histocompatibility matching has been felt to be of only minor importance in corneal transplantation surgery. Recent studies have been carried out to determine whether or not histocompatibility between the donor and recipient improves the success of corneal transplantation surgery (5, 12, 13). These studies seem to affirm the notion that while ABO blood group matching does not influence the success of corneal transplants, some improvement may be realized by matching donor and recipient HLA types, especially when grafts are carried out in vascularized corneas. In these situations, greater HLA incompatibility was associated with a higher risk of rejection (13), although other workers have found no significant difference in the number of clear grafts when HLA matching was attempted in patients with vascularized corneas (50). A definitive indication of the importance of HLA matching prior to corneal grafting awaits further investigation. However, a recent large study of 200 cases (5) demonstrated improved success when two HLA antigens were matched in patients with preoperatively vascularized corneas. This finding has been confirmed by Vannas (46), who reported a high success rate in keratoplasty when three of four loci were matched. Interestingly, a high rate of rejection occurred in keratoconus patients with avascular corneas who possessed HLA-B12 and HLA-B27 (47). These reactions occurred late and were triggered by nasopharyngeal infections. This phenomenon may reflect a hyperreactivity on the part of individuals with certain HLA types.

TYPES OF GRAFTS

Isografts are grafts between individuals who are genetically identical such as identical (monozygotic) twins or members of the same inbred strain of animal. This type of graft is the closest to the ideal and the least likely to be rejected. **Autografts** are grafts in which one individual is both the donor and the recipient. **Allografts,** once called **homografts,** are grafts between individuals of the same species who have different genetic constitutions. In this category fall the vast majority of human organ transplants. **Xenografts,** also called **heterografts,** are grafts between members of different species. These grafts are likely to fail quickly, because of extreme differences in histocompatibility. The type of rejection which occurs with heterografts is usually due to antibodies that are present in the recipient prior to grafting.

TYPES OF REJECTION

Hyperacute Rejection

Hyperacute rejection occurs within minutes or hours after transplantation of an organ. It is due to the presence of preexisting antibodies in the blood of the recipient which react with the donor tissue. Activation of the complement system and the clotting mechanism are involved and the lesions which occur are primarily vascular. When hyperacute rejection occurs in kidney transplants, IgG, complement, and sometimes IgM can be demonstrated in the walls of blood vessels. Biopsies of kidneys undergoing hyperacute rejection show infiltration by neutrophils and platelets, and fibrin deposition.

Acute Rejection

Acute rejection is a term applied to an initial immunologic rejection in the nonsensitized recipient. Acute rejection may occur at any time from several days to even years after the transplant. While both cellular and humoral immune mechanisms apparently play a role in acute rejection, cellular immune mechanisms appear to be most important. Direct killing of graft cells by T lymphocytes and the activation, by lymphokines, of macrophages which in turn act as aggressor cells, are the primary mechanisms in acute rejection. In addition, cytotoxic antibodies are formed in these rejections and may participate in cytotoxic reac-

tions. Histologically, grafts become infiltrated by mononuclear cells, predominantly immature lymphocytes but also plasma cells and macrophages. Infiltration by cells is particularly prominent around small and medium-sized blood vessels.

Chronic Rejection

Chronic rejection has a relatively late onset and involves the gradual loss of function in the transplanted organ. Pathologically, there is progressive vascular occlusion and ischemia of the graft. Chronic rejection is usually attributed to humoral immune mechanisms but the evidence to support this is scant. Both sensitized T cells and antibody directed against donor cells may be found in the blood of the transplant recipient. However, since chronic rejection can occur in a T-cell–depleted animal, chronic rejection is probably mediated primarily by antibody. Histologically, cellular infiltration is not impressive and immunoglobulins cannot always be demonstrated in the lesions.

Graft-versus-Host (GVH) Reaction

Graft-versus-host reactions occur following transplantation of a foreign graft containing viable lymphocytes into an immunodeficient recipient. This leads to an unopposed attack of histoincompatible cells on an individual who is unable to reject foreign cells.

IMMUNOPATHOLOGY OF CORNEAL TRANSPLANTATION

POSSIBLE MECHANISMS FOR GRAFT SURVIVAL AND REJECTION

The early studies of Medawar provided unequivocal evidence that the rejection of grafted tissues results from an immunologic reaction (28, 29). It became evident that histocompatibility matching between donor and recipient was necessary for the survival of most transplanted tissues. Corneal transplants, however, were often successful without matching. This fact led to the opinion that the cornea enjoyed an immunologic "privilege" not shared by other tissues (26, 27). Much speculation has taken place as to the reasons for the relative privileged existence of corneal transplants. Some hypotheses which might explain their survival include 1) a lack of antigenicity of the corneal elements; 2) rapid death of donor cellular elements and their replacement by the host before an active immune response could be stimulated; 3) the "adaptation" of the graft within the recipient, thereby preventing rejection even in the actively sensitized host; and 4) the presence of certain features of the corneal bed into which the graft is transplanted, especially its avascularity (41).

That corneal allografts can be rejected by immunologic mechanisms has been amply demonstrated (26, 27, 31). These mechanisms are now felt to account for many cases of corneal graft failure. In rejection situations, the usual privilege enjoyed by corneal grafts is lost for a variety of reasons. To understand the factors involved in rejection, we must first examine the possible mechanisms by which most corneal transplants can survive in a foreign host.

Early investigators suggested that corneal tissue was somehow less antigenic and therefore less likely to be rejected than other types of tissue. It soon became evident, however, that corneal tissue implanted in various vascularized regions of the body could induce rapid sensitization and undergo a specific rejection process (6, 17). The antigenicity of corneal tissue was further emphasized by the elegant experiments of Khodadoust and Silverstein, who showed that even individual cell layers of the cornea such as epithelium, stroma, or endothelium could initiate sensitization of the host and undergo subsequent rejection (19). It should come as no surprise that corneal tissue is antigenic, since every known nucleated cell studied thus far is endowed with a complete set of histocompatibility antigens on its surface.

A second possibility that was used to explain the prolonged survival of corneal allografts was the rapid replacement of donor tissue by comparable tissue from the host before the rejection process could take place. This notion, however, was proved incorrect by studies which demonstrated the long-term survival of donor keratocytes, identified by a sex-chromatin technique, in the cat (3) and in the rabbit (9). Similar evidence of long-term donor tissue survival was provided by labeling techniques using tritiated thymidine (14, 37). In addition, donor epithelium has been observed to undergo specific rejection as long as 6 months after corneal transplantation (18). The most convincing evidence for the long-term survival of donor tissue in corneal grafts comes from studies of heterografts in which the donor karyotype is so different from that of the recipient that there could be no question of the chimeric nature of the cornea (41). Thus it appears, at least in these experimental situations, that in the absence of the rejection process the grafted tissue is capable of surviving for an indefinite period of time. Clinically, allograft rejection may occur for the first time as long as 10–15 years after grafting, so it would appear that the donor material persists for as long as 15 years.

Another mechanism by which grafted tissue may survive indefinitely is the "adaptation" of the donor tissue to its new environment. This concept presumes that some change occurs in the donor tissue, and it should not be confused with immunologic tolerance, which is a property of diminished immunologic reactivity on the part of the host. The concept of adaptation was based on studies which showed long-term survival of grafts within the anterior chamber of the eye. Furthermore, it was observed that corneal allografts were less susceptible to rejection after a certain critical period of time (25). However, it is well known both clinically and experimentally that a corneal allograft may undergo immunologic rejection several months or even years after its initial acceptance by the host. It now seems more likely that the ultimate acceptance of grafted tissue is due to alterations in the host's immunologic mechanisms, rather than in the grafted tissue (2).

The mechanism now considered most important in explaining the privileged existence of corneal transplants is the nature of the recipient graft bed into which the transplant is placed. It has been recognized for some time that the avascularity of the cornea might well explain its peculiar suitability for the acceptance of grafted tissue (4, 6). Vascularization is often associated with a higher incidence of graft rejections in clinical and experimental situations (4, 32). The absence of blood vessels in the recipient corneal bed may prevent rejection of a graft in one of two ways: 1) The process of sensitization by which a host recognizes the foreign tissue may be prevented by the absence of contact between circulating host cells and the foreign antigen; and 2) sensitized host cells may be prevented from gaining access to the graft and initiating the rejection process.

The relative importance of the "afferent" sensitization process and the "efferent" rejection process has been considered.

The importance of the afferent process of sensitization has been amply demonstrated (25). In a series of successful penetrating keratoplasties in rabbits, Maumenee demonstrated that 90% of the corneal grafts were rejected by keratoplasty recipients who had first received skin grafts from the cornea donors. Sensitization by corneal tissue was absent in this situation, but was provided by identical antigens on the cells of the skin. The degree of sensitization by corneal grafts was also studied by observing the tempo of rejection of orthotopic skin allografts in rabbits that first received lamellar and penetrating corneal grafts (20). In these situations, rejecton of the skin grafts took place at the same rate as in control animals which had not undergone keratoplasty. Thus, it would seem that systemic sensitization by corneal grafting either does not occur or is insufficient to cause rejection of skin grafts. Still, it has been often observed that about 10% of successful avascular penetrating corneal grafts undergo spontaneous rejection despite the absence of vascularization (16). This implies that sensitization may in fact occur in the absence of vascularization; however, the mechanism by which this takes place is not known.

As early as 1953, Billingham and Boswell (6) concluded that the absence of blood vessels interfered with the efferent arc by which host cells could invade a foreign graft. This hypothesis, however, could not explain why some grafts survive despite the presence of vascularization. The efferent process of rejection does appear to be influenced to some extent by vascularization of the grafted tissue. In the absence of vascularization, lamellar grafts are virtually always spared, even when sensitization has been induced in the host (20, 23). In contrast, 90% of avascular penetrating grafts can be expected to undergo rejection after sensitization of the host by a skin graft (25), while 10% are not rejected. Khodadoust and Silverstein (20) found that induced sensitization led to rejection of 25% of avascular grafts and 100% of vascularized grafts. Vascularization clearly enhances the rejection process, presumably by providing a means by which host cells can be brought into contact with the foreign corneal tissue. It should be kept in mind that in a small percentage of avascular grafts, host cells will arrive on the scene and attack the graft by some unknown route. It may be that these sensitized cells escape from the host's capillary loops nearest the graft and migrate between the corneal lamellae. Alternatively, sensitized cells could reach the graft endothelium through iris vessels, especially if the iris is adherent to the cornea (15). During the rejection of corneal xenografts, draining lymphoid tissue undergoes hyperplasia and enlargement of germinal centers (35). These lymphoid changes are apparently stimulated by diffusion of corneal antigens from the donor tissue and may occur without the presence of blood vessels or lymphatics in the graft. It may be concluded that both the afferent and the efferent limb of the sensitization–rejection process are important for the efficient rejection of corneal transplants.

REJECTION OF DIFFERENT CELL LAYERS

It has been pointed out that rejection of a corneal transplant can be demonstrated in different cell layers of the graft and that rejection of each layer can be observed independently under experimental conditions (19). Epithelial rejection is characterized by congestion of circumcorneal vessels followed by a linear defect in the epithelium at the edge of the graft. This rejection line appears in the area adjacent to the vascularized portion of the cornea and migrates toward the center of the graft. The lin-

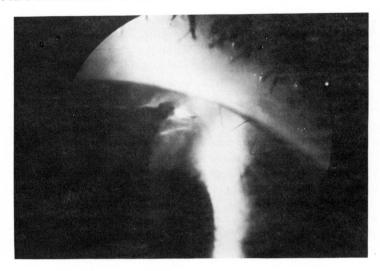

FIG. 11-2. Early corneal allograft rejection. Note keratic precipitates on endothelium.

ear defect is best observed when methylene blue stain is instilled in the eye. The rejected donor cells are rapidly replaced by recipient epithelial cells, and the rejection may be so subtle that it may be missed clinically. Histologically, the epithelium is infiltrated by lymphocytes and polymorphonuclear leukocytes.

Rejection of the corneal stroma also begins with congestion of the limbal blood vessels. A stromal haze appears at the edge of the graft nearest the vessels and a whitish band with ill-defined margins sweeps across the graft tissue. When the rejection process is completed, the haze resolves and the vessels in the graft regress. The inflammatory cell infiltrate consists mainly of plasma cells and neutrophils.

Rejection of the endothelium begins with congestion of the limbal blood vessels and the appearance of diffuse keratic precipitates over the donor endothelium nearest the blood vessels (Fig. 11-2). The keratic precipitates become larger over a few days' time and form a line at the extreme periphery of the graft. These keratic precipitates migrate toward the center of the graft, leaving a wake of destroyed endothelial cells behind (36). Endothelial rejection is the most important aspect of the rejection process, because of the crucial physiologic role played by the endothelial

monolayer. Rejection and consequent destruction of endothelial cells leads to edema, inflammation, and vascularization of the entire graft (Fig. 11-3), whereas rejection of the stroma or epithelium may be transient and inconsequential.

CELLULAR IMMUNE MECHANISMS IN GRAFT REJECTION

The immunologic mechanism by which solid tissue grafts are rejected is generally considered to involve cellular rather than humoral immunity (15, 32). This is based on the fact that destruction of grafts occurs after the passive transfer of cells but not of antiserum, and the fact that the acceptance of grafts follows treatment which interferes with cellular but not with humoral immunity. Transfer of sensitized lymphoid cells to the anterior chamber in the rabbit results in damage to the corneal endothelium (22). Pocklike areas of damaged corneal endothelium representing a developing focal graft-versus-host reaction (21, 22) may be observed. These studies indicate that the immunologic rejection of corneal allografts is mediated by the lymphoid cells contained in the passive-transfer inoculum. This picture of graft rejection differs from the picture that is usually observed in spontaneous corneal graft

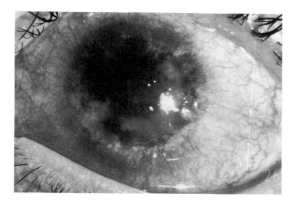

FIG. 11-3. Well-established corneal allograft rejection. Note opacification and early vascularization of the graft.

rejection, where a line of endothelial destruction works its way across the donor endothelium. These observations also suggest that the lymphocytes responsible for the destruction of the graft probably arise from vessels within the cornea itself. If they arose from the uveal tract, random focal destruction of the endothelium would be expected rather than a discrete rejection line.

Systemic cell-mediated sensitization can be measured by the leukocyte migration inhibition test by placing full-thickness corneal allografts centrally in human host corneas (24). Variable degrees of cellular immunity have been measured by the leukocyte migration inhibition test following xenografts in rabbits (49) and allografts in humans (1). In the latter experiments, the test became negative after the second postoperative month; however, it again became positive in three of seven patients with latent graft rejection. Migration inhibition factor (MIF) activity has recently been demonstrated in the anterior chamber following corneal allografts and xenografts in rabbits (40). The source of this MIF activity is not known.

The rejection process in a grafted rabbit eye can be halted by treatment with topical corticosteroids (34). This treatment is associated with a decrease in the number of leukocytes infiltrating the endothelium and with the destruction of lymphocytes. This direct cytolytic effect on the cell membrane of lymphocytes may be one mechanism by which steroid

treatment abrogates the cell-mediated immune rejection process. Corneal transplant rejection in rabbits can also be deterred by other forms of treatment which selectively impair cellular immunity. These include treatment of the animals with azathioprine (33) or with antilymphocyte serum (38, 48). In contrast, complete Freund's adjuvant given intradermally in the footpad and also subconjunctivally may lead to a more intense graft reaction than expected, possibly owing to nonspecific stimulation of cellular immune mechanisms (43).

HUMORAL IMMUNE MECHANISMS IN GRAFT REJECTION

The role of antibody in mediating corneal graft rejection is usually considered less important than the role of cellular immune mechanisms. Cytotoxic antibody may play a significant role in the hyperacute rejection of allogenic kidney grafts and in the rejection of solid tissue xenografts, but most investigators feel that cellular immunity, mediated by sensitized lymphoid cells, is the most significant factor in the acute rejection of solid tissue allografts (41)

The relationship between anticorneal antibodies and the development of graft rejection remains unclear. Anticorneal antibodies which are not usually present prior to keratoplasty can be demonstrated after grafting, both in animals and in humans (45). Some studies have demonstrated cytotoxic antibodies against corneal tissues in graft recipients (10, 11, 30). These antibodies may develop in response to tissue injury, and their importance in corneal graft rejection cannot yet be determined.

It has also been demonstrated that lymphocytotoxic antibodies may develop in patients whose graft rejection cannot be reversed by treatment, but are rarely found in patients with graft reactions that are treated successfully (44). In addition, some patients who have detectable lymphocytotoxins in their serum prior to surgery may have graft failure despite immunosuppressive therapy. The presence of lymphocytotoxic antibody prior to corneal grafting might therefore be considered an unfavorable prognostic sign.

Lysosomal constituents of neutrophils were

released during the second and third postoperative week in the host cornea and aqueous humor in 8 out of 23 rabbits undergoing keratoplasty. It was suggested that these protein constituents may be a factor in the development of a vascular response associated with corneal graft rejection (39).

THERAPY OF GRAFT REJECTION

Topical corticosteroids have been the mainstay of therapy in the prevention and treatment of corneal allograft rejection in humans. Systemic steroids are not necessary. Topical corticosteroids are generally started immediately after corneal transplant surgery. A great deal of individual variation exists with respect to the specifics of postoperative corticosteroid therapy. Steroids are sometimes continued until the time of suture removal, while some clinicians continue topical therapy in small doses for 1 or more years, and sometimes indefinitely. Patients must be alerted to the earliest symptoms of graft rejection, and intensive local corticosteroid treatment must be given early in the course of such a reaction. This usually consists of hourly applications of topical steroids and often periocular injections of depot preparations.

Other means of preventing graft rejection are continually being investigated. Drugs such as antilymphocyte serum and azathioprine have been used experimentally (33, 42, 48), but these drugs in general are considered too dangerous for use in clinical situations. One method of prolonging corneal allograft survival in rabbits involves the incubation of donor grafts with antilymphocyte serum or succinylated heterologous antilymphocyte antibodies. Pretreatment of corneal buttons with these preparations presumably allows noncytotoxic antibody to bind to and coat corneal cells, thus affording them protection from other cytotoxic antibodies (7, 8). This approach has not yet been adapted to the human situation.

While immunologic manipulation of the host and donor tissues holds promise for improved success in corneal grafting, other, non-immunologic, approaches are being pursued

as well. Undoubtedly, improved surgical techniques, better methods of examining the donor endothelium, and long-term storage of corneal tissue will ultimately improve the success of corneal grafting.

REFERENCES

1. Aviner Z, Henley WL, Okas S et al: Leucocyte migration test in patients after corneal transplantation. Can J Ophthalmol 11:165, 1976
2. Barker CF, Billingham RE: Immunologically privileged sites and tissues. In Corneal Graft Failures. Ciba Foundation Symposium, Amsterdam, Elsevier, 1973, p 79
3. Basu PK, Miller I, Ormsby HL: Sex chromatin as a biologic marker in the study of the fate of corneal transplants. Am J Ophthalmol 49:513, 1960
4. Basu PK, Ormsby H: Studies on the immunity with intralamellar corneal homografts in rabbits. Am J Ophthalmol 44:598, 1957
5. Batchelor JR, Casey TA, Gibbs DC et al: HLA matching and corneal grafting. Lancet 1:551, 1976
6. Billingham RE, Boswell T: Studies on the problem of corneal homografts. Proc R Soc Lond [Biol] 141:392, 1953
7. Chandler JW, Gebhardt BM, Kaufman HE: Immunologic protection of rabbit corneal allografts. I. Preparation and in vitro testing of heterologous "blocking" antibody. Invest Ophthalmol 12:646, 1973
8. Chandler JW, Gebhardt BM, Sugar J, Kaufman HE: Immunological protection of rabbit corneal allografts. Transplantation 17:146, 1973
9. Chi HH, Teng CC, Katzin HM: The fate of endothelial cells in corneal homografts. Am J Ophthalmol 59:186, 1965
10. D'Ermo F, Lanzieri M, Secchi AG: Anticorneal antibodies in rabbits after homologous and heterologous corneal grafts. Transplantation 4:512, 1966
11. D'Ermo F, Lanzieri M, Secchi AG: Anticorneal antibodies in rabbits after homologous and heterologous corneal grafts. Acta Ophthalmol (Kbh) 44:233, 1966
12. Ehlers N, Kissmeyer-Nielsen F: Influence of histocompatibility on the fate of the corneal transplant. In Corneal Graft Failure. Ciba Foundation Symposium, Amsterdam, Elsevier, 1973, p 307
13. Gibbs DC, Batchelor JR, Casey TA: The influence of HL-A compatibility on the fate of corneal grafts. In Corneal Graft Failure. Ciba Foundation Symposium, Amsterdam, Elsevier, 1973, p 293
14. Hanna C, Irwin ES: Fate of cells in the corneal graft. Arch Ophthalmol 68:810, 1962
15. Inomata H, Smelser GK, Polack FM: The fine

structural changes in the corneal endothelium during graft rejection. Invest Ophthalmol 9:263, 1970

16. Khodadoust AA: Penetrating keratoplasty in the rabbit. Am J Ophthalmol 66:899, 1968

17. Khodadoust AA, Silverstein AM: Studies on the heterotopic transplantation of cornea to the skin. Surv Ophthalmol 11:435, 1966

18. Khodadoust AA, Silverstein AM: The survival and rejection of epithelium in experimental corneal grafts. Invest Ophthalmol 8:169, 1969

19. Khodadoust AA, Silverstein AM: Transplantation and rejection of individual cell layers of the cornea. Invest Ophthalmol 8:180, 1969

20. Khodadoust AA, Silverstein AM: Studies on the nature of the privilege enjoyed by corneal allografts. Invest Ophthalmol 11:137, 1972

21. Khodadoust AA, Silverstein AM: Local graft-versus-host reactions within the anterior chamber of the eye: the formation of corneal endothelial pocks. Invest Ophthalmol 14:573, 1975

22. Khodadoust AA, Silverstein AM: Induction of corneal graft rejection by passive cell transfer. Invest Ophthalmol 15:89, 1976

23. Kornbleuth W, Nelken E: A study on donor-recipient sensitization in experimental homologous partial lamellar corneal grafts. Am J Ophthalmol 45:843, 1958

24. MacDonald AL, Basu PK: Systemic sensitization of corneal allograft recipients before the clinical onset of graft reaction. Can J Ophthalmol 12:60, 1977

25. Maumenee AE: The influence of donor-recipient sensitization on corneal grafts. Am J Ophthalmol 34:142, 1951

26. Maumenee AE: The immune concept: its relation to corneal homotransplantation. Ann NY Acad Sci 59:453, 1955

27. Maumenee AE: Clinical aspects of the corneal homograft reaction. Invest Ophthalmol 1:244, 1962

28. Medawar PB: Immunity to homologous grafted skin. I. The suppression of cell division in grafts transplanted to immunized animals. Br J Exp Pathol 27:9, 1946

29. Medawar PB: Behaviour and fate of skin autografts and skin homografts in rabbits. J Anat 78:176, 1946

30. Nelken E, Nelken D: Serologic studies in keratoplasty. Br J Ophthalmol 49:159, 1965

31. Paufique L, Sourdille GF, Offert G: Les Greffes de la Cornée (Kératoplasties). Paris, Masson, 1948

32. Polack FM: Histopathological and histochemical alterations in the early stages of corneal graft rejection. J Exp Med 116:709, 1962

33. Polack FM: Modification of the immune graft response by azathioprine. Surv Ophthalmol 11:545, 1966

34. Polack FM: Lymphocyte destruction during corneal homograft reaction. A scanning electron microscopic study. Arch Ophthalmol 89:413, 1973

35. Polack FM, Gonzales CE: The response of the lymphoid tissue to corneal heterografts. Arch Ophthalmol 80:321, 1968

36. Polack FM, Kanai A: Electron miscroscopic studies of graft endothelium in corneal graft rejection. Am J Ophthalmol 73:711, 1972

37. Polack FM, Smelser GK, Rose J: Long-term survival of isotopically labeled stromal and endothelial cells in corneal homografts. Am J Ophthalmol 57:67, 1964

38. Polack FM, Townsend WM, Waltman SR: Antilymphocyte serum and corneal graft rejection. Am J Ophthalmol 73:52, 1972

39. Ranadive NS, Basu PK: Role of lysosomal constituents of neutrophils in corneal graft reaction. Can J Ophthalmol 10:377, 1975

40. Sher NA, Doughman DJ, Mindrup E et al: Macrophage migration inhibition factor activity in the aqueous humor during experimental corneal xenograft and allograft rejection. Am J Ophthalmol 83:858, 1976

41. Silverstein AM, Khodadoust AA: Transplantation immunobiology of the cornea. In Corneal Graft Failure. Ciba Foundation Symposium, Amsterdam, Elsevier, 1973, p 105

42. Smolin G, Hyndiuk RA: Suppression of corneal graft reaction by antilymphocyte serum. III. Effect of pretreatment of donor animals. Arch Ophthalmol 85:451, 1971

43. Smolin G, Stein MR: Potentiation of the corneal graft reaction by complete Freund's adjuvant. Arch Ophthalmol 87:60, 1972

44. Stark WJ, Opelz G, Newsome D et al: Sensitization to human lymphocyte antigens by corneal transplantation. Invest Ophthalmol 12:639, 1973

45. Tsutsui J, Watanabe S: Clinical evaluation of the precipitin test in the postoperative course of keratoplasty. Arch Ophthalmol 65:375, 1961

46. Vannas S: Histocompatibility in corneal grafting. Invest Ophthalmol 14:883, 1975

47. Vannas S, Vannas A, Tiilikainen A: Corneal transplantation reaction in avascular keratoconus patients due to HLA–associated immune aberration against infection. Invest Ophthalmol 16:644, 1977

48. Waltman SR, Faulkner HW, Burde RM: Modification of the ocular immune response. I. Use of antilymphocytic serum to prevent immune rejection of penetrating corneal homografts. Invest Ophthalmol 8:196, 1969

49. Wang HS, Basu PK: Cellular immunity to xenogeneic corneal grafts in rabbits. Can J Ophthalmol 10:263, 1975

50. Watson PG, Joysey VC: Difficulties in the use of tissue typing for corneal grafting. In Corneal Graft Failure. Ciba Foundation Symposium, Amsterdam, Elsevier, 1973, p 323

TWELVE TWELVE TWELVE ocular tumors

TUMOR IMMUNOLOGY

ETIOLOGIC FACTORS

The search for etiologic agents in cancer began nearly 200 years ago with the discovery that chimney sweeps who were chronically exposed to hydrocarbons had a high incidence of scrotal carcinoma (83). It is now recognized that environmental factors are responsible for the vast majority of human cancers (43). The role of cigarette smoking and industrial exposure to various substances is well established. Oils and coal tars, dye stuffs, and chemicals such as vinyl chloride are among the ever-increasing list of chemical carcinogens. Environmental stimuli such as ultraviolet light and X-irradiation have been implicated in the development of skin tumors.

Viruses can produce a broad spectrum of tumors in animals, ranging from leukemias to osteogenic sarcomas. Viruses have been suspected of causing a number of human tumors, including Burkitt's lymphoma and nasopharyngeal carcinoma (Epstein–Barr virus), cervical carcinoma (herpes simplex type 2) (69), Kaposi's sarcoma (cytomegalovirus), acute myelogenous leukemia (type C oncornavirus), and breast cancer (type B oncornavirus) (85). The common denominator among oncogenic viruses appears to be their ability to merge their genetic complement with that of the host.

TUMOR ANTIGENS

Two categories of tumor antigens can be distinguished: those which form part of the tumor cell surface and those which do not (80). The latter, which are located intracellularly, may be products of viral genes, and although such antigens elicit an immune response which can be demonstrated serologically, they do not play any part in the rejection of tumor cells. Tumors can be rejected much as transplants are rejected, and it appears that T lymphocytes are of key importance in this process. The antigens which are responsible for the rejection of tumors, and which are more relevant to the immunotherapy and immunodiagnosis of tumors, are located on the cell surface where they make the cell vulnerable to attack by humoral and cellular immune responses. These antigens are known as tumor-specific transplantation antigens (TSTAs) (see Tumor Antigens, Ch. 1). Chemically induced tumors possess unique TSTAs, while virus-induced tumors, whatever their histologic type, typically share TSTAs with all other tumors caused by that virus.

Antigens on most tumors are capable of eliciting both humoral and cell-mediated immune responses. Circulating antibodies to tumor cell surface antigens have been identified in a variety of tumors (44, 59, 76, 101). Humoral antitumor immunity may in some cases actually be harmful, since antibody

295

which serves as a blocking factor (see that section) may be produced.

Certain antigens, such as carcinoembryonic antigen (CEA), elicit an antibody response which is a good indicator for the presence of malignancy, but serves no known protective function. Histocompatibility antigens have also been demonstrated on the surface of tumor cells. Generally, there is an inverse relation between the concentration of histocompatibility antigens and tumor antigens.

Fetal Antigens

Fetal antigens may be found on the surface of tumor cells but are easily shed into the environment. The most widely studied fetal antigens are CEA and α-fetoprotein. CEA, which is present in the gut, liver, and pancreas of the human fetus, is found in adenocarcinomas of the human digestive tract (40). It is useful in the diagnosis and monitoring of patients with cancer of the gastrointestinal tract. Elevated levels of CEA are found in a majority of patients with entodermally derived neoplasms. Recently, CEA has been studied in patients with intraocular tumors and has proven helpful in distinguishing primary from metastatic lesions (71-73). In metastatic tumors of entodermal origin, the level of CEA is usually greater than 20 ng/ml and may be as high as 4000 ng/ml (23). α-Fetoprotein is detectable in the blood of most patients with hepatomas and in some patients with embryonal carcinoma. It is also found in high concentrations in cord blood.

IMMUNE SURVEILLANCE

The concept of immune surveillance is used to explain the organism's ability to differentiate between "nonself" and "self." Malignant cells are thought to arise constantly in all animals but are normally eliminated by the immune system because they are recognized as nonself. If a defect in immune surveillance develops— for example, if the immune system is unable to recognize tumor antigens—a tumor may grow too large for the cellular immune system to destroy it effectively. Individuals who are immunosuppressed by drugs or who are born with congenital immunodeficiencies have a high incidence of tumors, presumably because of a defect in immune surveillance. (See also Immune Surveillance, Ch. 2.)

BLOCKING FACTORS

Blocking factors have been found in the serum of tumor patients and may prevent tumor destruction despite the presence of adequate cell-mediated immune responses. Blocking factors are usually soluble tumor antigens or antigen–antibody complexes. They can act directly on tumor cells or on sensitized lymphocytes. Blocking factors may be formed by humoral immune respones to tumors.

CELL-MEDIATED CYTOLYSIS

Cellular immunity is the main mechanism by which tumor cells are destroyed. Four possible cell-mediated responses to tumors have been proposed. 1) Cytotoxic T lymphocytes may come into intimate contact with tumor cells, establish a firm adhesion to the cells, and cause lysis by creating an osmotic disequilibrium (3). 2) Antibody-dependent lymphocyte cytotoxicity may occur when target tumor cells are coated with specific antitumor antibody. Nonimmune lymphocytes could interact with cell-bound antibodies and cause tumor cell lysis. These nonimmune effector lymphocytes are not T lymphocytes; however, their true identity remains unknown. 3) Activated, or armed, macrophages may recognize and destroy tumor cells. This type of cytotoxicity is nonspecific and may affect local "bystander" cells as well as tumor cells. 4) Macrophages may participate in a nonspecific way in T cell responses against tumors. They are frequently found in close association with lymphoid cells, although their exact function remains unclear.

IMMUNOTHERAPY

Several approaches to immunotherapy have been investigated. These include nonspecific immunotherapy, active specific immunotherapy, adoptive immunotherapy, and the use of tumor-specific transfer factor (48).

Nonspecific immunotherapy is induced by

stimulation of the immune system with adjuvants which nonspecifically enhance the patient's ability to respond to his own tumor. The contact sensitizer dinitrochlorobenzene (DNCB) has been used in the treatment of malignant melanomas and cutaneous lymphomas, and BCG, the attenuated form of the live human tubercle bacillus, has been administered systemically and also injected locally in treating melanomas of the skin. The mode of action of BCG is uncertain and there has been concern that it may stimulate the formation of blocking factors. Other nonspecific immunizing agents include *Corynebacterium parvum* and MER, a methanol-extracted residue of the tubercle bacillus.

Levamisole, an antihelminthic agent, enhances phagocytosis and *in vitro* lymphocyte function in animals. It augments macrophage chemotaxis in man and restores T cell function to normal levels in certain patients. It has been used in a wide variety of immunologic diseases. However, its efficacy in cancer therapy is still controversial.

Active specific immunotherapy consists of immunization with a vaccine containing an appropriate tumor antigen. While this form of therapy appears to be useful in certain experimentally-induced tumors, its clinical potential remains to be fully evaluated.

Adoptive immunotherapy, using nonsensitized or sensitized lymphocytes has not proven successful. The lymphoid cells are rapidly rejected, often before reaching the site of the tumor. Alternatively, a graft-versus-host reaction can take place in immunologically compromised patients who are not able to kill the foreign cells.

Transfer factor has been used in the treatment of a variety of tumors and is currently being evaluated in a number of clinical trials. This molecule transfers cell-mediated immune responses to host lymphocytes. Tumor-specific transfer factor endows host lymphocytes with specific antitumor activity.

LEUKEMIAS

Leukemias are neoplastic proliferations of white blood cells and their precursors throughout the body. They are usually classified on the basis of their clinical course and the cell type undergoing malignant transformation. Acute leukemias are seen more often in middle-aged and older people. Visual symptoms and ocular findings are common in patients with leukemia. Leukemic cells can infiltrate various ocular tissues and produce hemorrhage, exudates, proptosis and papilledema.

Immunopathology

The cause of leukemia in man is unknown. Recent evidence has implicated viruses, as well as genetic and environmental factors. Viruses have been shown to produce leukemia in mice, cats, fowl, and nonhuman primates. These viruses may be passed to the offspring in the genetic material or in the colostrum. RNA virus particles have been found within human leukemic cells and may play a role in the development of human leukemia.

Antibodies which are cytotoxic for acute lymphocytic or acute myelogenous leukemia cells and for cultured lymphoid cell lines are found in about 15% of patients with acute leukemia. Immunoglobulins can be detected on the cell membranes of human leukemia cells; these may be derived from serum antibody which has adsorbed to the tumor cells. Leukemia-associated antigens can also be detected on leukemic cell membranes by immunofluorescent techniques. These antigens produce lymphoblastic changes in lymphocytes from normal subjects and from patients who are in remission.

Leukemia cells in acute lymphocytic leukemia can be characterized by their surface markers and their ability to form rosettes. In 80% of patients, these cells are neither T nor B lymphocytes but, rather, "null" cells which lack features of both subpopulations. The remaining 20% of children with acute lymphocytic leukemia have leukemic T cells. These patients are somewhat older, have a higher incidence of mediastinal thymic tumors, and have a poorer prognosis. High levels of antileukemia antibody and of leukemia-associated antigens, and reduced lymphocyte activation by phytohemagglutinin, all indicate a poor prognosis.

In chronic lymphocytic leukemia, the leukemic cell is a B lymphocyte in about 98% of cases and a T cell or null cell in the remainder. The surface immunoglobulins detectable on B cells may be a single L chain or H chain type or a monoclonal IgM. Immunoglobulin deficiencies associated with recurrent infections are often seen in chronic lymphocytic leukemia. In addition, monoclonal or biclonal proteins are often found.

Clinical Features

General. Acute leukemia may present with fever, weight loss, fatigue, weakness, sternal tenderness, lymphadenopathy, hepatosplenomegaly, or bleeding tendencies. Chronic leukemias may present in the same way; however, the prognosis is considerably better.

Ocular Findings. The eye is said to be affected at any one time in nearly all leukemic patients some time during the course of the disease (2). Eye findings are four times more common in acute leukemia than in chronic leukemias. It is not possible, however, to distinguish between the different forms of leukemia on the basis of the ocular examination (41). Hemorrhage and leukemic infiltration of the conjunctiva may be an early sign in myelogenous leukemic (87). The choroid, optic nerve, and orbit may be infiltrated by leukemic cells. Sudden hemorrhage into the orbit may occasionally lead to prominent exophthalmos. Funduscopic changes are among the most striking abnormalities seen in leukemia. Retinal veins may be engorged and tortuous, and may exhibit sheathing. Hemorrhages may be intraretinal, subretinal, or preretinal. The intraretinal hemorrhages, which have a white center, are commonly termed **Roth spots.** Hard exudates, representing focal accumulations of leukocytes, and cotton-wool spots are often seen. Retinal capillary microaneurysms and retinal neovascularization have also been described in leukemia (34, 52). Generalized retinal edema and nodular masses of leukemic cells are sometimes found on the retina.

Optic nerve changes suggestive of papilledema are frequently seen in leukemia. These alterations are thought to be due to direct infiltration of the retina and optic nerve by leukemia cells or they may be secondary to increased intracranial presure (77).

Treatment

Chemotherapeutic drugs are used for all types of leukemia, while the patient's impaired bone marrow status is supported with transfusions of blood cells and platelets. Boosting the immune response with BCG has also been effective in some situations. When the optic nerve is involved, irradiation of the eye and the administration of cytotoxic drugs is usually the most successful therapy (27).

RETICULUM CELL SARCOMA

Reticulum cell sarcoma is characterized by proliferation of cells in the central nervous system which are probably derived from the monocyte-macrophage series. It affects older individuals, especially males, and may present with lymphoid proliferation, abnormal cells in the blood, and sometimes a uveitis.

Immunopathology

The reticulum cell contains many long cytoplasmic projections and multiple ribosome–lamella complexes in the cytoplasm. Because of the surface features of the reticulum cell this sarcoma is sometimes termed "hairy-cell leukemia." The cells adhere to surfaces and are capable of phagocytosis. They probably belong to the monocyte-macrophage series; however, in some instances the cells appear to be B lymphocytes. A selective IgA depression is sometimes found in patients with this disorder.

Clinical Features

General. Elderly males are most often affected. They may present with lymphadenopathy, splenomegaly, pancytopenia, abdominal discomfort, fatigue, malaise, or infection. From 30% to 60% of the cells in the peripheral blood may be abnormal.

Ocular Findings. Reticulum cell sarcoma is a rare cause of chorioretinitis. The tumor may be primary in the eye or secondary to generalized disease with involvement of the central nervous system. Tumors that produce ocular symptoms may arise from the meninges or the base of the brain (47). Uveitis may be the initial sign in reticulum cell sarcoma. Examination typically shows a perivascular pattern of tumor areas with hemorrhagic necrosis, a fluffy outline, and in some instances a grayish green color (87). Reticulum cell sarcoma should be considered in the differential diagnosis of chronic uveitis or deep retinal or choroidal infiltrates of unknown etiology. A recent case presented with a ring scotoma and involved the ciliary body, producing neovascular glaucoma (99).

Treatment

The prognosis for reticulum cell sarcoma is relatively good. Splenomegaly and pancytopenia can be treated by splenectomy with excellent results. Chemotherapy is of uncertain value and can be associated with a high mortality rate. This may be due to the precarious state of the bone marrow or its massive infiltration by abnormal cells. Treatment with chemotherapeutic agents has been associated with regression of intraocular tumors in some instances (99) but not in others (8).

LYMPHOMAS

Lymphomas are malignant tumors of the reticular stem cells and their derivatives. They represent solid tumors of the immune system and are commonly associated with immunologic abnormalities. Lymphomas may be broadly divided into Hodgkin's disease and the more common non-Hodgkin's lymphomas. Lymphomas may also be classified by the immunologic nature of their main cell type. Thus, T cell lymphomas may be differentiated from B cell lymphomas, histiocytic lymphomas, and those with undefined cell types. The orbit and conjunctiva are involved in about 3% of patients with lymphomas.

Immunopathology

Hodgkin's disease is distinguished by the presence of Reed–Sternberg cells, large, polypoid mesenchymal cells with multiple, large nucleoli. Immunoglobulin levels are usually normal, as is the ability to mount a primary and secondary antibody response to common antigens. Cell-mediated immunity is depressed in one-half to two-thirds of Hodgkin's disease patients when the disease is present at multiple sites (12). Defective cellular immunity also exists in the early stages of Hodgkin's disease. Anergy to common skin test antigens is present (74), and it is difficult to sensitize patients with dinitrochlorobenzene. Skin allografts are rejected poorly or not at all. Some individuals with Hodgkin's disease will retain cellular immune responses to antigens encountered before the onset of the disease but are unable to react to new antigens. *In vitro* responses, such as lymphocyte transformation in response to mitogens, antigen, and allogeneic cells, are often abnormal. The impaired delayed hypersensitivity responses of Hodgkin's disease may be due to an inadequate quantity of functioning lymphocytes (12). Administration of chemotherapeutic drugs may further impair delayed hypersensitivity responses. In advanced Hodgkin's disease, an excess of suppressor lymphocytes is found despite an overall depletion of lymphocytes.

A number of antigens have been isolated from patients with Hodgkin's disease by tissue culture of their lymphoid tissue (24). These antigens have been designated F and S antigens on the basis of their fast and slow electrophoretic mobilities. The F antigen has recently been identified as ferritin. A third antigen, known as PL antigen, is a constituent of normal peripheral lymphocytes. Splenic tissue synthesizes increased levels of IgG in 91% of patients with Hodgkin's disease. The spleen may be responding with humoral antibody to an antigen that is associated with lymphocytes.

The exact nature of this antigen, however, has not been determined.

Mycosis fungoides is an uncommon chronic and often fatal disease which may begin in the reticuloendothelial system of the skin. This condition may remain localized to the skin for many years but may eventually involve the lymph nodes and internal organs. The tumors are composed primarily of lymphocytes, plasma cells, and atyptical mononuclear cells (mycosis cells). A less severe form of cutaneous T cell lymphoma is known as **Sézary syndrome.** This is a primary cutaneous lymphoma which is associated with chronic leukemia and generalized erythroderma. Sézary cells are large mononuclear cells which are diagnostic features of the syndrome. They are felt to be abnormal T cells. Both mycosis fungoides and Sézary syndrome are considered to be part of a larger spectrum of cutaneous lymphomas involving T lymphocytes. Another T cell lymphoma, known as **convoluted lymphocyte syndrome,** arises in the thymus and is associated with diffuse proliferation of immature cells which infiltrate lymph nodes and other organs.

Burkitt's lymphoma occurs in tropical areas where malaria is endemic. It has been suggested that persistent immunologic stimulation by malarial infection and consequent lymphoreticular hyperplasia may be an important factor in the development of this malignancy (79). A constant association between Burkitt's lymphoma and the Epstein–Barr virus (EBV) has been noted. Burkitt cells harbor virus particles and many investigators feel that EBV may be the first proven human cancer virus (59). EBV is also felt to be the etiologic agent in infectious mononucleosis, and the anti-EBV antibody observed in mononucleosis is identical to that found in patients with Burkitt's lymphoma.

Angioimmunoblastic lymphadenopathy is thought to represent an abnormal hyperimmune response of B cells rather than a true lymphoma. It is associated with a hypergammaglobulinemia and a high incidence of autoimmune hemolytic anemia. **Immunoblastic sarcoma** may arise *de novo* or secondary to another immunologic disorder. In this disease, cells known as immunoblasts undergo progressive proliferation.

Clinical Features

General. Histologic classification in Hodgkin's disease is based on the presence of Reed–Sternberg cells, lymphocytes, plasma cells, histiocytes, and fibrous tissue. The current classification includes four types: type 1, lymphocyte predominance; type 2, nodular sclerosis; type 3, mixed cellularity; and type 4, lymphocyte depletion. This classification has diagnostic and prognostic significance, with lymphocyte predominance and nodular sclerosis representing a strong immune response to the lymphoma, and lymphocyte depletion representing failure of the immune response.

Mycosis fungoides classically progresses through three stages: eczema, plaque, and tumor. In addition, exfoliative erythroderma or psoriatic dermatitis may also be present. In Sézary syndrome the skin lesions are exfoliative and may develop into plaques. Intense itching is common, but the fever, malaise, weakness, and weight loss seen in other lymphomas are uncommon.

Burkitt's lymphoma often presents with tumors of the face or jaw. Angioimmunoblastic lymphadenopathy presents with fever, sweating, weight loss, rash, lymphadenopathy, and hepatosplenomegaly.

Ocular Findings. The ocular manifestations of Hodgkin's disease involve primarily the orbit, lids, and lacrimal gland. Bilateral granulomas of the conjunctiva (27) (Fig. 12–1), corneal infiltration, uveitis, episcleritis, and funduscopic changes may be observed. Papilledema may be present owing to direct invasion of the optic nerve or involvement of the apex of the orbit (87).

In mycosis fungoides, the lids and conjunctiva are most likely to be affected. Intraocular lesions have also been reported (31, 32, 38, 57). Retinal hemorrhages, edema, venous stasis, and perivascular granulomas may be observed.

In Burkitt's lymphoma, the maxillary and orbital tumors which originate from the marrow space are usually painless. Proptosis is

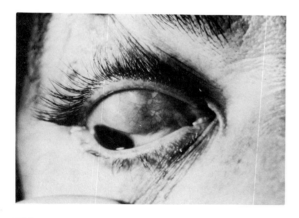

FIG. 12-1. Episcleral infiltrates in patient with lymphoma. (Courtesy of Dr. J. Michelson)

common when the maxillary bones are involved. Central nervous system involvement is also common. The globe may be invaded by tumor but this is relatively rare (30, 54).

Treatment

Treatment of Hodgkin's disease requires complete staging of the lymphoma to determine the extent of involvement. In stages I, II, and III, in which the disease is confined to the lymph nodes, radiation therapy is often curative. If the tumor is found in the bone marrow, liver, or lung (stage IV) the patient is treated with chemotherapy. Patients with unfavorable histologic types of tumor are treated with chemotherapy in addition to radiation, even when the disease is confined to the lymph nodes. Advanced Hodgkin's disease responds well to multiple drug chemotherapy. The "MOPP" therapy regimen (mechlorethamine, vincristine [Oncovin], procarbazine, and prednisone) is associated with remission rates of up to 80%. Mycosis fungoides may be treated with radiotherapy and systemic chemotherapy (57). Burkitt's lymphoma is extremely sensitive to radiotherapy or methotrexate.

Surgery is frequently used to establish the diagnosis of an ocular lymphoma. If the lesion is producing severe exophthalmos, a Krönlein procedure may be indicated. Following surgical excision, postoperative irradiation is usually advisable. [Lymphomas of the orbit are usually quite sensitive to radiation.]

PARAPROTEINEMIAS (PLASMA CELL DYSCRASIAS)

This group of disorders is distinguished by the uncontrolled proliferation of plasma cells. An abnormal or malignant clone of plasma cells continually synthesizes a single immunoglobulin product which can be detected in the serum or urine. These abnormal proteins are most frequently associated with multiple myeloma or macroglobulinemia.

MULTIPLE MYELOMA

Multiple myeloma is the most common of the plasma cell proliferative disorders. It is characterized by lytic lesions of bone, anemia, and the production of a serum or urine paraprotein. The paraprotein is the result of proliferation of a single clone of plasma cells. Ocular involvement is common and may consist of a primary lesion in the orbit or secondary involvement of adjacent ocular structures. The cornea, ciliary body, retina, and optic nerve may be affected in some cases.

Immunopathology

A key diagnostic feature in multiple myeloma is the demonstration of paraproteins in the serum or urine by electrophoresis. These proteins are found in the urine of about half of multiple myeloma patients, and roughly 20% demonstrate Bence Jones proteinuria without abnormal serum proteins. Bence Jones protein consists of monoclonal κ or λ light chains. They are observed after heating the urine of myeloma patients to 50°–60°C. If Bence Jones proteins are present, a white precipitate will appear. When the temperature is raised to boiling, the precipitate redissolves. The most common types of serum paraproteins are IgG (50%) and IgA (25%). Rarely, IgD and IgE myeloma proteins will be found. About 90% of IgD myeloma patients excrete Bence Jones protein, most of which is the λ light chain form. The frequency of the various immunoglobulin types found in myeloma patients reflects the normal levels of immunoglobulins in the serum. This relationship suggests that the neoplastic process results from random proliferation of a single clone of plasma cells.

Serum levels of nonmyeloma immunoglobulins are usually lower than normal in myeloma patients. The primary antibody response to new antigens is also poor, although the secondary response to previously encountered antigens is usually intact. Myeloma patients are generally more susceptible to bacterial infections than are normal individuals.

Defects in cellular immunity are also found in multiple myeloma patients. Deficient delayed hypersensitivity and a diminished lymphocyte stimulation with phytohemagglutinin have been noted. Defects in macrophage and granulocyte function have also been found.

Clinical Features

General. Clinical manifestations are variable in multiple myeloma. Patients typically present with bone pain, anemia, hypercalcemia, and renal insufficiency. The bone pain is due to plasma cell proliferation within the ribs, sternum, spine, shoulder, and skull. Lytic "punched-out" bone lesions may be seen radiographically and these increase in size and number as the disease progresses. Anemia occurs because of the encroachment of the plasma cell tumor on the bone marrow's erythropoietic capacity. As mentioned, increased susceptibility to infection is common in patients with multiple myeloma. Pneumonia, pyelonephritis, and septicemia are probably due to depression of the immune system. Polyneuropathy may be caused by direct infiltration of the nervous system by the tumor or may be due to deposition of amyloid. A rheumatoid like arthropathy of unknown etiology may precede the onset of other findings.

Some features of multiple myeloma are due to the presence of the myeloma protein (81). Coagulation disturbances result from the capacity of some myeloma proteins to bind fibrinogen, prothrombin, and clotting factors V and VII (63). Hyperviscosity and cryoprecipitability are also due to the presence of myeloma protein (11).

Bone marrow examination shows increased numbers of plasma cells. These cells may be arranged in sheets and show signs of immaturity.

Ocular Findings. Primary orbital or extraosseous myeloma of the orbit may be an initial finding in multiple myeloma (21). The eye may also be affected secondary to a primary focus in the cranial bones, paranasal sinuses, nose, nasopharynx, or mucous membranes of the upper respiratory tract. The bones of the cranium are said to be involved at some time in over 70% of patients with myeloma (9). Compression of the cranial nerves may lead to loss of vision or to extraocular muscle palsies (6). Proptosis can result from orbital bone involvement (89). Pars plana cysts are often found and these may be so large that they relax the zonular fibers and displace the lens anteriorly (7). Iridescent crystals may be deposited in the cornea and conjunctiva of patients with multiple myeloma (5). Funduscopic abnormalities include microaneurysms, retinal hemorrhages and exudates, tortuous vessels, and central retinal vein thrombosis. These findings seem to be related to secondary hematologic complications such as anemia and thrombocytopenia. Ocular infections, including metastatic bacterial endophthalmitis, have been reported, and these may be the result of the depressed humoral and cellular immunity which accompanies multiple myeloma (7).

Treatment

Local irradiation may be used to control pain and reduce the tumor mass, but chemotherapy is the mainstay of treatment in multiple myeloma. Melphalan, with or without prednisone, is the usual drug of choice for initial treatment. Cyclophosphamide is also widely used. Other treatment of multiple myeloma requires general supportive measures such as control of pain with analgesics, adequate fluid intake, blood transfusions, and treatment of recurrent infections. Complications due to hypercalcemia, renal failure, spinal cord compression, and hyperviscosity must also be treated.

WALDENSTROM'S MACROGLOBULINEMIA

In Waldenstrom's macroglobulinemia, there is a monoclonal increase in immunoglobulin of the IgM class. Clinical findings are directly attributable to the excess IgM and a consequent hyperviscosity syndrome. Hematologic and clotting abnormalities are generally found. Ocular findings include sludging and congestion of the conjunctival and retinal blood vessels, vascular occlusions and hemorrhages, and infiltration of the lacrimal gland and orbit.

Immunopathology

The paraprotein in Waldenstrom's macroglobulinemia belongs to the IgM class. It may be the entire 19S immunoglobulin but a significant portion consists of 7S monomeric units. This suggests a possible defect in assembly of the 19S molecule. Bence Jones protein is found in approximately 10% of patients.

Several factors contribute to the hyperviscosity syndrome, including the abnormal serum concentration of IgM, polymer or aggregate formation, cryoprecipitation, abnormal shape of the IgM molecule, antibody activity against serum proteins,and abnormalities of red cells and blood vessels. Unlike the case in multiple myeloma, the levels of normal immunoglobulins and the humoral and cellular immune responses are not severely impaired.

Clinical Features

General. Two-thirds of all patients with macroglobulinemia are males and 80% are over age 50 (67). Early symptoms include fatigue, weakness, and weight loss. The type of skeletal lesion that is seen in multiple myeloma is uncommon in marcroglobulinemia. Hepatosplenomegaly and lymphadenopathy are often seen and anemia may occur secondary to an increased plasma volume, decreased erythropoiesis, and hemolysis (81). A hemorrhagic diathesis may lead to purpura or epistaxis. The function of platelets may be altered, possibly due to their interaction with an abnormal protein (63). Hyperviscosity of the blood leads to

an increased resistance of blood flow and to hypervolemia. The cardiac workload increases and circulatory failure can occur (96). This may lead to headaches, lightheadedness, vertigo, stupor, coma, generalized seizures, postural hypotension, and deafness.

Although the clinical course varies, the disease may be present for many years before symptoms develop. Some patients have a rapid downhill course and eventually develop reticulum cell sarcoma.

Ocular Findings. Ocular findings in Waldenstrom's macroglobulinemia are common. Sludging of the conjunctival blood stream can be observed, and can be exaggerated by application of ice to the closed lids prior to observation (1). Retinopathy may be severe, with diffuse hemorrhages, cotton-wool spots, retinal microaneurysms, neovascularization, and dilated, tortuous retinal veins. As the retinal veins continue to dilate, they develop the appearance of huge strings of sausage. Retinal vein occlusion, exudative retinal detachment, vitreous hemorrhage, glaucoma, and rubeosis iridis may eventually develop and permanently impair vision. The retinopathy may diminish markedly when the patient is treated with plasmapheresis to decrease blood viscosity (14). Papilledema is an uncommon finding in Waldenstrom's macroglobulinemia.

Treatment

Plasmapheresis often produces dramatic reversal of symptoms and is usually well tolerated (82). The treatment of choice in Waldenstrom's macroglobulinemia, it removes excess IgM and restores the plasma volume to normal. Patients with severe hyperviscosity may require plasmapheresis for several days at a time. Chlorambucil can be given in low doses on a daily basis; it requires monitoring of the blood count and bone marrow status.

AMYLOIDOSIS

Amyloidosis includes a group of disorders which result from deposition of a proteinaceous, amorphous substance in certain tissues. Deposition of amyloid may be primary, secondary to other diseases, or familial. Virtually any organ can be involved, including the eye. Several protein constituents have been identified in amyloid, including portions of immunoglobulin molecules (39).

Immunopathology

Two major types of amyloid have been distinguished. One of these, known as the AL protein, is structurally related to immunoglobulin light chains (51). The other, termed AA protein, is structurally unrelated to any other known serum protein (10). The protein related to light chains is the major and perhaps the sole component of amyloid fibrils in primary amyloidosis and in the type of amyloidosis that is associated with myeloma. It is found in smaller amounts in secondary and some familial types of amyloidosis. The nonimmunoglobulin AA protein is the major component of the secondary forms and in other familial forms of amyloidosis. This component has also been found in patients with primary amyloidosis and in myeloma-associated amyloidosis by some investigators (50), but not by others (36).

The reason for amyloid production is unknown. It may represent a disorder of serum proteins, a disorder of protein metabolism, an abnormality of the reticuloendothelial system, the result of chronic immunologic stimulation, a disorder of delayed hypersensitivity, or a combination of these defects (94). Amyloid appears to be deposited in the tissues under circumstances in which the immune response is overwhelmed by an antigenic load or in which the lymphoid system undergoes neoplastic transformation.

The role of cellular immunity in amyloidosis has been investigated. T cell depletion by thymectomy, X-irradiation, or antimetabolite administration favors the reduction of amyloid deposition. Amyloidosis is often found in patients with Hodgkin's disease, lepromatous leprosy, and multiple myeloma, all diseases in which delayed hypersensitivity responses are impaired. In multiple myeloma, prolonged antigenic stimulation leads to the development of plasmacytomas and probably impairment of T cell function and of immune surveillance. Lymphocyte transformation studies in amyloid patients have shown a selective depression of T cell responses to concanavallin A but normal responses to other mitogens (94). These studies suggest that a selective defect in a subpopulation of T lymphocytes may be important in the pathogenesis of amyloid disease.

Homogenous amyloid consists of characteristic long fibrils. It is not known whether the fibrils are synthesized as such or if they are the result of degradation of intact protein molecules. It has been suggested that lysosomal proteolytic digestion of light chains by macrophages could result in amyloid formation (39).

Clinical Features

General. Many classifications of amyloidosis exist; however, the simplest and most widely used one is based on the four major categories described by Reimann *et al* (88): 1) Primary amyloidosis occurs in the absence of coexistent or antecedent disease. Mesenchymal tissues including those of the heart, muscle, or almost any other organ can be involved. Bence Jones protein may be present in the urine. 2) Secondary amyloidosis usually follows chronic diseases such as neoplasms, infections, or connective tissue disorders, especially rheumatoid arthritis. The kidney, liver, spleen, and intestine are often affected. Bence Jones protein is usually absent. Amyloidosis associated with multiple myeloma and other plasma cell dyscrasias is characterized by homogeneous proteins in the serum and urine. Amyloid deposits have also been found in small amounts in post-mortem examinations of various tissues. 3) Tumor-forming amyloid is an isolated mass of amyloid that appears in the skin, eye, or urinary tract. 4) Familial types of amyloidosis affect different organ systems and have different patterns of inheritance. The most common is associated with familial Mediterranean fever, seen mostly in Sephardic Jews.

Virtually any organ system can be affected in amyloidosis. Kidney involvement is potentially the most serious manifestation of the disease and is usually the major cause of death. Cardiac amyloid may be asymptomatic but on occasion leads to congestive heart failure. The gastrointestinal system is frequently affected; symptoms include obstruction, ulceration, malabsorption, hemorrhage, and protein loss. Diagnosis depends on biopsy of the involved tissues. The rectum, conjunctiva, or gingiva may be biopsied and stained with Congo red or viewed with a polarizing microscope for a characteristic green birefringence.

Ocular Findings. The skin of the eyelids is a frequent site of amyloid deposition. Small papules with a waxy, yellowish appearance are typical. Conjunctival nodules are rarely seen; however, large deposits may follow trachoma and other forms of conjunctivitis.

Amyloid may be deposited in response to a preexisting chronic corneal disease and has been demonstrated in the corneal epithelium of a patient with retrolental fibroplasia (97). It has also been detected in the corneas of seven unsuspected cases of amyloidosis showing corneal scarring and opacification (68). Corneal involvement is characterized by the presence of cobblestone masses of yellowish pink material, which stain bright salmon pink with 0.2% Congo red. Familial amyloidosis of the cornea has been described (98) and may be associated with cataracts (which do not contain amyloid) (98). Lattice dystrophy of the cornea is considered a localized form of amyloidosis in which deposits of amyloid are found in the corneal stroma (70). It has been reported in association with systemic amyloidosis (70).

Amyloid may be deposited in the iris secondary to chronic infection (86), and may be found in the vitreous, where it has a characteristic grey, glass-wool appearance. Most patients with amyloid in the vitreous have familial amyloidosis, although some had no family history of the disease. Vitreous opacities may be unilateral, or asymmetric in the two eyes, and may be in contact with the posterior lens surface. Pupillary abnormalities are not uncommon in familial amyloidosis. The irides may show segmental paralysis (100), light-near dissociation (61) and inequality of the pupils (25), and even heterochromia (4).

Scalloped pupils are a characteristic feature of familial amyloidosis and may be a helpful clue in making a correct diagnosis (4, 64). This pupillary abnormality may be due to infiltration of the sphincter or nonadjacent ciliary nerves with amyloid. Orbital involvement may be seen in amyloidosis and may lead to proptosis (93). Lacrimal gland involvement has also been described (60). The extraocular muscles may be infiltrated with amyloid.

Treatment

In amyloidosis associated with plasma cell tumors, treatment is directed at the tumor; however, regression of the amyloid lesion may be slow or imperceptible. Primary amyloidosis should not be treated with antitumor chemotherapy unless definite evidence of a neoplasm is found (35). Treatment of an infection or an inflammatory process may cause mobilization of systemic amyloid. Colchicine may abort the febrile episodes of familial Mediterranean fever, a disease often accompanied by amyloidosis. This drug can also prevent the development of amyloidosis in mice (56), and may be useful in far-advanced human cases. Various other agents including steroids, ascorbic acid, and immunosuppressive agents have also been tried without clear-cut benefit.

The vitreous deposits associated with amyloidosis may be removed by vitrectomy (55); however, redeposition tends to occur. Corneal transplanation may be necessary in advanced corneal lattice dystrophy or for the localized form of corneal amyloidosis.

MALIGNANT MELANOMA

Malignant melanoma of the uveal tract is the most common primary intraocular tumor (87). Despite numerous studies of ocular melanomas, the diagnosis and management of these tumors remain problematic. Immunologic studies have concentrated on distinguishing choroidal melanomas from lesions that are similar in appearance. Immunologic defects in patients with these tumors have also been studied, as have methods of therapy which enhance immune responses.

Immunopathology

As discussed previously (see Tumor Antigens), the evidence for tumor-associated antigens is now well established. Antibodies to tumor cell surface antigens have been identified in melanoma (76, 101). Cellular immune responses to melanomas have also been studied (20, 53), and it is this type of immunity which seems to be important in the body's defense against tumors.

Humoral Immunity. Early studies, using several serologic techniques including gel diffusion, hemagglutination, and complement fixation, were unable to detect antibodies to ocular melanomas (49). Subsequently, complement-dependent cytotoxic antibodies were found in the serum of some patients with uveal melanomas (84). These antibodies were directed against the surface antigen of the patient's own tumor cells grown in tissue culture (84). More recently, circulating antitumor antibodies have been found in the serum of many patients with ocular melanomas (13, 28, 101). Antitumor antibodies of the IgM class that were directed against antigens of allogenic choroidal melanomas could be detected in the serum of 91% of patients with primary choroidal melanomas (101). Such antibodies could also be detected in metastatic choroidal melanomas and in a late orbital recurrence of the tumor. These antibodies, identified by the indirect immunofluorescent technique, reacted with cytoplasmic antigens found in choroidal melanomas of different histologic types and could be absorbed with melanoma tissue taken from other patients.

IgM antibody could also be found in patients with conjunctival and iris melanomas. IgG antibodies to tumor-associated antigens have also been found in some patients with primary choroidal melanomas. Circulating antibodies to cytoplasmic melanoma antigens have been demonstrated in several patients but most do not cross react with other melanomas.

Antibodies directed against surface membrane antigens appear early in the course of the tumor. They possess complement-dependent cytotoxicity against cutaneous and uveal melanoma cells (65, 66). They disappear from the blood prior to dissemination of the tumor and may influence the growth and metastasis of the tumor by reacting with accessible antigens. These antibodies are not found in the serum of patients with larger tumors, possibly because they are not produced in advanced disease or cannot be demonstrated because of blocking factors. Antibodies to cytoplasmic antigens are found in the serum of most melanoma patients. They are thought to appear as a result of destruction of tumor cells and generally appear after antibodies to cell surface antigens. They do not seem to have any prognostic significance.

Fetal Antigens. Carcinoembryonic antigen (CEA), as discussed earlier (see under Tumor Immunology), is found in association with tumors of entodermal origin (40). In patients with nonpigmented choroidal masses which may represent a metastatic tumor or an amelanotic melanoma, a highly elevated level of CEA may indicate that the lesion is metastatic and of entodermal origin (71).

Cellular Immunity. Several lines of evidence point to the importance of cellular immune mechanisms in the host's response to melanomas. Lymphocytes from patients with cutaneous melanomas have a cytotoxic effect on autochthonous and allogeneic melanoma cells (45). Delayed hypersensitivity skin reactions can be elicited from patients with cutaneous melanomas (26) and with uveal melanomas (19) by use of a soluble melanoma antigen. Cellular reactivity to tumor-associated antigens can be demonstrated in patients with uveal melanomas by use of the leukocyte migration inhibition assay (20). This *in vitro* assay has been used to distinguish choroidal melanomas from similar appearing choroidal lesions (15).

Clinical Features

Malignant melanomas of the choroid may present in a variety of ways. Typical melanomas are pigmented, have a dome-shaped or mushroom-shaped configuration (Figs. 12-2 and 12-3) and often have orange pigment on their surface. Occasionally, a yellow halo can be seen around the margin. It may be difficult to distinguish choroidal melanomas from choridal nevi, hemangiomas, and metastatic tumors. The history as well as a thorough medical and ophthalmic examination may be helpful in making a proper diagnosis. In addition, other diagnostic methods may be of use, including contact lens examination, transillumination, fluorescein angiography, visual field examination, ultrasonography, and the radioactive phosphorus uptake test (95).

Treatment

When the visual acuity is significantly decreased by a sizable tumor, enucleation is indicated. In patients with small melanomas not affecting visual acuity, close serial examinations without therapeutic intervention appear to be safe until growth is observed (18). Other modes of therapy include photocoagulation, radiotherapy, cryotherapy, diathermy, and local resection (95).

Immunotherapy has recently been used in the treatment of cutaneous melanomas (75). BCG (bacillus Calmette–Guérin) vaccine has caused regression of skin melanomas when injected into the lesion. BCG has also been used for the treatment of disseminated malignant melanomas. The value of this vaccine in the therapy of primary ocular melanomas is unknown; however, small amounts of BCG

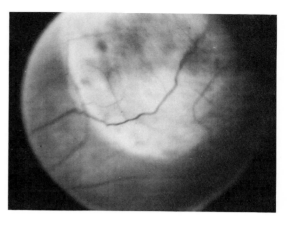

FIG. 12-3. Fundus photograph of malignant melanoma of the choroid. (Courtesy of Dr. J. Michelson)

can safely be administered subconjunctivally in the rabbit (91). Inoculation of BCG into experimentally induced conjunctival melanomas in hamsters has slowed or completely prevented tumor growth in 56% of treated eyes (92). Other approaches to immunotherapy of melanomas include immunization with vaccines made from tumor cells (22), adoptive immunotherapy through the transfer of sensitized lymphoid cells or their extracts (78), and passive immunotherapy with antiserum. Recently, repeated plasmapheresis has been used to remove antibodies which block cell-mediated immunity in patients with disseminated melanomas (46). This procedure increases cell-mediated cytotoxicity, presumably by the removal or alteration of circulating immune complexes in the serum. It is not known whether this improves the patient's immune response against the tumor; however, the procedure is well tolerated and may be a useful adjunct in the treatment of advanced melanomas.

RETINOBLASTOMA

Retinoblastoma is the most common intraocular malignancy of childhood. It arises from the nuclear layers of the retina, developing from multiple foci in one or both eyes. As in other kinds of tumors, cell-mediated immune responses to tumor-associated antigens are

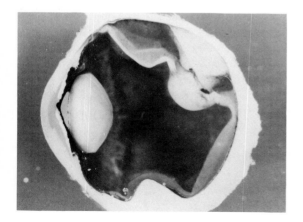

FIG. 12-2. Malignant melanoma of the choroid in enucleated eye. (Courtesy of Dr. J. Michelson)

thought to be important in resistance to retinoblastomas. The high rate of spontaneous regression of this tumor has also led to speculation that immunologic factors are particularly important in this tumor. Retinoblastoma may be due to a somatic mutation which is not hereditary, a germinal mutation which is autosomal-dominantly inherited, or a deletion of the long arm of chromosome 13 (33).

Immunpathology

Cellular immune responses in patients with retinoblastomas have been studied both *in vivo* and *in vitro* (16, 17). Eleven of fourteen patients with retinoblastomas had increased levels of cytotoxicity against a tissue culture line derived from retinoblastoma when compared with control subjects (16). This cytotoxicity appeared to be specific for the retinoblastoma cell line, since cytotoxicity against a breast carcinoma line was not increased. Whether this cell-mediated immune response was directed against retinoblastoma tumor antigens, other retinal antigens, fetal antigens, or virus-coated antigens, remains uncertain. When retinoblastoma patients are skin-tested with a crude membrane extract of the tumor, they demonstrate a positive skin test response which is not present in control subjects (17). No difference was seen in response to common skin test antigens when retinoblastoma patients were compared with normal subjects. While skin testing with a tumor extract and the *in vitro* cytotoxicity test may one day serve as valuable diagnostic tools, currently these tests are not widely used.

Retinoblastoma has a much higher spontaneous rate of regression than other human malignancies have. There have been several well-documented cases of spontaneous regression of retinoblastoma, both in bilateral and unilateral cases (58). It has been suggested that the development of immunity may be a significant factor in this form of tumor rejection. It has been postulated that this tumor may possess high antigenicity which incites an immune response, causing the tumor to regress (62). If retinoblastoma tumor cells are injected into the anterior chamber of "athymic" nude mice, which possess a severe defect

in cellular immunity, the tumor grows in some of the animals. No significant cell-mediated response and only a mild humoral immune response to the tumor can be demonstrated. A markedly positive antibody response was discovered in laboratory personnel who had come in contact with the tumor cell line. Cells from the Y-79 retinoblastoma cell line demonstrated much greater invasiveness than did freshly removed surgical specimens of retinoblastoma (37). Retinoblastoma tumor cells survive for varying periods of time in the anterior chamber of normal mice; however, they show little growth. The nude mouse seems to provide a good *in vitro* system for maintaining retinoblastoma cells for a relatively long period through serial transplantation.

Clinical Features

Retinoblastoma occurs in 1 out of every 14,-000–23,000 births (87). The average age at the time of diagnosis is 18 months; however, cases have been reported in patients 29–62 days old. About 30% of cases are bilateral but usually the disease is much more advanced in one eye than the other. Multiple independent foci of tumor cells are frequently found in the affected retina. The more differentiated tumors show photoreceptor differentiation toward rosettes and fleurettes, and such tumors are more resistant to radiation than the anaplastic variety. The tumor has a predilection for in-

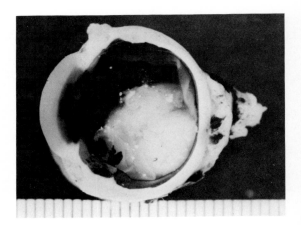

FIG. 12-4. Large retinoblastoma in enucleated eye. (Courtesy of Dr. J. Michelson)

vading the optic nerve but may also extend into the choroid and orbit.

Retinoblastoma may present in several ways, the most common being leukocoria (Fig. 12-4). Less often the patient develops an esotropia, an exotropia, or a red, painful eye. The single most important instrument in the diagnosis of retinoblastoma is the indirect ophthalmoscope. Other useful diagnostic tools include ultrasonography, computerized axial tomography (42), aqueous humor cytology (90), and aqueous humor enzyme patterns (29). Levels of both lactate dehydrogenase and phosphoglucose isomerase may be higher in the aqueous than in the serum of retinoblastoma patients.

Treatment

The type of treatment depends on the size of the tumor and the extent of the ocular and systemic involvement. Enucleation is indicated for advanced unilateral cases; a generous section of optic nerve should be removed. Bilateral enucleation is performed only when the disease is so extensive that no vision can be saved by any means and enucleation is necessary to prevent a fatal outcome. Irradiation with radon seeds or orthovoltage has proven to be a useful therapeutic measure. Chemotherapy with nitrogen mustard, triethylenemelamine (TEM), fluorouracil, cyclophosphamide, vincristine, and adriamycin has been employed. Cryotherapy and photocoagulation have also been used in the treatment of retinoblastoma.

REFERENCES

1. Ackerman A: The ocular manifestations of Waldenstrom's macroglobulinemia and its treatment. Arch Ophthalmol 67:701, 1962
2. Allen RA, Straatsma BR: Ocular involvement in leukemia and allied disorders. Arch Ophthalmol 66:490, 1961
3. Allison AC, Ferluga J: How lymphocytes kill tumor cells. N Engl J Med 295:165, 1976
4. Andrade C: A peculiar form of peripheral neuropathy: familial atypical generalized amyloidosis with special involvement of peripheral nerves. Brain 75:408, 1952
5. Aronson S, Shaw R: Corneal crystals in multiple myeloma. Arch Ophthalmol 61:541, 1959
6. Ashton N: Ocular changes in multiple myelomatosis. Arch Ophthalmol 73:487, 1965
7. Baker TR, Spencer WH: Ocular findings in multiple myeloma. Arch Ophthalmol 91:110, 1974
8. Barr CC, Green WR, Payne JW et al: Intraocular reticulum cell sarcoma. Surv Ophthalmol 19:224, 1975
9. Bayrd ED, Heck FJ: Multiple myeloma. JAMA 133:147, 1947
10. Benditt EP, Eriksen N: Chemical classes of amyloid substances. Am J Pathol 65:231, 1972
11. Bloch KJ, Maki DG: Hyperviscosity syndromes associated with immunoglobulin abnormalities. Semin Hematol 10:113, 1973
12. Brown RS, Haynes HA, Foley HT et al: Hodgkin's disease. Immunologic, clinical, and histologic features of 50 untreated patients. Ann Intern Med 67:291, 1967
13. Brownstein S, Sheikh KM, Lewis MG: Immunological studies in patients with malignant melanoma of the uvea. Can J Ophthalmol 12:16, 1977
14. Carr R, Henkind P: Retinal findings associated with serum hyperviscosity. Am J Ophthalmol 56:23, 1963
15. Char DH: Inhibition of leukocyte migration with melanoma-associated antigens in choroidal tumors. Invest Ophthalmol Vis Sci 16:176, 1977
16. Char DH, Ellsworth R, Rabson AS et al: Cell-mediated immunity to a retinoblastoma tissue culture line in patients with retinoblastoma. Am J Ophthalmol 78:5, 1974
17. Char DH, Herberman RB: Cutaneous delayed hypersensitivity responses of patients with retinoblastoma to standard recall antigens and crude membrane extracts of retinoblastoma tissue culture cells. Am J Ophthalmol 78:40, 1974
18. Char DH, Hogan MJ: Management of small elevated pigmented choroidal lesions. Br J Ophthalmol 61:54, 1977
19. Char DH, Hollinshead A, Cogan DG et al: Cutaneous delayed hypersensitivity reactions to soluble melanoma antigen in patients with ocular malignant melanoma. N Engl J Med 291:274, 1974
20. Char DH, Jerome L, McCoy JL, Herberman RB: Cell-mediated immunity to melanoma-associated antigens in patients with ocular malignant melanoma. Am J Ophthalmol 79:812, 1975
21. Clarke E: Plasma cell myeloma of the orbit. Br J Ophthalmol 37:543, 1953
22. Currie GA, LeJeune F, Fairley G: Immunization with irradiated tumor cells and specific lymphocyte cytotoxicity in malignant melanoma. Br Med J 2:305, 1971
23. Denslow GT, Kielar RA: Metastatic adenocar-

cinoma to the anterior uvea and increased carcinoembryonic antigen levels. Am J Ophthalmol 85:363, 1978

24. Eshar Z, Order SE, Katz DH: Ferritin, a Hodgkin's disease-associated antigen. Proc Natl Acad Sci USA 71:3956, 1974

25. Falls HF, Jackson J, Carey JH et al: Ocular manifestations of hereditary primary systemic amyloidosis. Arch Ophthalmol 54:660, 1955

26. Fass L, Herberman RB, Zieglar JL, Kiryabwire J: Cutaneous hypersensitivity reactions to autologous extracts of malignant melanoma cells. Lancet 1:116, 1970

27. Faulborn J: Malignant lymphogranulomatosis of the conjunctiva. Klin Monatsbl Augenheilkd 156:409, 1970

28. Federman JL, Lewis MG, Clark WH Jr et al: Tumor-associated antibodies in the serum of ocular melanoma patients. Trans Am Acad Ophthalmol Otolaryngol 78:784, 1974

29. Felberg NT, McFall R, Shields JA: Aqueous humor enzyme patterns in retinoblastoma. Invest Ophthalmol 16:1039, 1977

30. Feman SS, Niwayama G, Hapler RS, Foon KF: "Burkitt tumor" with intraocular involvement. Surv Ophthalmol 14:106, 1969

31. Foerster HC: Mycosis fungoides with intraocular involvement. Trans Am Acad Ophthalmol Otolaryngol 64:308, 1960

32. Francesschetti A: Miscosi fungoide con manifestazioni oculari (un caso con retinopatia disorcia). Ann Ottalmol Clin Ocul 76:413, 1950

33. François J: Genetics of retinoblastoma. Mod Prob Ophthalmol 18:165, 1977

34. Frank R, Ryan S: Peripheral retinal neovascularization with chronic myelogenous leukemia. Arch Ophthalmol 87:585, 1972

35. Franklin EC: Amyloidosis. Bull Rheum Dis 26:832, 1976

36. Franklin EC, Rosenthal CJ, Pras M, Levin M: Recent progress in amyloid. In Beers RF Jr, Bassett EG (eds): The Role of Immunological Factors in Autoimmune Processes. New York, Raven, 1976

37. Gallie BL, Albert DM, Wong JJY et al: Heterotransplantation of retinoblastoma into the athymic "nude" mouse. Invest Ophthalmol 16:256, 1977

38. Gartner J: Mycosis fungoides mit Beteiligung der Aderhaut. Klin Monatsbl Augenheilkd 131:61, 1957

39. Glenner GG, Terry WD, Isersky C: Amyloidosis: its nature and pathogenesis. Semin Hematol 10:65, 1973

40. Gold P, Freedman SO: Demonstration of tumor specific antigens in human colonic carcinomata by immunological tolerance and absorption techniques. J Exp Med 121:439, 1965

41. Goldbach L: Leukemic retinitis. Arch Ophthalmol 10:808, 1933

42. Goldberg L, Danziger A: Computed tomographic scanning in the management of retinoblastoma. Am J Ophthalmol 84:380, 1977

43. Heidelberger C: Chemical carcinogenesis. Cancer 40:430, 1977

44. Hellström I, Hellström KE, Pierce G, Bill AH: Demonstration of cell bound and humoral immunity against neuroblastoma cells. Proc Natl Acad Sci USA 60:1231, 1968

45. Hellström I, Hellström KE, Sjögren H, Warner GA: Demonstration of cell-mediated immunity to human neoplasms of various histological types. Int J Cancer 7:1, 1971

46. Hersey P, Edwards A, Adams E et al: Antibody-dependent cell-mediated cytotoxicity against melanoma cells induced by plasmapheresis. Lancet 1:825, 1976

47. Hogan MJ, Spencer WH, Hoyt WF: Primary reticuloendothelial sarcomas of the orbital and cranial meninges: ophthalmologic aspects. Am J Ophthalmol 61:1146, 1966

48. Holmes EC, Morton DL, Eilber FR: Immunotherapy of cancer (Medical Progress). West J Med 126:102, 1977

49. Howard GM, Spalter HF: Study of autoimmune serologic reactions to ocular melanoma. Arch Ophthalmol 76:399, 1966

50. Husby G, Sletten K, Michaelson TE, Natvig J: Amyloid fibril protein subunit, Protein AS: distribution in tissue and serum in different clinical types of amyloidosis including that associated with myelomatosis and Waldenstrom's macroglobulinemia. Scand J Immunol 2:395, 1973

51. Isersky C, Ein D, Page DL et al: Immunochemical cross reactions of human amyloid proteins with immunoglobulin light chains. J Immunol 108:486, 1972

52. Jampol L, Goldberg M, Busse B: Peripheral retinal microaneurysms in chronic leukemia. Am J Ophthalmol 80:242, 1975

53. Jehn UW, Nathanson L, Schwartz RS, Skinner M: In vitro lymphocyte stimulation by a soluble antigen from malignant melanoma. N Engl J Med 283:329, 1970

54. Karp LA, Zimmerman LE, Payne T: Intraocular involvement in Burkitt's lymphoma. Arch Ophthalmol 85:295, 1971

55. Kasner D, Miller GR, Taylor WH et al: Surgical treatment of amyloidosis of the vitreous. Trans Am Acad Ophthalmol Otolaryngol 72:410, 1968

56. Kedar I, Ravid M, Sohar E et al: Colchicine inhibition of casein induced amyloidosis in mice. Isr J Med Sci 10:787, 1974

57. Keltner JL, Fritsch E, Cykiert RC, Albert DM: Mycosis fungoides. Arch Ophthalmol 95:645, 1977

58. Khodadoust AA, Roozitalab HM, Smith RE, Green WR: Spontaneous regression of retinoblastoma. Surv Ophthalmol 21:467, 1977

59. Klein G, Clifford P, Klein F et al: Membrane

immunofluorescence reactions of Burkitt lymphoma cells from biopsy specimens and tissue cultures. J Natl Cancer Inst 39:1027, 1967

60. Knowles DM II, Jakobiec FA, Rosen M, Howard G: Amyloidosis of the orbit and adnexae. Surv Ophthalmol 19:367, 1975

61. Königstein H, Spiegel EA: Muskelatrophie bei Amyloidose. Neurol Psychiatr (Bucur) 88:220, 1924

62. Kravetz AI, Harnett NM, Gallie BL: Immunobiology of reinoblastoma. (Quoted by Basu PK). Am J Ophthalmol 84:438, 1977

63. Lackner H: Hemostatic abnormalities associated with dysproteinemias. Semin Hematol 10:125, 1973

64. Lessell S, Wolf PA, Benson MD, Cohen AS: Scalloped pupils in familial amyloidosis. N Engl J Med 293:914, 1975

65. Lewis MG: Tumour-specific antigens in melanoma. Seventh Natl Cancer Conf Proc. Am Cancer Soc, 1973, pp 77–83

66. Lewis MG, Ikonopisov RL, Nairn RC et al: Tumour-specific antibodies in human malignant melanoma and their relationship to the extent of the disease. Br Med J 3:547, 1969

67. McCallister BD, Bayrd ED, Harrison EG Jr, McGuckin WF: Primary macroglobulinemia. Am J Med 43:394, 1967

68. McPherson SD, Kiffney TG Jr, Freed CC: Corneal amyloidosis. Am J Ophthalmol 62:1025, 1966

69. Melnick JL, Adam E, Rawls WE: The causative role of herpesvirus type 2 in cervical cancer. Cancer 34:1375, 1974

70. Meretoja J: Comparative histopathological and clinical findings in eyes with lattice corneal dystrophy of two types. Ophthalmologica 165:15, 1972

71. Michelson JB, Felberg NT, Shields JA: Carcinoembryonic antigen. Its role in the evaluation of intraocular malignant tumors. Arch Ophthalmol 94:414, 1976

72. Michelson JB, Felberg NT, Shields JA: Evaluation of metastatic cancer to the eye. Arch Ophthalmol 95:692, 1977

73. Michelson JB, Felberg NT, Shields JA, Foster L: Carcinoembryonic antigen-positive metastatic adenocarcinoma of the choroid. Arch Ophthalmol 93:794, 1975

74. Miller DG: The immunologic capability of patients with lymphoma. Cancer Res 28:1441, 1968

75. Morton DL, Eibler FR, Malmgren RA, Woos WC: Immunological factors which influence response to immunotherapy in malignant melanoma. Surgery 68:158, 1970

76. Morton DL, Malmgren RA, Holmes EF, Ketcham AS: Demonstration of antibodies against human malignant melanoma by immunofluorescence. Surgery 64:233, 1968

77. Murray KH, Paolino F, Goldman JM et al: Ocular involvement in leukemia. Report of three cases. Lancet 1:829, 1977

78. Nadler SH, Moore GE: Immunotherapy of malignant melanoma. Geriatrics 23:150, 1968

79. O'Connor GT: Persistent immunologic stimulation as a factor in oncogenesis, with special reference to Burkitt's tumor. Am J Med 48:279, 1970

80. Oettgen HF: Immunotherapy of cancer. N Engl J Med 297:484, 1977

81. Osterland CK, Espinoza LR: Biological properties of myeloma proteins. Arch Intern Med 135:32, 1975

82. Perry MC, Hoagland HC: The hyperviscosity syndrome. JAMA 236:392, 1976

83. Pott P: Cancer of the scrotum. In Chirurgical Observations. London, Hawkes, Clarke & Collins, 1775, pp 63–68

84. Rahi AHS: Autoimmune reactions in uveal melanoma. Br J Ophthalmol 55:793, 1971

85. Rapp F, Reed CL: The viral etiology of cancer. A realistic approach. Cancer 40:419, 1977

86. Ratnaker KS, Mohan M: Amyloidosis of the iris. Can J Ophthalmol 11:256, 1976

87. Reese AB: Tumors of the Eye. Hagerstown, Harper & Row, 1976

88. Reimann HA, Koucky RF, Eklund CM: Primary amyloidosis limited to tissue of mesodermal origin. Am J Pathol 11:977, 1935

89. Rodman H, Font R: Orbital involvement in multiple myeloma. Arch Ophthalmol 87:30, 1972

90. Rodriguez A: Diagnosis of retinoblastoma by cytologic examination of the aqueous and the vitreous. Mod Probl Ophthalmol 18:142, 1977

91. Rugard J, Frenkel M, Peyman GA et al: Ocular tolerance of Bacillus Calmette-Guerin organisms. Arch Ophthalmol 95:2210, 1977

92. Rutgard J, Peyman GA, Frenkel M, Saks S: Calmette-Guerin Bacillus treatment of experimental conjunctival malignant melanoma. Arch Ophthalmol 95:2214, 1977

93. Sarino PJ, Schatz NJ, Rodrigues MM: Orbital amyloidosis. Can J Ophthalmol 11:252, 1976

94. Scheinberg MA, Cathcart ES: Casein induced experimental amyloidosis. III. Responses to mitogens, allogeneic cells and graft versus host reactions in the murine model. Immunology 27:953, 1974

95. Shields JA: Current approaches to the diagnosis and management of choroidal melanomas. Surv Ophthalmol 21:443, 1977

96. Somer T: Hyperviscosity in plasma cell dyscrasias. In Advances in Microcirculation Vol 6. Basel, S Karger, 1975

97. Stafford WR, Fine BS: Amyloidosis of the cornea. Report of a case without conjunctival involvement. Arch Ophthalmol 75:53, 1966

98. Stock EL, Kielar R: Primary familial amyloidosis of the cornea. Am J Ophthalmol 82:266, 1976

99. Sullivan SF, Dallow RF: Intraocular reticulum cell sarcoma: its dramatic response to systemic chemotherapy and its angiogenic potential. Ann Ophthalmol 9:401, 1977

100. Walsh FB, Hoyt WF: Clinical Neuro-ophthalmology, 3rd ed. Baltimore, Williams & Wilkins, 1969, p 811

101. Wong IG, Oskvig RM: Immunofluorescent detection of antibodies to ocular melanomas. Arch Ophthalmol 92:98, 1974

index